Occupational Therapy Approaches to Stro

Occupational Therapy Approaches to Stroke

Ann Allart Wilcock DipOT(Derby)
Lecturer, Department of Occupational Therapy,
The South Australian Institute of Technology,
Adelaide, Australia

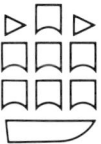

CHURCHILL LIVINGSTONE
MELBOURNE EDINBURGH LONDON AND NEW YORK 1986

CHURCHILL LIVINGSTONE
Medical Division of Longman Group Limited

Distributed in Australia by Longman Cheshire Pty, Limited,
Kings Gardens, 95 Coventry Street, South Melbourne, 3205,
and by associated companies, branches and representatives
throughout the world.

First published 1986

ISBN 0-443-03267-X

British Library Cataloguing in Publication Data
Wilcock, Ann Allart
    Occupational therapy approaches to stroke.
    1. Cerebrovascular disease — Patients —
    Rehabilitation   2. Occupational therapy
    I. Title
    616.8′1065152   RC388.5

Library of Congress Cataloging in Publication Data
Wilcock, Ann Allart.
    Occupational therapy approaches to stroke.
    Includes index.
    1. Cerebrovascular disease — Patients — Rehabilitation.
2. Occupational therapy. I. Title. [DNLM: 1. Cerebro-
vascular Disorders — rehabilitation. 2. Occupational
Therapy — methods. WL 355 W6670]
RC388.5.W466   1986   616.8′1   85–13221

Produced by Longman Group (FE) Ltd
Printed in Hong Kong

Preface

For many years I have felt the need for a text designed for occupational therapy students, to bring together traditional and current intervention procedures which have been found effective in the treatment of stroke.

The many facets of behaviour and sensory motor skills which may be impaired by stroke, and the complex, varied and often conflicting approaches to treatment propounded in textbooks written for those involved in stroke rehabilitation, may confuse undergraduates when no specific reference about the application of these approaches to their own profession is available.

For example, different neurophysiological treatment techniques are based on known (as currently understood) neuro-mechanisms. Those who have expounded, and those who have followed, specific methods of treatment have expressed belief in their clinical efficacy. No study of which I am aware has proved conclusively that one form of treatment is more effective than another, and some experts believe that an eclectic approach may provide therapists with a greater range of skills for the wide variety of disorders which may occur. It would certainly seem reasonable that an awareness of procedures which recognised authorities have found to be effective will be useful tools on which to build clinical expertise, so that future beliefs are not based solely on fashion and prevailing attitudes.

The need to integrate neurophysiological approaches with neuropsychological, social and emotional approaches further complicates treatment planning for the occupational therapist who needs to prescribe individual programs to meet future life-style requirements of individual patients.

This book discusses practical suggestions to integrate the many aspects of treatment and applies approaches to meet the needs of those who fit into usual rehabilitation programs, those who are selected out of those programs and discharged to dependent care facilities, and those who experience good recovery and attempt to resume former life-styles.

Details of different approaches are not discussed in depth as this information is available at original sources; rather, the book introduces suggestions of how different techniques may be integrated into occupational therapy practice. It is hoped that this will encourage students to further study, referring to original texts, or attending courses, and progressively developing ideas to implement improved treatment procedures and to evaluate and record results.

I have not presumed to describe the roles of other professionals working in the rehabilitation team, nor made great mention of the importance of a 'team approach', but have assumed that wherever a team is available the members will work together for patient neurophysiological and neuropsychological re-education, social resettlement, and to meet individual priorities and goals. Sharing evaluation, discussing, and, if necessary, adapting treatment objectives so that an ultimate learning experience is provided for each patient must be considered of primary importance by any treatment team. Working towards an integrated approach, which will be flexible to meet individual goals, requires ongoing understanding, adaptability, and review. This will be less effective, and slower in development and growth, if any member advocates rigid adherence to a single approach.

The ongoing debate amongst occupational therapists as to whether purposeful activity or other intervention techniques should be the principal component in occupational therapy approaches is addressed. The accepted definition of W.F.O.T. still maintains that activity is the specific treatment medium of the occupational therapist. How confusing it must be for students basing career choices on such information, if other media are stressed in their education without specific application to activity. In an attempt to lessen confusion, I have chosen as the starting point to quote the W.F.O.T. definition before reviewing the development of occupational therapy intervention in stroke, and have suggested in Chapter 4 a model where purposeful activity of significance to each individual is combined with or facilitated by other techniques. That purposeful activity may be used effectively for physical and psychological gains cannot be doubted; however, facilitating activity of significance to each individual by use of other techniques aimed at maximizing central nervous system function, and possibly speeding up recovery seems logical and appropriate, particularly if patients are able to understand and be taught to self-apply successful facilitatory procedures. By doing so cortical, sub-cortical, and peripheral stimulation may be used in combination to enhance and normalize responses.

There is some repetition within the text as approaches and techniques are applicable to different situations and problems, but need re-stating to promote awareness of varied uses or slight changes in emphasis. My years in student education have reinforced my appreciation of repetition being essential to learning. They have also made me aware that few students find time to read a text from cover to cover, but use sections for course, clinical, or assignment work, possibly missing important aspects as a result, unless they are reiterated throughout the text.

I have chosen to use photographs of students during practical training sessions, rather than line drawings, to illustrate the text, because I believe they show more detail and because I would like to encourage students to practise use of themselves as therapeutic tools before trying out their skills on patients. The techniques illustrated and discussed have been used successfully with stroke patients, and whilst photographs of patients may be desirable there are several disadvantages in their use; for example, respect for privacy and confidentiality must be a prime consideration, particularly at a time of crisis and when central nervous system dysfunction may allow agreement to photographs which later may be regretted, and because taking the photographs can be time-consuming, fatiguing, and cause undesirable affective responses.

I have tried to record a reasonable cross-section of approaches, techniques and ideas which occupational therapists have used and found effective over the years, although there is no possibility of complete coverage, in the belief that a basic appreciation of what is possible may lead to greater experimentation, research, review and development of new, more effective, procedures.

I would like to thank The South Australian Institute of Technology for granting study leave to start this work; to Audio Visual Services, S.A.I.T. and to Brad Jeffrey for assistance with the photographs and illustration; to Derek Wilcock for manuscript typing; to my work colleagues for their support and encouragement; and to clinical colleagues, students and patients.

Adelaide, 1986   A.A.W.

Contents

Basis to approaches

1

A review of occupational therapy in stroke rehabilitation

DEEINITION

Occupational therapy is assessment and treatment through the specific use of selected activity. This is designed by the occupational therapist and undertaken by those who are temporarily or permanently disabled by physical or mental illness, by social or by developmental problems. The purpose is to prevent disability and to fulfil the person's needs by achieving optimum function and independence in work, social and domestic environments (W.F.O.T., Paris, 1976).

HISTORIC OVERVIEW

Activity has been seen as a medium for restoring physical and psychological well-being for centuries. Early in this century experimentation and study of the use of activity for therapeutic intervention began, and results justified training courses in the scientific analysis and application of activity to the treatment of dysfunction.

Most of the patients initially treated through this medium were restricted to institutions, and the major aims were restoration of function through the appropriate choice of activity for its physical and psychological components, and alleviation of emotional disturbance caused or increased by institutional inactivity. The types of activity most suited to the needs of that time were of a creative nature, from simple to complex, which could stimulate interest, motivate continuing activity, and provide specific gains for individual problems. It proved more economic in staff and equipment, where possible, to group patients together in a workroom. Automatically this provided social interactions and stimulations which therapists used in their treatment formula and which thus established their role as environmental therapists. They created an environment with people and activity which stimulated endeavour, interaction, mobilisation, and pleasure.

TRADITIONAL APPROACHES

The legacy of individual creative activity in a group situation is with us today. Many people have the idea that this remains our major role in health care, although unfortunately Departments actually offering this as part of their treatment regime are becoming scarce. This type of program offered to stroke patients:

(a) The opportunity to be involved in enjoyable activity which, by demanding their attention, decreased anxiety because time available for introspection was lessened; made use of cognitive skills such as planning, memory, concentration, and sequential processes; assisted the maintenance of self-esteem through

3

achievement, and promoted pleasure and expression through simply 'doing'.

(b) The opportunity to work towards overcoming their motor deficit through the use of individually adapted activities and specially designed equipment which facilitated specific movement patterns, prolonged use of the body in co-ordinated activity, and normal sequence and timing of movement.

(c) The opportunity to achieve despite dysfunction, thereby retaining and improving self-esteem and the remaining physical and cognitive skills.

(d) The opportunity to do things with other people thus providing the chance to ventilate, without undue pressure, their feelings with others who had shared similar experiences; the chance to share in common activity, to be in a non-dependent role, and to improve their communication skills.

(e) The opportunity to have a more normal daily time cycle which promoted physiological well-being, natural relaxation, and fatigue, and decreased the occurrence of problems associated with inactivity.

SUBSEQUENT DEVELOPMENT

1. Activities of daily living

As health care workers became more skilled in rehabilitation techniques, home care activities began to expand to meet the needs of patients returning to the community. This resulted in the development of programs within rehabilitation units to retrain skills for independent living. A.D.L. approaches were mainly adaptive and sought to find answers to the difficulties patients with residual disabilities experienced when performing functional tasks. Occupational therapists designed and made in their own workshops special aids and equipment to overcome individual problems.

Departments developed special facilities to assess and retrain A.D.L. skills. Traditionally assessment and retraining took place in these special units and not in wards. Home visits were made and retraining was based on the reality of the home situation to which the patient was returning.

Gradually functional A.D.L. retraining became a major component of Occupational Therapy intervention in stroke rehabilitation. Techniques, equipment, and aids were developed to compensate for lack of mobility, bilaterality, balance, and dexterity. Everyday tasks were analysed, simplified, and adapted to compensate for problems in planning and understanding, and to overcome fatigue. Emphasis was placed on making full use of remaining abilities and on the patient being as independent as possible as soon as possible.

Functional retraining involved dressing, showering, bathing, hygiene tasks, hair care, eating, cooking, shopping, managing transport, household tasks, night self-care, transfer techniques, and mobility around the home. One well-defined program following an adaptive approach is that described in 'The Newcastle Method of Managing Hemiplegia in the Elderly' (Mort, 1976). This method was part of a total co-ordinated management program and patients were selected for it because of multiple problems rather than because they had rehabilitation potential.

The method incorported:

(a) Regular normal daily tasks as a basis for retraining

(b) Repetition throughout the day by all treatment personnel to reinforce learning.

(c) Emphasis on abilities rather than disabilities

(d) Familiarity with tasks and equipment which motivated achievment and reduced fear of the unknown

(e) Carry over of techniques into the home by family training and a comprehensive domiciliary service also using the same approach to maintain gains.

Currently in many hospitals occupational therapists carry out assessment and retraining of A.D.L. within the normal ward routine, including utilisation of the ward bathing facilities and meal arrangements. Domiciliary care services assist activities of daily living in the home. A.D.L. indexes are sometimes used as a measurement of recovery in research studies.

2. Neurophysiological approaches

The work of Sherrington (1906) on spinal reflexes,

stretch and reciprocal inhibition stimulated hypotheses and research on rehabilitation of the nervous system. Theories and rationales for intervention which may modify dysfunction have been developed, many by physiotherapists. Some occupational therapists have included techniques from these approaches in their treatment programs to enhance patients' functional achievement and to reinforce sensory motor retraining by repetition and continuity of treatment approaches.

Harris (1980) suggests in his discussion of facilitation techniques that 'therapists contemplate the full range of procedures available for application in therapeutic exercise activities' and that those who 'incorporate this entire armament of procedures in an eclectic fashion, rather than being exclusive devotees of any one method will be best equipped to deal effectively with the infinite neurological symptoms encountered in rehabilitation practice'.

(a) Proprioceptive Neuromuscular Facilitation (P.N.F.)

P.N.F. was first developed at the Kabat Kaiser Institute by Herman Kabat, and expanded by the physiotherapists Margaret Knott and Dorothy Voss (1956 & 1968).

P.N.F. techniques aim to promote or hasten the response of neuromuscular mechanisms through stimulation of the proprioceptors. Basic to all techniques are mass movement patterns which are considered a characteristic of normal motor activity and can be used as facilitators of normal movement. These facilitatory movement patterns are spiral and diagonal, and closely resemble the movements of sport and work activities. The techniques are superimposed on developmental sequence.

Other components of P.N.F. include manual contact, verbal command and communication, stretch, traction and approximation, normal timing, maximal resistance, reinforcement, and the use of cold and heat as facilitatory tools.

The movement patterns are an integral part of some activities, including those of daily living, used in occupational therapy. Their performance may be facilitated and enhanced by use of the other components advocated.

(b) The Brunnstrom approach

The approach was designed by Signe Brunnstrom (1970), physical therapist, specifically for the treatment of hemiplegia and follows the stages of recovery as described by Twitchell (1951). It makes use of reflex activities and synergies including those caused by irradiation following resistance of the sound side, to facilitate early movement. Reflex movement is gradually refined until it is cortically controllable, by using tactile sensory input and relaxation.

(c) The Rood approach

In the approach developed by Margaret Rood, physical and occupational therapist, and described by Trombly and Scott (1977), a functional developmental sequence is hypothesised, and the importance of sensory input to promote motor output is stressed. Treatment is progressed through stages of unskilled light work (full range, gross reciprocal movement), heavy work holding (co-contraction of muscle for stability), heavy work movement (movement superinposed on co-contraction) and skilled light work (co-ordinated movement). Discrete cutaneous stimulation is used to modify tone and promote contraction of underlying muscles by increasing stretch receptor sensitivity. Purposeful movement is used to draw attention to a goal, making movement subcortical whenever possible, and repetition is considered necessary for learning.

(d) The Bobath approach

The Bobath approach developed by Karl and Berta Bobath (1970 & 1978) is a neurodevelopmental approach to patients with neuromuscular disorder and applied specifically to adult hemiplegia. It hypothesises that in normal neuromuscular development primitive reflex behaviour is inhibited prior to the development of normal automatic reactions and voluntary activity. When part of the central nervous system is destroyed, as in stroke, it causes a 'release' of reflex activity from mature control.

Techniques of treatment are based on inhibition of reflex activity to facilitate normal movement patterns; the sensory experience of movement; and the prevention of overuse or effort of the sound side which may reinforce and perpetuate abnormal patterns and lead to an increase in spasticity. Components of the treatment technique include the use of reflex inhibitory positions and patterns of movement; facilitation of equilibrium and righting reactions; ontogenetic sequence; cutaneous and proprioceptive stimulation.

(e) Sensory approaches

A sensory integrative approach for use with children, was developed by Dr Jean Ayres, occupational therapist (1972) who hypothesised that treatment should include controlled sensory input in a situation conducive to integration, and adaptive response to it.

Other occupational therapists (Farber, 1982; Ranka & Chappara, 1982) following sensory approaches also based their treatment on the facilitation of motor responses by sensory modalities. Modalities are usually used in the sequence in which they appear developmentally. Tactile and vestibular stimulation are therefore early modalities to be used and are the basis for the development of co-ordinated motor activity and higher level auditory and visual skills. The interdependence of the sensory system is emphasised in the belief that stimulation of one system influences another and may facilitate a response.

3. Advances in neuropsychology

The term neuropsychology is of relatively recent origin apparently first mentioned in 1949 by Hebb. It is defined by Kolb and Whishaw (1980) as 'the study of the relations between brain function and behaviour.' The rapid expansion of neuroscience in the last two decades and the use of micro techniques in animal studies has greatly expanded accuracy of knowledge about the human nervous system and behaviour, and has initiated new hypotheses and areas of research.

Since the work of Broca and Wernicke in the latter half of the nineteenth century on the location of language function, hemispherical differences and the possibility of specific localization for physio-

logical and cognitive processes has been energetically pursued (Kolb & Whishaw, 1980). The impact of such studies upon occupational therapy has been to increase the awareness of specific sensory, perceptual, and cognitive functions, how they inter-relate with each other and with motor behaviour, and how they affect activity processes. Programs have been developed to evaluate and attempt to retrain dysfunction when higher cortical abilities have been impaired by stroke. More accurate information on location and specificity of lesion sites may lead to the development of techniques to improve dysfunction or to circumlocate impaired areas.

CURRENT APPROACHES AND ISSUES

Approaches, techniques, and priorities differ from service to service, apparently the result of individual development, economic restrictions and the attitudes and expertise of the personnel employed by them. The major components currently used by occupational therapists include evaluation and retraining of:
- perceptual and cognitive skills
- activities of daily living
- sensory motor abilities by neurophysiological developmental or functional approaches
- affective and social skills by structured group therapy for education, relaxation, support, and counselling
- vocational skills
and maintenance therapy through appropriate use of community agencies.

Most occupational therapists seem to include evaluation and treatment of perceptual disorders, and some method of treating sensory motor impairment; but often there appears to be a tendency to use either a neurophysiological, or an A.D.L. adaptive approach. Despite having found one method useful, many therapists appear defensive if other techniques are suggested; perhaps this is because limited study opportunity makes it difficult to keep up to date with the many and varied approaches which sometimes seem to contraindicate each other. On the other hand, trying to keep up with prevailing attitudes and treatment 'fashion' may lead to anxiety about adequacy of treatment, particularly as there is sometimes disputation between therapists, especially those who 'become fanatical adherents of a single method or devotees of a particular expositor' (Harris, 1980).

It should be remembered that all the approaches described have proven successful in some measure and for some patients, and as Mossman (1976) says 'if any method were flawless there would not be so many'. He suggests that most therapists borrow techniques from many approaches and should carefully scrutinize the methodology, its neurophysiologic basis, the limitations, and the results. Harris (1980) suggests that a technique properly applied ought to work if it considers the anatomical organisation and functional principles of the nervous system, and that therapists should be willing to try new techniques, even if the neural mechanisms behind them are not currently understood. As we do not at present have a treatment vehicle guaranteeing 100% success, we should be receptive to new approaches which may extend the scope and effectiveness of individual treatment, closely observing and recording results, and modifying activity if undesirable responses occur.

Recent publications (Carr & Shepherd, 1982; Cotton & Kinsman, 1983) have suggested the study and application of theories of learning, and active involvement of patients in their own treatment at a cognitive level. They emphasize the need to combine neurophysiological and functional activity, and to break activity down into component parts for evaluation and retraining purposes.

Carr and Shepherd (1982) describe their approach as a motor relearning program for stroke and hypothesise that effectiveness of this approach, which uses functional rather than abstract exercise activity, is dependent upon accurate recognition and analysis of the problem preventing normal movement, clear explanation to the patient by speech and demonstration, accurate feedback, evaluation of effectiveness throughout each treatment, achievement before progression, consistency of practice and the provision of an enriched environment to assist motivation and recovery of both mental and physical abilities.

Cotton and Kinsman (1983) describe conductive education for adult hemiplegia, based on the approach developed by Professor Peto at the Institute for the Motor Disabled in Budapest, as aiming to facilitate function by developing patients' adaptive and learning abilities changed by cerebral dysfunction. Patients work in groups for motivation, development of initiative, learning of motor skills, vicarious learning through watching others, stimulation, and social interaction. Everything within the system is designed to facilitate: for example, words spoken before movement, and counting or dynamic speech which continues as movement is carried out (known as *rhythmical intention*), is seen as important in the learning of tasks or task parts, and in the reduction of fatigue because of the slow rhythmic tempo of the work. Use of dynamic speech utilises the hypothesis that initial verbal instruction is gradually modified to become internal speech for task modification.

Many of these principles have been inherent components of traditional occupational therapy programs. The need to consider theories of learning as a basis for rehabilitation was a necessary part of traditional approaches in which patients were taught creative activities to redevelop impaired skills.

Activity analysis, simplification and repetition of techniques so that achievement promotes progression, and patient motivation through active cognitive participation in programs and appropriate choice of tasks, appear as necessary for current approaches as for traditional. Fordyce (1971) suggests that some reduction in learning efficiency is the most likely functional consequence of brain damage, but that it is often the rate of learning rather than the ability to learn that is affected. He recommends in treatment the use of rehearsal (practice and repetition), clear signals (appropriate cueing), and adequately paced increments (treatment graded and progressed with achievement).

The benefits of patients working in groups for affective and social gains is well recognised although, as treatment methods have become increasingly specific, it is becoming common practice to treat on a one-to-one basis for a short time daily. This is more labour intensive, requiring greater numbers of staff to see fewer patients than when individual activity took place in group situations. Economic restraints are curtailing staff growth and this, together with the changes to one-to-one treatment, necessitates selection of patients for rehabilitation from all of those who survive stroke.

Those selected out by non-referral often include those with apparently limited potential who are disposed of to long-term care institutions early post stroke, patients being treated privately, and those with rapid return of function but who may have some residual problems. From a comparative survey of four general hospitals it also appears that more women than men may be excluded (Wilcock & Hall, 1982). Therapists may not be aware of how many patients are excluded from the benefits of retraining programs, and that many research studies are only on those subjects who fulfil the selection criteria for rehabilitation and do not include every C.V.A. patient.

As Mossman (1976) reminds us 'we can all remember patients who were discharged to nursing homes, before neurologic return, within 3 weeks of onset of their strokes' who much later made dramatic recoveries, after being found and referred for rehabilitation. Those excluded from rehabilitation programs, would benefit from treatment.

One hospital whose criteria for rehabilitation, contrary to the norm, selects those with limited potential and multiple problems of both a medical and social nature, despite an older population than the other hospitals in the survey conducted by Wilcock and Hall (1982), sent more people home and fewer to institutions. If, however, some patients are likely to be discharged early after onset of stroke, it is important that some treatment to facilitate recovery of impaired function has commenced, especially that which will help patients to be aware of their body and the position of dysfunctional parts.

Most authorities emphasise the importance of early treatment. Gersten (1975) cites several studies which support the belief that the time between the occurrence of stroke and the start of treatment is an important factor relating to prognosis. Poorer results are evidenced following long-standing untreated dysfunction, and the achievement of good results is more likely following immediate or early treatment. Swenson (1980) suggests that patients should be out of bed as soon as possible to promote early mobilization and neurological reintegration, and in the case of an uncomplicated stroke due to infarction this should be within 2–3 days. Patients with strokes secondary to subarachnoid haemorrhage may need to remain in bed for up to 14 days, and those with associated myocardial infarction may need to stay in bed for several weeks.

Johnstone (1980) states that it is 'urgently necessary for rehabilitation to begin immediately after the onset of disability', and Carr and Shepherd (1982) suggest that treatment should commence in the first few days after onset, to prevent psychological and perceptual-motor deterioration, non-use of the affected side being learned, and to stimulate physical and psychological learning abilities.

As occupational therapists have an important role in the re-education of sensory inattention and perceptual impairment necessary for adaptive motor responses, as well as concern about how each patient feels, early intervention by occupational therapists is indicated.

Economic and community concerns

The expense of lengthy hospitalization and of institutional care has led to economic rationalization of bed use and pressure for early discharge. This has influenced the development of community-based medical and ancilliary services. Because long, intensive therapy may be required, stroke patients may be discharged to long-term care institutions which are less expensive for the community.

Treatment procedures tend to lag behind community concerns. For example, awareness of differences between ethnic groups is increasing. Maintaining the differences as well as integrating cultures is encouraged, but in treatment situations the social requirements of patients may not be considered of sufficient importance to affect approaches and goals significantly. There is also growing awareness in the community of the need for a well-balanced lifestyle. This has led to consideration of pre-retirement planning and the importance of leisure pursuits, but this awareness does not seem to be adequately reflected in treatment.

Emphasis in treatment should reflect the real needs of each patient as part of the community in which they live or to which they will be discharged. It should include attention to their daily living requirements, home and institutional cultural skills, personal and social expectations and leisure pursuits.

SUMMARY

Occupational therapists have developed treatment procedures for rehabilitation of stroke from the use of creative activity for specific physical and psychological benefits, the use of group therapy within structured environments, the adaptive and remedial use of activities of daily living, and the inclusion of techniques to maximise neurophysiological and neuropsychological functioning. Current practice, which should start as soon as possible after onset of stroke, may include any of these procedures.

It is important for occupational therapists to retain what has been useful in the past, to keep pace with new developments, and to incorporate what is relevant into the activity programs of the future.

REFERENCES

Ayres J 1972 Sensory integration and learning disorders Western Psychological Services, Los Angeles

Bobath B 1970 and 1978 Adult hemiplegia: evaluation and treatment. William Heinemann Medical Books Ltd, London

Brunnstrom S 1970 Movement therapy in hemiplegia: a neurophysiological approach. Harper and Row, New York

Carr J, Shepherd R 1982 A motor relearning programme for stroke. William Heinemann Medical Books Ltd, London

Cotton E, Kinsman R 1983 Conductive education for adult hemiplegia. Churchill Livingstone, Edinburgh

Farber S D 1982 Neurorehabilitation a multisensory approach. Saunders, Philadelphia

Fordyce W E 1971 Psychological assessment and management. In: Krusen F H, Kottke F J, Ellwood P M (eds) Handbook of physical medicine and rehabilitation, 2nd edn. W B Saunders, Philadelphia

Gersten J W 1975 Rehabilitation potential. In: Licht S (ed) Stroke and its rehabilitation. Waverly Press, Baltimore

Harris F A 1980 Facilitation techniques in therapeutic exercise. In: Basmajian J V (ed) Therapeutic exercise student edition. Williams and Wilkins, Baltimore

Hebb D O 1949 The organisation of behaviour; a neuropsychological theory. John Wiley and Sons, New York

Johnstone M 1980 Home care for the stroke patient; living in a pattern. Churchill Livingstone, Edinburgh

Kolb B, Whishaw I Q 1980 Fundamentals of human neuropsychology. W H Freeman, San Francisco

Knott M, Voss D E 1968 Proprioceptive neuromuscular facilitation, 2nd edn. Harper and Row, New York

Mort M 1976 The Newcastle method of managing hemiplegia in the elderly, a handbook to supplement the film of the same title. William Lyne Community Service Fund, Newcastle N.S.W.

Mossman P L 1976 A problem-oriented approach to stroke rehabilitation. Charles C Thomas, Springfield, Illinois

Ranka J, Chappara C 1982 Workshop on sensory integrative techniques for stroke patients. Australian Association of Occupational Therapists 12th Federal Conference, Adelaide

Sherrington C S 1906 The integrative action of the nervous system. Yale University Press, New Haven

Trombly C A, Scott A D 1977 Occupational therapy for physical dysfunction. Williams and Wilkins, Baltimore

Twitchell T E 1951 The restoration of motor function following hemiplegia in man. Brain 74: 443–480

Wilcock A A, Hall R E 1982 Disposal of post acute C.V.A. patients, discussion of a statistical comparative study. Australian Occupational Therapy Journal 29:4: 161–177

World Federation of Occupational Therapists 1976 Minutes of Council Meeting, Paris

RECOMMENDED READING

Bobath B 1978 Adult hemiplegia: evaluation and treatment. William Heinemann Medical Books Ltd, London

Brunnstrom S 1970 Movement therapy in hemiplegia: a neurophysiological approach. Harper and Row, New York

Carr J, Shepherd R 1982 A motor relearning programme for stroke. William Heinemann Medical Books Ltd, London

Gersten J W 1975 Rehabilitation potential. In: Licht S, (ed) Stroke and its rehabilitation. Waverly Press, Baltimore

Harris F A 1980 Facilitation techniques in therapeutic exercise. In: Basmajian J V (ed) Therapeutic exercise student edition. Williams and Wilkins, Baltimore

Knott M, Voss D E 1968 Proprioceptive neuromuscular facilitation, 2nd edn. Harper and Row, New York

Trombly C 1983 Occupational therapy for physical dysfunction. Williams and Wilkins, Baltimore.

Twitchell T E 1951 The restoration of motor function following hemiplegia in man. Brain 74: 443–480

Stroke, causes and effect

DEFINITION

Stroke is:

> A condition of sudden onset caused by acute vascular lesions of the brain, such as haemorrhage, embolism, thrombosis, or rupturing aneurysm, which may be marked by hemiplegia or hemiparesis, vertigo, numbness, aphasia and dysarthria; it is often followed by permanent neurological damage. Called also cerebrovascular accident. (Dorland, 1974)

BLOOD SUPPLY

1. Arterial system

The brain receives its blood supply from two pairs of arteries.

(i) The internal carotid arteries which, after they divide into the middle and anterior cerebral arteries, supply the superior anterior portion of the cerebrum (Fig. 2.1).

(ii) The vertebral arteries which join at the level of the pons to become the basilar artery and divide at the Circle of Willis into two posterior cerebral arteries. They supply the inferior posterior portion of the cerebrum (Fig. 2.1).

It is at the level of the Circle of Willis that the arteries serving the cerebrum arise, and this is important clinically as damage to vessels above this point will be specific to the cerebral area served by the middle, anterior, or posterior arteries.

Below the Circle of Willis are the arteries serving the cerebellum and brain stem. These are the superior, anterior inferior, and posterior inferior cerebellum arteries.

The Circle of Willis is a meeting place of the major cerebral arteries (Fig. 2.2). It is a polygonal anastomosis (Dorland 1974)—an anastomosis being a connection between vessels allowing intercommunication, in this case of blood flow. It is formed by the internal carotid, the middle,

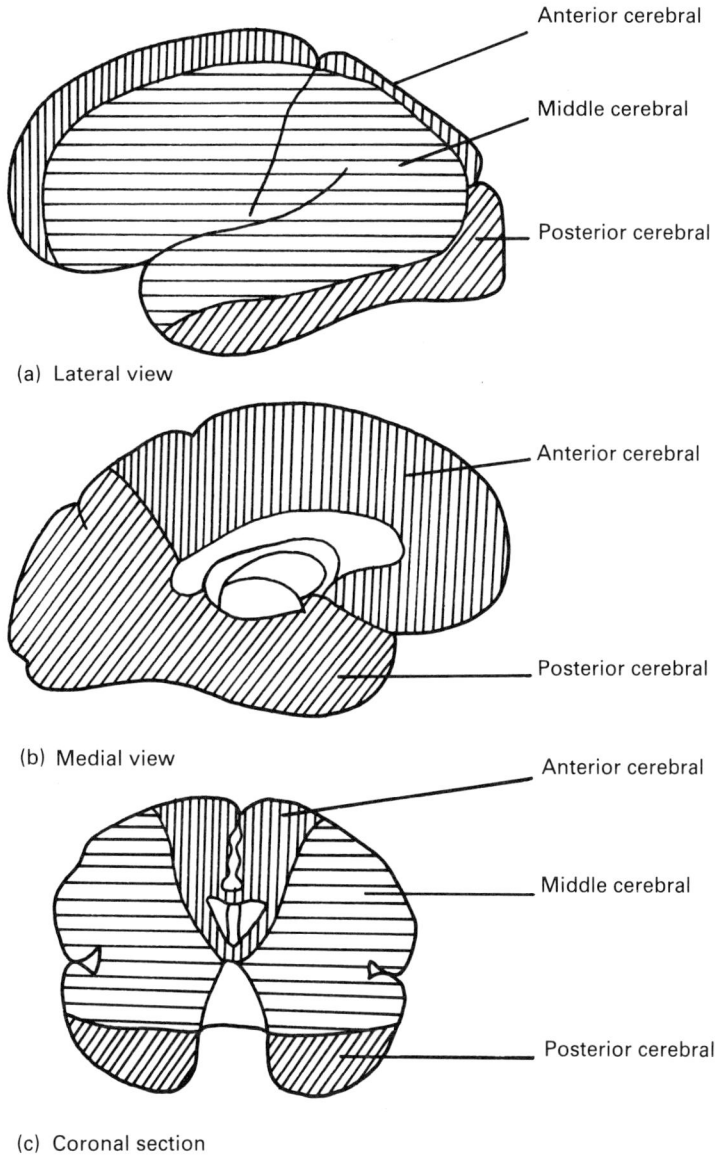

Fig. 2.1 Areas of the cerebrum served by the middle, anterior and posterior arteries.

anterior, and posterior cerebral arteries, and communicating arteries, one anterior and two posterior.

The basilar artery divides into the posterior cerebral arteries at the junction of the posterior communicating arteries.

Blood flow in the communicating arteries shows no particular tendency to go one way or the other, because blood flow up both vertebral and internal carotid arteries equalises the pressure between them (Goldberg, 1974)

The formation of the Circle of Willis may allow the blood an alternative route to an infarcted zone should one of the major vessels be blocked.

2. Venous system

The cerebrovenous system does not correspond to

Anterior
cerebral

Anterior
communicating

Middle
cerebral

Posterior
communicating

Posterior
cerebral

Internal carotid

Basilar

Vertebral

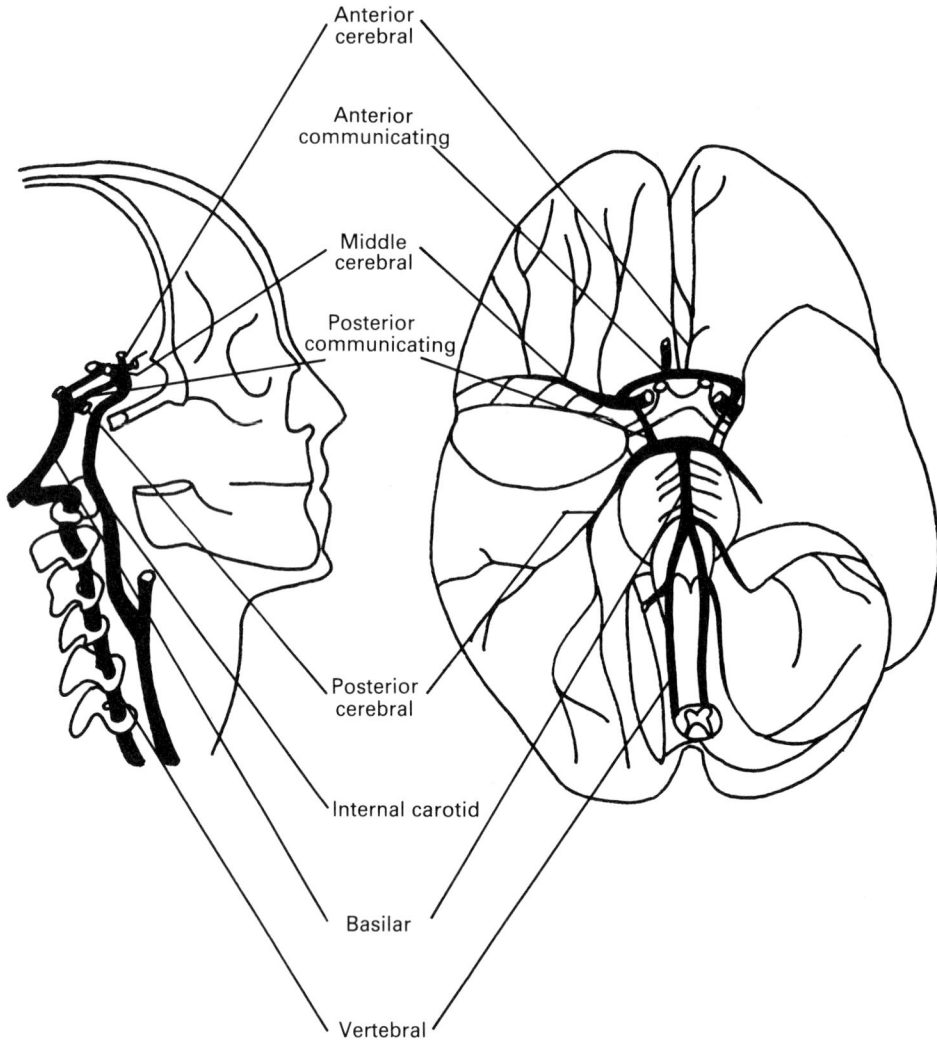

Fig. 2.2 The Circle of Willis looking (a) laterally and (b) ventrally.

the arterial system as in other parts of the body. Venous return is via sinuses draining the dura, leaving the brain by the internal jugular vein. The vessels are known as the internal and external veins and cerebellar veins.

CAUSES OF INTERRUPTION TO BLOOD SUPPLY

1. Stenosis (narrowing) or occlusion of a vessel

Arterial stenosis or occlusion may have several causes.

(a) Hypertensive disease of the small vessels of the brain which stenose and gradually occlude penetrating end branches which often lead deeply into cerebral hemispheres, pons and cerebellum.

(b) Arterial disease of the major vessels leading to the brain, namely the carotid and vertebral arteries, causing thrombosis or embolic occlusion in intra-cranial arteries. Major sites are shown in Figure 2.3.

(c) Emboli from other parts of the body particularly as a result of cardiac or (less commonly) pulmonary disease occlude intracranial vessels.

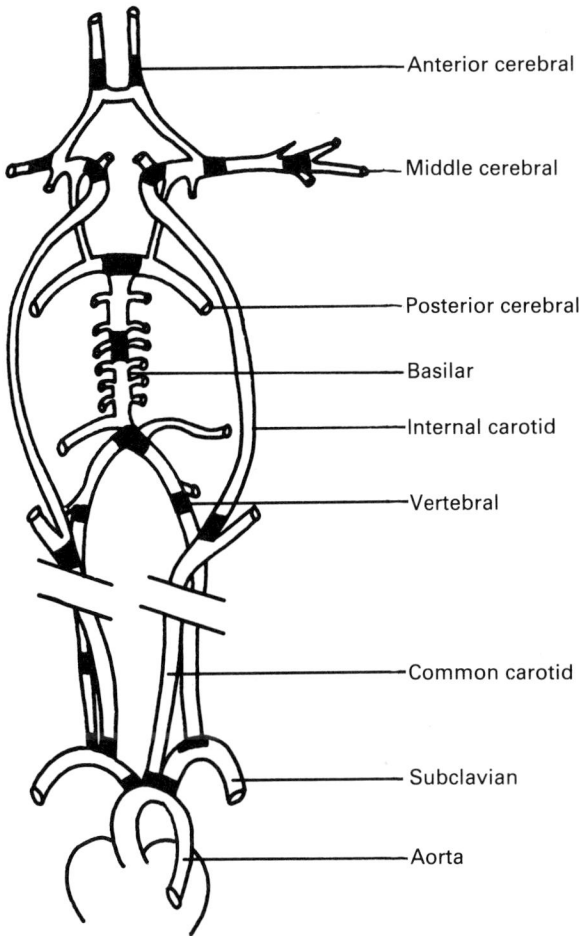

Fig. 2.3 Major sites of arterial disease (Dunphy & Way, 1981).

(d) Atheroma and secondary local thrombi occlude middle, anterior and posterior cerebral arteries (Burrow, 1983).

If episodic occlusion occurs producing brief focal disturbance, the term 'transient ischaemic attack' (T.I.A.) is used. Medical treatment (e.g. anticoagulant therapy) or surgical procedures (e.g. arterial bypass) to prevent the occurrence of a major stroke are necessary.

As a result of the circulatory obstruction an area of coagulation necrosis is formed which is known as an *infarct*.

Approximately 85% of completed strokes are due to cerebral infarctions, with embolism being probably the major pathogenic factor, the other 15% being due to haemorrhage. (Weller et al, 1983)

2. Cerebral haemorrhage, aneurysms, angiomas

Cerebral haemorrhage may result from several causes.

(a) Hypertension, particularly when atheroma is present, results in the rupture of small intracranial arteries. The internal capsules, narrow pathways of descending motor fibres and ascending sensory fibres, are commonly infarcted by haemorrhage of the small anterior choroidal and striate arteries. Other common sites of haemorrhage are in the thalamus, the pons, and the cerebellum.

(b) Rupture of an aneurysm or, less frequently, an angioma (arteriovenous malformation) may cause leaking or flooding of the blood into the subarachnoid space (subarachnoid haemorrhage). Aneurysms are common around the Circle of Willis (Fig. 2.4).

(c) Other causes may be trauma, haemorrhage into tumour, or a bleeding abnormality.

EFFECTS OF INTERRUPTION TO BLOOD SUPPLY

1. Infarction

Within six to twelve hours of infarction, ischaemic changes to neurons and cell degeneration can be seen histologically. After 2–3 days the whole area becomes oedematous with swelling extending beyond the lesions which, if extensive, may lead to death due to transtentorial herniation, midbrain compression, and haemorrhage. The oedema starts to subside after 7–10 days with softening of the infarcted tissue. There is increased blood flow around the edges of the infarct and after about 4 days macrophages, which ingest other cells, become the most prominent cells within the lesion, gradually removing dead tissue, a process which may take many years depending on the necrosed area. A cystic, fluid filled cavity remains (Weller et al, 1983).

2. Haemorrhage

Cerebral haemorrhage produces a space occupying lesion of sudden occurrence, resulting in increased

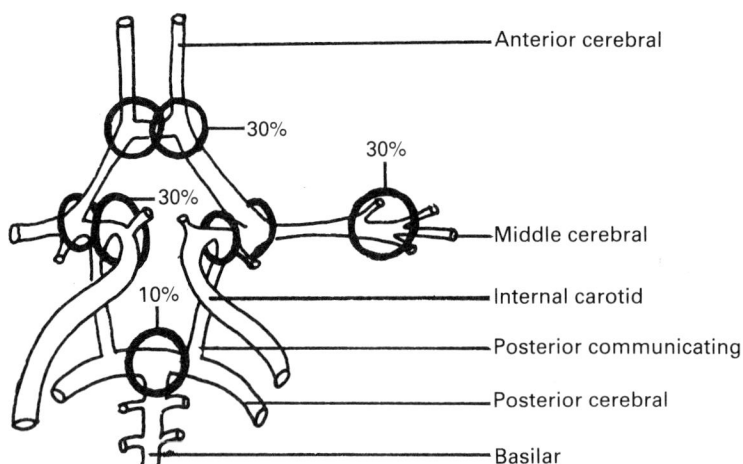

Fig. 2.4 Distribution and sites of berry aneurysms (McKissock et al, 1960; Rubenstein & Wayne, 1980).

intracranial pressure, displacement of brain, and oedema. Death is more common following haemorrhage than infarction.

In patients who survive, absorption of the haematoma occurs by action of macrophages. Good recovery is possible because haemorrhages may disrupt the white matter but may not necessarily cause extensive destruction.

The clinical features of stroke depend upon the location and the extent of the lesion (Weller et al, 1983).

RELEVANT FUNCTIONAL TOPOGRAPHY OF THE BRAIN

The two hemispheres of the cortex, divided for convenience into the anatomical regions known as the frontal, parietal, temporal and occipital lobes, have been loosely attributed with different functions:

- the frontal lobe with motor function
- the parietal lobe with somatosensory function
- the temporal lobe with auditory function, and
- the occipital lobe with visual function.

Motor and sensory fibres are, however, apparent in all areas. (Kolb & Whishaw, 1980) Specific research techniques have enabled the construction of topographical maps of the cortex. Cytoarchitechtonic maps are constructed by grouping areas of similar neuronal structure, such as by the distribution, size, and shape of the cells. Brod-

mann (1909) analysed and numbered in random order new conformations of cells as he found them. The numbered areas of the cytoarchitechtonic map he constructed have subsequently been found to have a close relationship with different functions, the primary motor and sensory areas appearing to have particularly distinct boundaries (Fig. 2.5) (Kolb & Whishaw, 1980).

Areas not numbered in this map (Fig. 2.5) are currently called association or tertiary areas, because it is believed that they perform integrative and association functions rather than those of a specific motor or sensory nature.

The primary motor and somatosensory strip are responsible for specific points of the body (Fig. 2.6). Representation of body parts is not identical in motor and somatosensory strips or indicative of the anatomical size of body parts; for example, projections related to hands and mouth occupy a much larger area of the cortex than does the trunk, reflecting the complex and refined motor functions and somatosensory importance of these areas. It should be noted that the lower limb is represented within the cortex supplied by the anterior cerebral artery and the rest of the body in the cortex supplied by the middle cerebral artery.

There is lateralization or asymmetry of hemispherical function. The left hemisphere is mainly concerned with behaviour relating to language and the analysis and interpretation of symbols, and the right hemisphere with processing non verbal and

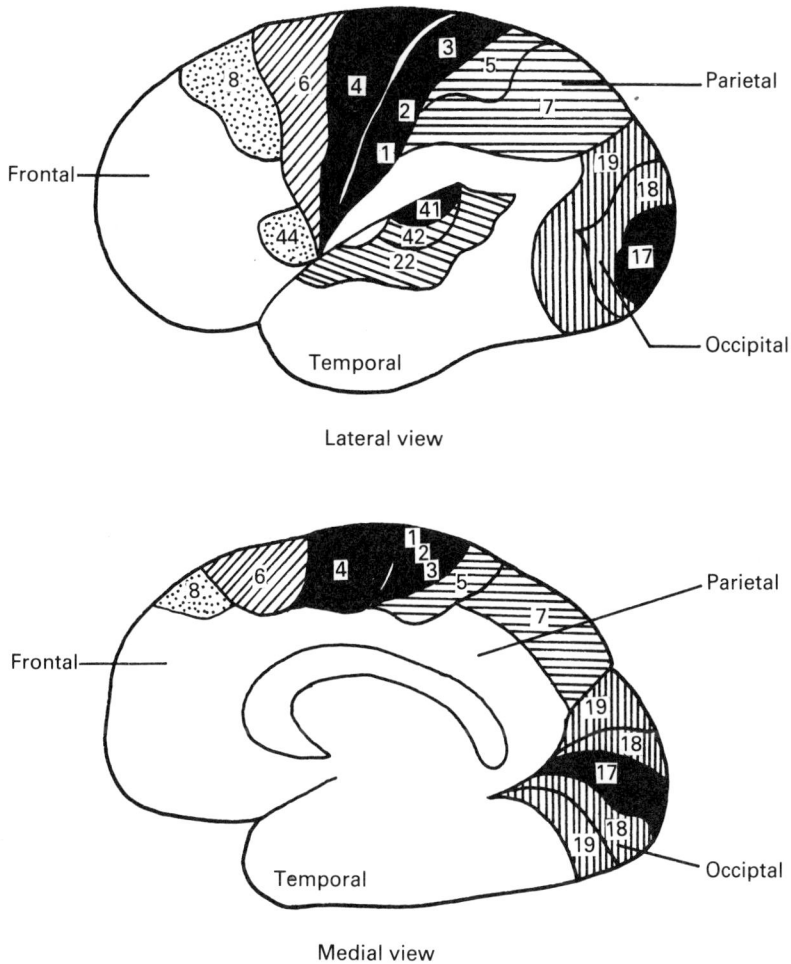

Lateral view

Medial view

Motor:	Primary 4, Secondary 6, Eye movement 8, Speech 44
Somatosensory:	Primary 1, 2, 3, Secondary 5, 7
Auditory:	Primary 41, Secondary 42, 22
Visual:	Primary 17, Secondary 18, 19

Fig. 2.5 The cerebral lobes with the primary and secondary areas of brain function, as mapped by Brodmann. (Adapted from Elliot H 1969 Textbook of Anatomy. Lippincott)

spatial material. Motor and sensory systems are organized in a functional hierarchy performing symmetrically at the lowest levels and asymmetrically at the highest cortical levels, the association areas. Sensory information is received, conveyed to, and interpreted by the primary and secondary sensory cortex of either side, before being transmitted to the association areas for integration and understanding. These highest levels of the sensory system are sometimes known as *gnostic* areas, from the Greek 'to know'. Dysfunction is known as *agnosia*. The left and right gnostic areas tend to specialize in either symbol or spatial analysis, so functioning is asymmetrical. The processed sensory information is transmitted to the highest cortical levels of the motor system where appropriate action and movement is planned. Skilled movement is known as *praxis* from the Greek for 'action', therefore dysfunction is known as *apraxia*. The left hemisphere is usually more

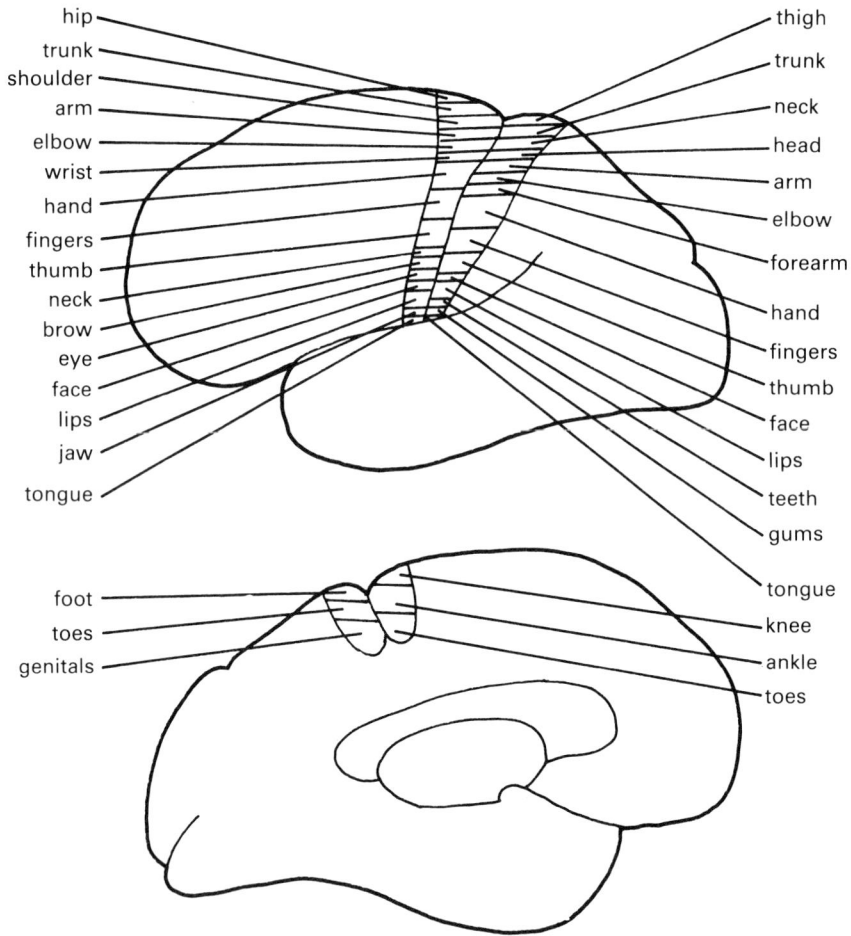

Fig. 2.6 Localization of motor and somatosensory functions.

concerned than the right with the production of skilled movement, so the highest motor levels are also seen to be asymmetrical. Below this level the motor system appears symmetrical (Fig. 2.7) (Kolb & Whishaw, 1980). This implies that lesions affecting the sensory and motor systems to the level of the primary and most of the secondary cortex will cause the same dysfunction in either contralateral side, and lesions which affect the left or right association areas are likely to cause different disorders. However, despite asymmetry of association areas, this is relative rather than absolute, with considerable functional overlap being evidenced between hemispheres.

1. The frontal lobes

The frontal lobes, which are served by the middle and anterior cerebral arteries, are often described as the *motor cortex*. Within them are the primary motor cortex (Brodmann's area 4) which is concerned with the execution of motor activity, including fine motor control, and speed and strength of movements; the secondary motor areas (Brodmann's areas 6 and 8), which appear to affect the smoothness and fluidity of movement; parts of Brodmanns's area 8 and 9 which affect movements of the frontal visual field; and Brodmann's area 44 which is concerned with expressive or motor

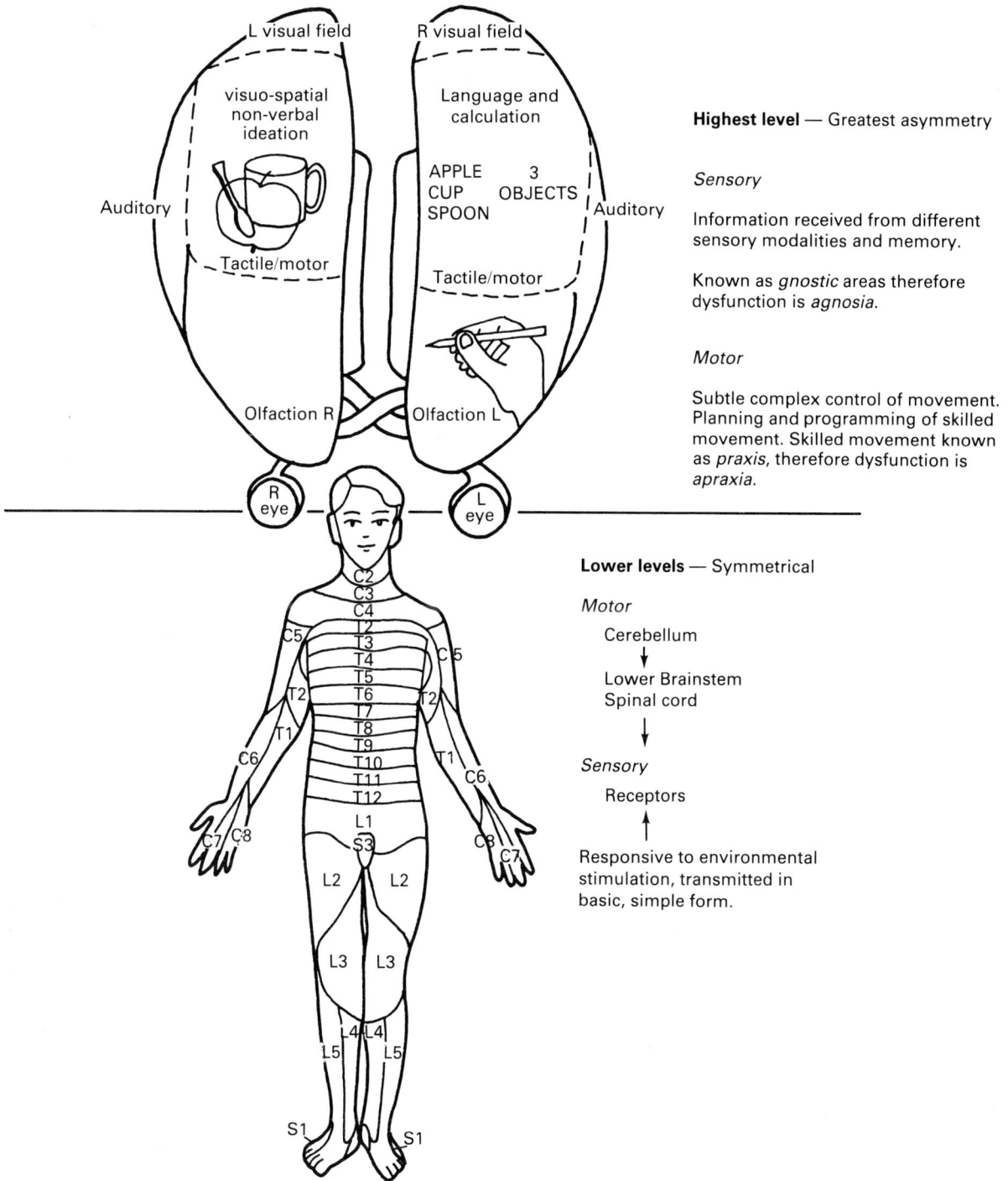

Fig. 2.7 Hierarchical organizational of sensory and motor systems demonstrating symmetry of lower level functioning of central nervous system, and asymmetry of secondary and tertiary cortical functioning (Kolb & Whishaw, 1980).

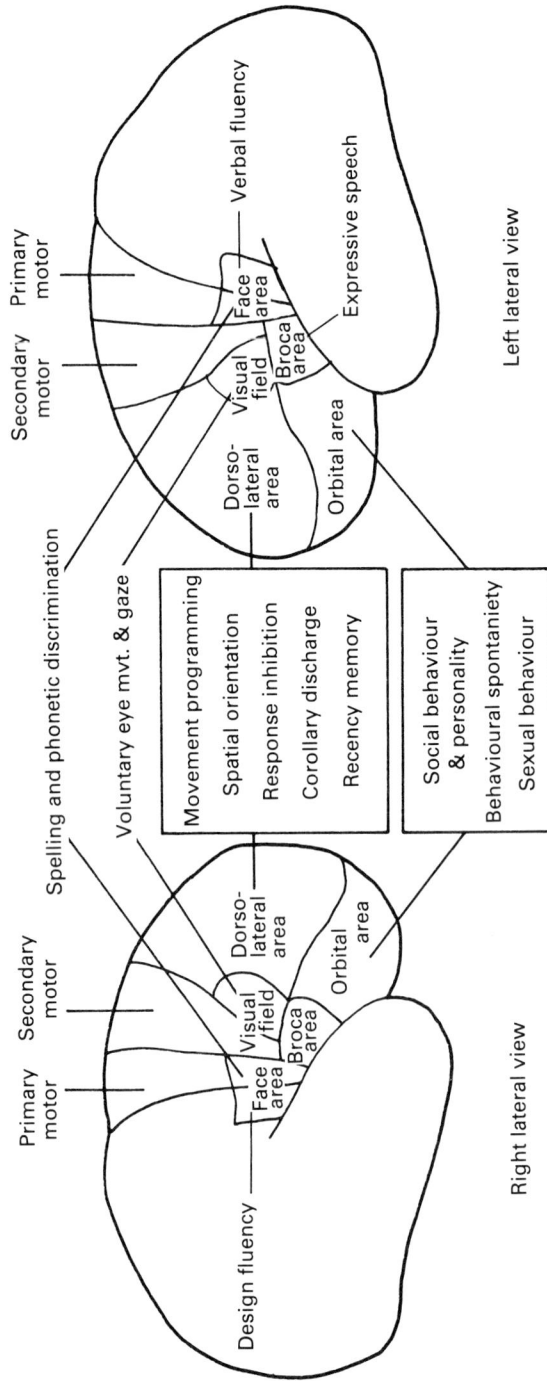

Fig. 2.8 Specific functions attributed mainly to the frontal lobes (Kolb & Whishaw, 1980).

speech. In addition, the pre-frontal cortex or association area controls overall motor programs and modification of behaviour so that it is appropriate to different circumstances, adding flexibility to motor output. The frontal association areas also appear to control basic affect, and emotional and social behaviour. Specific functions that have been attributed through research findings of effect of lesions to the frontal lobe (Fig. 2.8) include:

(a) Motor activity
(b) Spontaneous expressive speech (Brown, 1972)
(c) Response inhibition to changing demands (which prevents perseveration) and flexibility of behaviour (Milner, 1964; Perret, 1974)
(d) Voluntary eye movement and gaze (Teuber, 1964; Tyler, 1969)
(e) Memory for order of events (Milner, 1974)
(f) Initiative and spontaneity of behaviour (Hecaen & Albert, 1975)
(g) Verbal and design fluency (Milner, 1964; Jones-Gotman & Milner, 1977)
(h) Movement planning and sequencing (Luria, 1973; Kolb & Milner 1980)
(i) Spatial orientation of personal space (which indicates the presence of sensory fibres in the frontal lobe) (Semmes et al, 1963)
(j) Social behaviour and personality (Blumer & Benson, 1975)
(k) Sexual behaviour (Walker & Blumer, 1975)
(l) Phonetic discrimination and spelling (Taylor, 1979)
(m) Corollary discharge to other cortical areas indicating occurrence of movement to facilitate sensory adaptation (Teuber, 1964)

Lesions to the frontal lobe, depending on the side, site, and extent, may affect any of the above functions, resulting in possible impairment or change to motor ability, social and affective behaviour, and communication.

The variety of functions of the frontal lobes is reflected in its numerous connections, with afferent fibres received from the visual, auditory and somatosensory areas via the parietal lobe, the thalamus, hypothalamus and amygdala; efferent fibres project to the parietal and temporal association areas, cingulate cortex, basal ganglia, thalamus, hypothalamus, hippocampus, amygdala and lower brain stem (Kolb & Whishaw, 1980).

2. The parietal lobes

The parietal lobes which are served by the middle and anterior cerebral arteries contain the primary and secondary somatosensory areas. The primary area (Brodmann 1,2,3) receives projections from the thalamus, its neurons being very specific and responsive to exact points of the body. The secondary areas are mainly modality specific, being in control of identification and understanding of somatosensory inputs. This information is collected from sensory receptors in the body and transmitted through the spinal cord, the reticular formation of the brain stem, the cerebellum, and the thalamus to the cortex, as shown in Figure 2.9. The posterior regions of the parietal lobes are the association areas responsible for the integration and analysis of sensory information from the somatic, visual, and auditory zones, making it possible to understand inputs and to relate them to past experience. This integrative function extends into the posterior zone of the temporal lobes (Brodmann's area 37). Asymmetry of function is evident with the left (usually) parietal temporal region specializing in processing symbolic analytic information such as language and mathematics, and the right having a special role in spatial processes; however there is some overlap of functions between hemispheres. Specific functions that have been attributed through research studies of the effects of lesions to the parietal lobe (Fig. 2.10) include:

(a) Tactile sensation (Semmes et al, 1960)
(b) Visual and tactile gnosia (Brown, 1972; Hecaen & Albert, 1978)
(c) Praxis of proximal limb movements (Geshwind, 1965; Brown, 1972)
(d) Constructional praxis (Piercy et al, 1960)
(e) Language (Hecaen & Albert, 1978)
(f) Calculation skills (Hecaen, 1969)
(g) Cross-modal matching (Butters & Brody, 1968)
(h) Contralateral awareness and body image (Heilman & Watson, 1977; Hecaen & Albert, 1978)
(i) Short term (working) memory (Warrington & Weiskrantz, 1973)
(j) Right/left discrimination (Benton, 1959; Semmes et al, 1960)

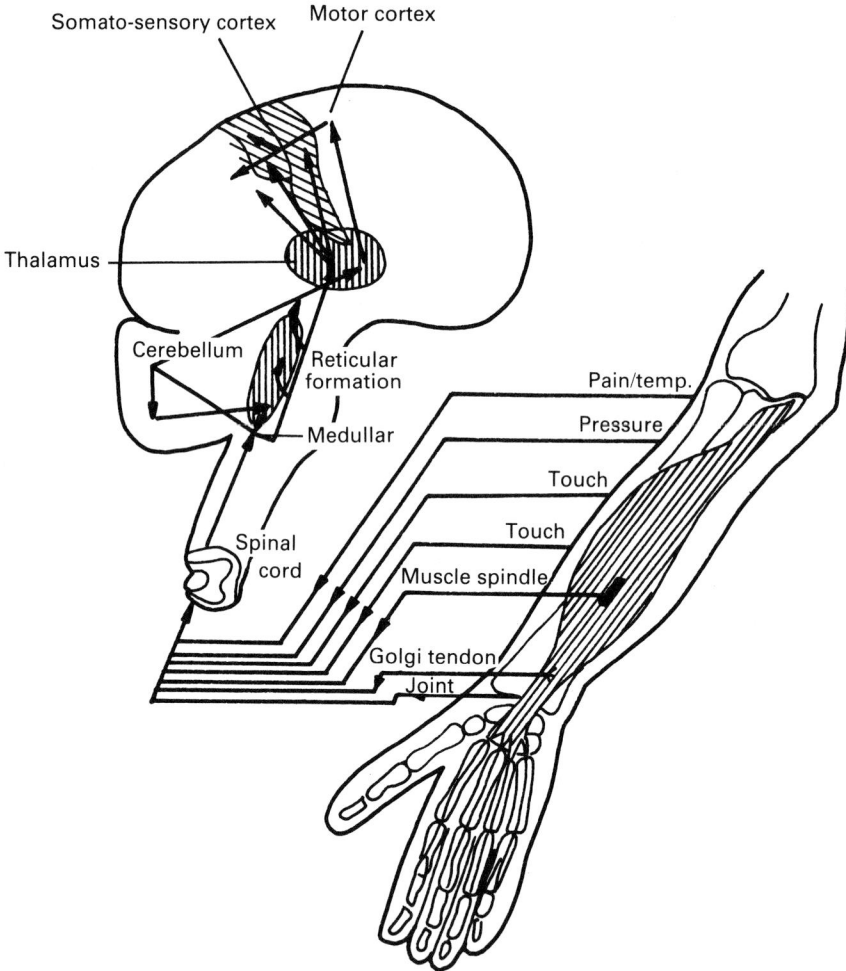

Fig. 2.9 Transmission of information from the sensory receptors to the somatosensory cortex. (Adapted from Guyton A C 1981 Basic Human Neurophysiology, Fig. 6.2. Saunders.)

(k) Spatial skills (Semmes et al, 1963; Benton, 1969)

(l) Drawing skills (Warrington, et al, 1966)

Lesions to the parietal lobes, depending on the side, site and extent, may affect any of the above functions resulting in possible impairment to somatosensation, visual spatial perception, body awareness, and communication. Evidence of praxic functions in the parietal lobe indicates the presence of motor fibres.

Afferent connections are received from all primary and secondary sensory areas, the frontal association areas, the thalamus and hypothalamus; the efferent fibres project to the frontal and temporal association areas, thalamus, basal ganglia, mid brain, and spinal cord.

3. The temporal lobes

The temporal lobes, which are served by the posterior and middle cerebral arteries, include the auditory and limbic cortex as well as association areas, and are concerned with auditory sensations, auditory and visual perception, the neural mechanisms for storage and retrieval of information and sensory input analysis. Sensory input analysis associates motivational and emotional significance to input, preventing all stimuli being treated as

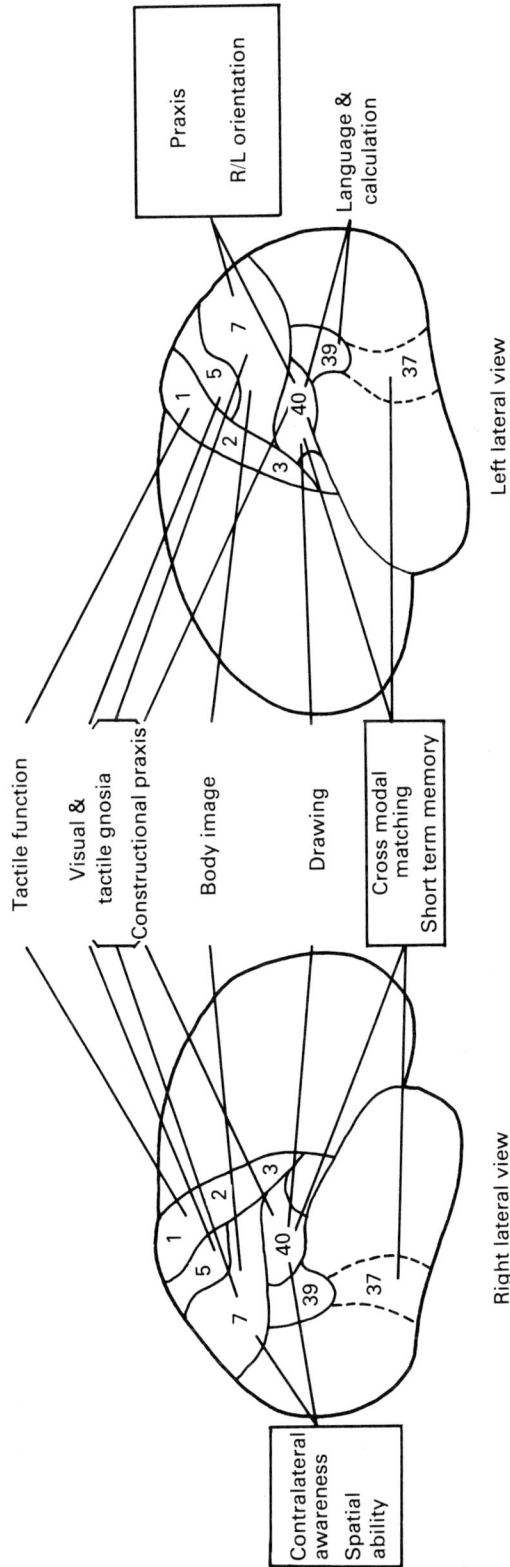

Fig. 2.10 Specific functions attributed mainly to the parietal lobes (Kolb & Whishaw, 1980).

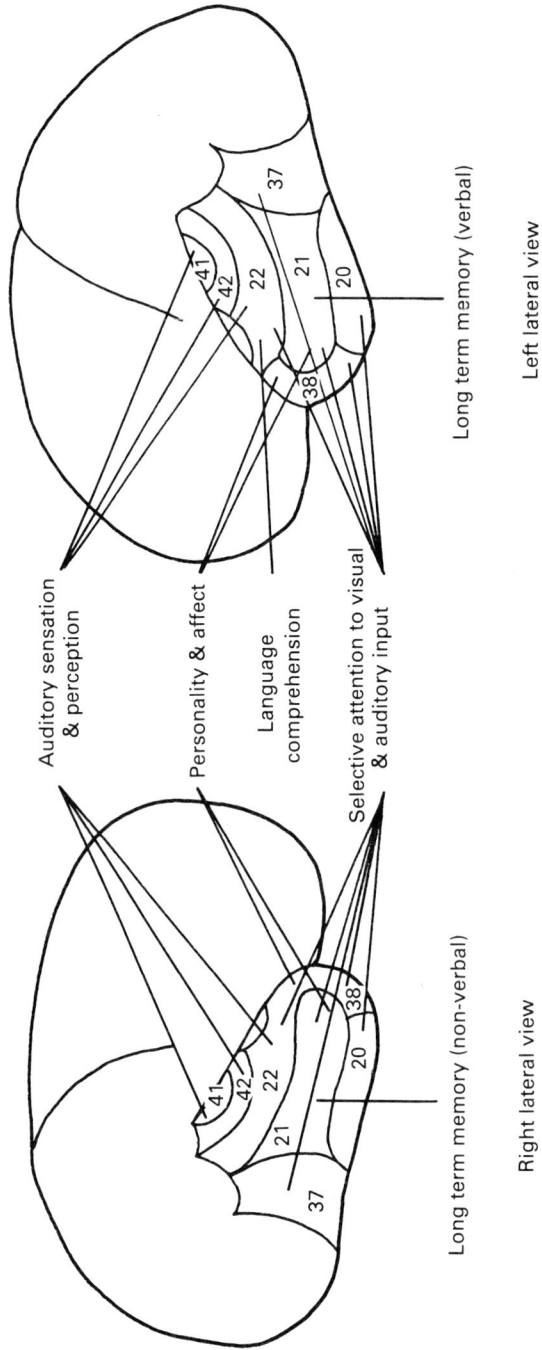

Fig. 2.11 Specific functions attributed mainly to the temporal lobes (Kolb & Whishaw, 1980).

equal, and allowing behaviour to be modified by experience.

The limbic system is currently thought to be involved in many aspects of behaviour including learning, memory, inhibition, organisation of movement, and spatial orientation (Kolb & Whishaw, 1980). Asymmetry is evident in memory functions, with the left hemisphere being involved in verbal memory and the right in non-verbal, and there is also some evidence of differences in affect and personality functions between hemispheres. However, despite some left and right specialisation there is substantial functional overlap. Specific functions that have been attributed to temporal lobes (Fig. 2.11) from research findings through effects of lesions and surgery include:

(a) Auditory sensation and perception (Vignolo, 1969; Hecaen & Albert, 1978)
(b) Selective attention to visual and auditory input (Dorff et al, 1965; Milner, 1970; Sparks et al, 1970)
(c) Language comprehension (Hecaen & Albert, 1978)
(d) Long term verbal and non-verbal memory (Milner, 1958)
(e) Personality and affect (Pincus & Tucker, 1974; Blumer & Benson, 1975)
(f) Sexual activity (Walker & Blumer, 1975)

Lesions to the temporal lobes, depending on the side, site and extent, may affect any of the above functions, resulting in possible impairment to communication, comprehension, visual and auditory perception, and changes in behaviour.

Afferent connections are received from the sensory systems and efferent fibres project to the parietal and frontal association regions and the basal ganglia.

4. The occipital lobes

The occipital lobes, which are served by the posterior cerebral artery, contain the primary and secondary visual cortex, the association areas for vision being located in the temporal lobes (Brodmann's areas 20 and 22), and integration with other sensory information occurring in the parietal lobes. A unilateral lesion in the occipital lobes may produce homonymous hemianopia with macular sparing. Small lesions often produce scotomas,

which are tiny blind spots in the visual field. Cortical blindness, with denial or impaired perception of blindness, occurs with bilateral lesions (Mossman, 1976). The visual system is composed (Kolb & Whishaw, 1980) of two anatomical routes: the tectopulvinar system, which does not project through the occipital lobes, specializing in locating visual stimuli; and the geniculostriate system which specializes in the perception of form, colour, and patterns. These systems converge on the visual association areas of the temporal lobe and, although separate, are not mutually exclusive, as some degree of either function is spared in lesions affecting one or other system (Fig. 2.12).

More complex visuoperceptual dysfunction results from lesions beyond the primary visual cortex. Probable sites for visual gnostic activity are shown in Figure 2.13.

5. Cortical connections

Cortical connections, which transmit information between areas of the brain, are currently being evaluated to determine whether and what functional impairment may result as a direct consequence of specific damage. Geschwind (1965) has theorized that apraxia, agnosia, and alexia may be the result of disconnection syndromes.

There are three major types of connection within the cerebrum:

(a) The projection fibres which link cortical areas with the rest of the body via subcortical structures. Nearly all the fibres of the motor and somatosensory systems cross, so that each hemisphere is mainly responsible for the sensory/motor activity of the contralateral side of the body;
(b) The commissural fibres which connect the two hemispheres, principally the corpus callosum, anterior commissure, and the hippocampal commissure;
(c) The association fibres which connect various regions of each hemisphere. These are responsible for the transmission of information required for integration, response, and action.

If lesions affect cortical connections, impairment is likely to reflect that of areas they connect, as transmission of information needed for appropriate

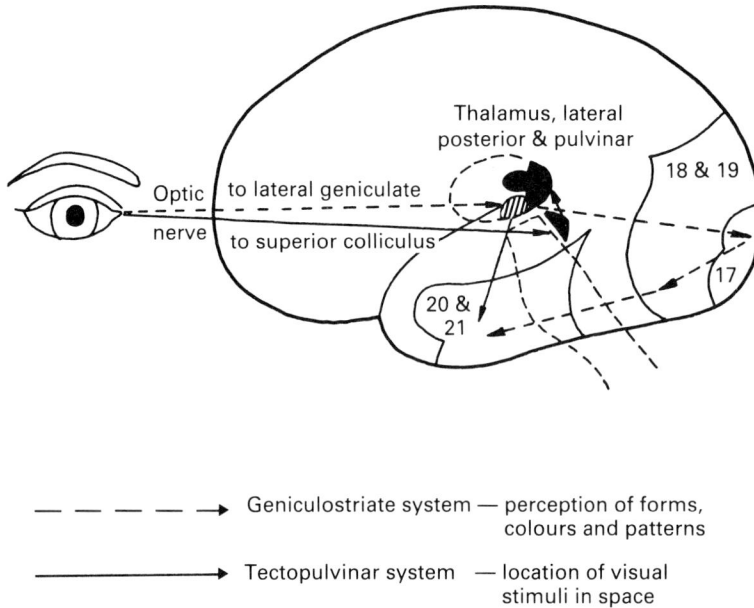

Fig. 2.12 The geniculostriate and tectopulvinar routes of the visual system (Kolb & Whishaw, 1980).

function is prevented or retarded (Kolb & Whishaw, 1980).

6. The thalamus

The thalamus, which is served by branches of the posterior cerebral, posterior communicating, and internal carotid arteries, connects many areas of the brain, acting as a sensory relay and integrative centre (Fig. 2.14). Ascending sensory fibres pass through the brain stem, synapse in the thalamus, then pass through the internal capsules to reach the cerebral cortex.

Lesions may produce the thalamic syndrome with loss or impaired sensation contralaterally, or overactive sensory responses, with pain and discomfort (Noback & Demarest, 1977).

Descending motor fibres pass through the internal capsule then by-pass the thalamus to reach the brain stem.

7. The internal capsule, brain stem and cerebellum

The internal capsule, which is served by the middle, anterior, and posterior cerebral arteries is the point at which the fibres from the motor, somatosensory, visual, and auditory areas converge to enter the brain stem.

Lesions of the internal capsule will result in dysfunction which reflects the cortical areas that the damaged fibres project to or from. Small bilateral lesions may produce the condition known as *pseudobulbar palsy*.

The brain stem, which is served by the vertebrobasilar artery, continues to carry the motor and sensory fibres to and from the spinal cord. It also is responsible for controlling many neuronal circuits (including those of vital functions, equilibrium, and support of the body against gravity) and is the exit site for the twelve cranial nerves.

Lesions may produce a variety of symptoms such as contralateral and ipsilateral signs (because not all tracts have crossed), cranial nerve disorders, dysarthria and dysphagia.

Posterior-superior to the brain stem is the cerebellum which has direct communication with the motor cortex and the brain stem. It is responsible for the continuous monitoring of movement and for correcting and adjusting motor activity, including relatively independent movement of the limbs and fingers.

Lesions in the cerebellum cause ipsilateral loss of co-ordination and tone. The cerebellum is an

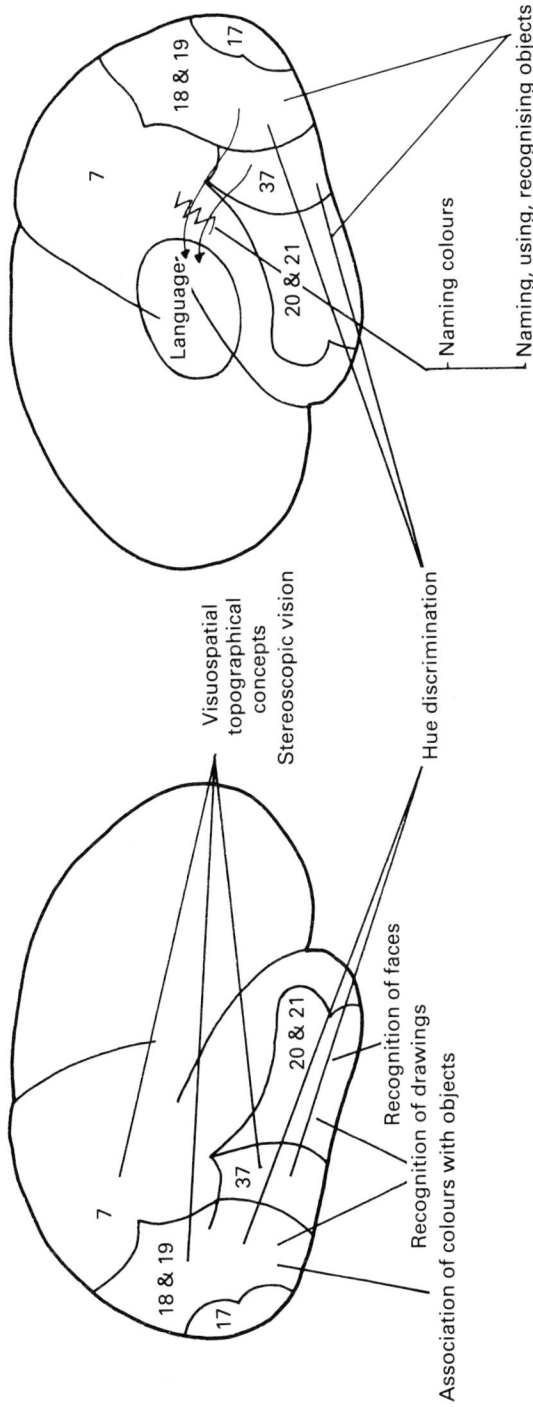

Fig. 2.13 Probable sites for specific visual gnostic functions (Kolb & Whishaw, 1980).

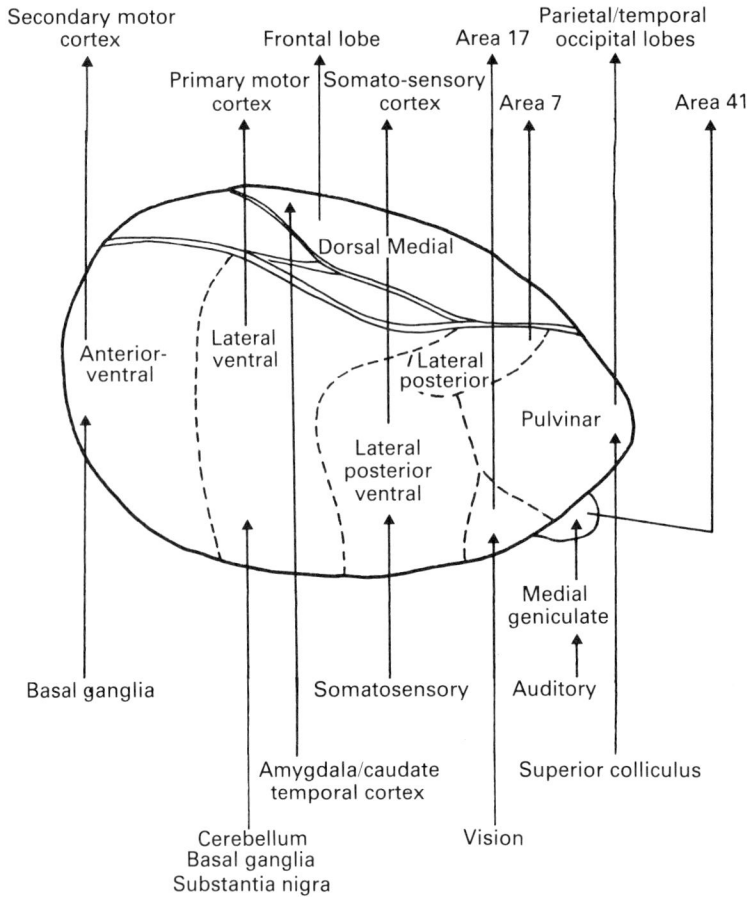

Fig. 2.14 Connections of the thalamic nuclei. (Adapted from Kolb B, Whishaw I Q 1980 Fundamentals of human neuropsychology. Freeman.)

uncommon site of infarction, lesions usually occurring in conjunction with lesions of the brain stem. (Levy, 1975).

EFFECTS OF LOCATION OF LESION

1. The internal carotid system

The internal carotid artery, which divides into the middle and anterior cerebral arteries, supplies the major cerebral areas responsible for motor and somatosensory function. Occlusion of one internal carotid which does not extend intracranially, often produces only slight neurological deficits as the cortex is still supplied by co-lateral anastomosis.

When disease spreads intracranially, causing occlusion in both the middle and anterior cerebral arteries, the following areas of the brain are affected: the frontal, parietal, and temporal lobes; the internal capsule; and the optic nerve. The effects of such an infarct are contralateral hemiplegia, sensory loss, homonymous hemianopia, aphasia (if the speech dominant hemisphere is involved), and perceptual dysfunction.

Middle cerebral artery occlusion can affect the frontal, parietal, and temporal lobes, and also the internal capsule, a very common site, and the anterior thalamus. The effects of occlusion here, therefore, may be contralateral hemiplegia (particularly upper limb and facial weakness), sensory loss, homonymous hemianopia, perceptual problems, aphasia if the speech dominant hemisphere is involved, and contralateral neglect if the other hemisphere is affected (Fig. 2.15).

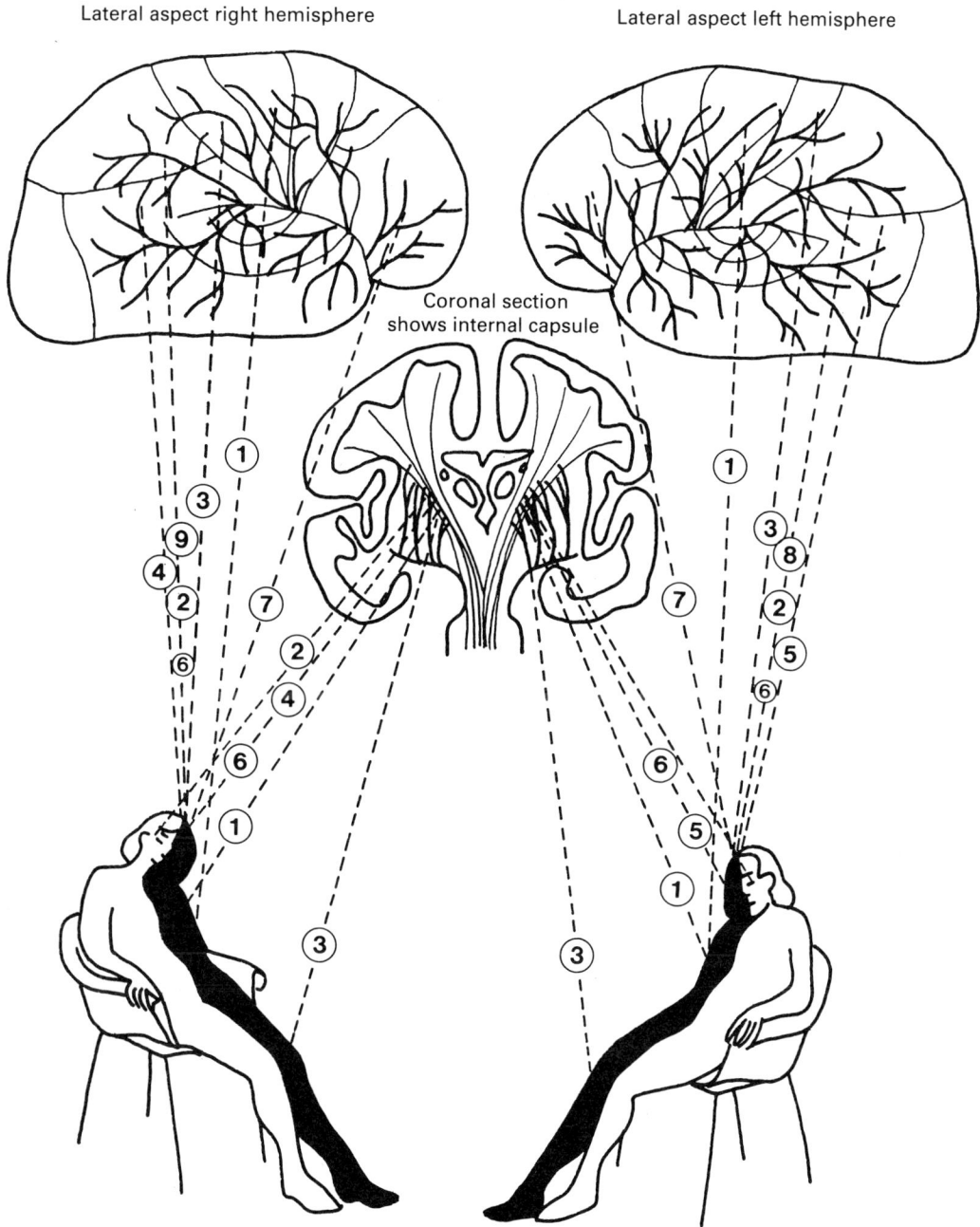

Lateral aspect right hemisphere

Lateral aspect left hemisphere

Coronal section shows internal capsule

1 Contralateral hemiplegia particularly UL & face
2 Perceptual problems
3 Somatosensory impairment
4 Contralateral neglect/Spatial disorders
5 Language disorders

6 Homonymous hemianopia
7 Affect and behaviour changes/Apraxia
8 Apraxia
9 Constructional apraxia

Fig. 2.15 Clinical profile of middle cerebral artery stroke. A general indication of dysfunction which may be caused by infarction in either cortex or internal capsule.

If there are bilateral infarcts within both internal capsules, brain stem symptoms such as difficulties with speech, swallowing, mastication, tongue and facial movements may result; emotional lability may also be evident. This syndrome ('pseudo bulbar palsy') is not truly a disorder of the brain stem but of the tracts leading to the cranial nerve nuclei from the cortex.

Anterior cerebral artery occlusion can affect the medial surface of the frontal and parietal lobes and the junction of the occipital lobe. It also supplies the anterior part of the internal capsule. Manifestations of occlusion may be contralateral lower limb paralysis and hypesthesia (decreased sensation), facial weakness, sensory loss, homonymous hemianopia, or, if the ophthalmic artery is involved, homolateral amaurosis (ipsilateral blindness).

2. The vertebro-basilar system

The vertebral arteries join to form the basilar artery from which branches leave to service the brain stem and cerebellum. The basilar artery then divides into the posterior arteries which supply the medial and inferior aspects of the temporal lobe, the occipital lobe and the visual cortex, and the posterior and lateral parts of the thalamus and subthalamus. Occlusion of one vertebral artery alone affects the brain stem but because of the continuation of supply to the basilar artery by the other vertebral artery good recovery is usual (Bladin, 1976). However, complete basilar artery occlusion is often fatal because of the brain stem's controlling function of vital systems. Incomplete lesions affect balance and proprioception. There may be ataxia, decreased tendon reflexes on the affected side, asthenia (muscle fatigability), intention tremor, nystagmus, and difficulties with speech, swallowing, mastication, and facial, tongue, and eye movements.

Posterior cerebral artery occlusion, because it supplies the occipital lobe and visual association areas of the temporal lobe, can result in homonymous hemianopia (with macular sparing), problems of visual recognition and, because of its medial temporal (hippocampal) supply, can affect memory.

When there is occlusion to the thalamus there may be loss of contralateral sensation, unpleasant distortions of cutaneous sensation with burning pain occurring spontaneously, and ataxia. There may also be contralateral hemiplegia and hemianaesthesia (Levenson, 1971; Guyton, 1981).

PROCESSES IN RECOVERY

The prognosis is dependent upon the nature and extent of the lesion although intervention procedures during rehabilitation affect eventual qualitative functional status.

1. Anatomical considerations

The risk of death following basilar artery occlusion with subsequent brain stem infarction is great; but partial occlusion within the vertebrobasilar circulation may lead to reasonable recovery of sensory motor and dysphagic disorders, because intellectual functioning, apart from possible short-term memory loss, remains intact (Mossman, 1976).

When, as is more frequent, the internal carotid system suffers infarction, wide ranging dysfunction may occur which affects the outcome, particularly when there is loss of higher intellectual skills which may retard relearning.

Some disorders thought to indicate a poor prognosis are: diffuse cortical involvement, prolonged flaccidity or spasticity, gross somatosensory and visual defects, asomatognosia, and gross visuospatial or praxic disturbance (Levenson, 1971; Gersten, 1975). The presence of any of these factors does not imply unsuitability for rehabilitation programs, as individual variables are great and other factors may effect recovery.

2. Etiological considerations

Because of increased intracranial pressure resulting from haemorrhagic strokes, death or initially diffuse and life threatening neurological impairment is more likely than with thrombotic or embolic strokes. There is also more cerebral oedema surrounding the area of dead tissue.

These factors affect recovery time schedules; embolic or thrombotic strokes usually have most significant recovery gains during the first three months, and haemorrhagic strokes experience gains between six to twelve months after C.V.A., often achieving reasonable function.

3. Spontaneous recovery

For those who survive there is some spontaneous remission from the extent of symptoms apparent at the time of C.V.A. Probable factors are the reduction of oedema and ischaemic penumbra surrounding the area of destroyed tissue, which temporarily extend the size of the lesion, and the gradual recovery from cerebral functional shock which may have caused a temporary disruption of neural transmission and integration processes (Laurence & Stein, 1978).

Recovery from brain damage is widely recognised as progressing from a period of shock or diaschisis, through a period of recovery, which tends to follow an ontogenetic developmental sequence, to the state of chronic impairment which reflects the locus and extent of the tissue destroyed (Kolb & Whishaw, 1980). There are many theories about possible mechanisms for recovery of brain function but it is still uncertain whether regeneration or alternative neuronal organization occurs.

There has been some research into the sequence of motor recovery. Twitchell (1977) reports that initial flaccidity is followed by increased reflex activity, followed by flexor and extensor synergies, followed by voluntary motor return. He suggests that recovery can be divided into three stages, the first being dominated by proprioceptive responses, and the second by contactual stimulation, with vision being facilitatory in both. In the third stage movement is apparent in response to will, and is independent of external stimuli, gradually ceasing to require vision to monitor control. Recovery can be retarded or stop at any of these levels.

If somatosensory function does not recover, alternative intact cognitive and sensory skills may develop to counteract the loss and give the appearance of some return of function.

Recovery of contralateral neglect appears to pass through two stages. In the first the patient begins to respond to stimuli (notably verbal) on the left side but as if it were happening on the right. This is known as *allesthesia*. In the second stage the patient responds to stimuli on the left side but not if a simultaneous stimulus is applied to the right side. Response occurs to stimuli on the sound side alone. This known as *simultaneous extinction* (Kolb & Whishaw, 1980).

4. Psychological and social factors

Psychological and social factors may also affect recovery processes and increase motivation, concentration, and participation in the re-education programs. Two known positive factors are acceptance and understanding of the disability, and the presence of a spouse in the home (Gersten, 1975).

CLINICAL PROFILE

The symptoms most commonly seen are those of the motor system, notably hemiplegia and impaired balance; the somatosensory system, notably tactile and proprioceptive sensory loss and impaired body awareness; the visual system, notably homonymous hemianopia and visuospatial agnosia; impaired communication and cognitive skills, and altered affect and behaviour.

1. Motor dysfunction

(*a*) *Hemiplegia*: defined as paralysis of one side of the body on the side contralateral to the lesion. The paralysis may be incomplete (paresis), the amount of motor dysfunction varying considerably according to the level, size, and type of infarction. Hemiplegia is the major observable sign of stroke, and has therefore received more attention than other symptoms which may be equally dysfunctional.

Impairment causes malfunctioning of central nervous system control, resulting in loss of voluntary movement due to changes in postural tone, and disinhibition of primitive reflex activity (Bobath, 1978). Normal tone, which is reflex in nature, maintains muscles in slight contraction even at rest. When reflex activity is released from cerebral control following damage to the motor system, hypotonicity (flaccid hemiplegia) is evident during the period of cerebral shock, and sometimes persists permanently. Hypotonicity is usually followed by increasing hypertonicity (spastic hemiplegia) in an exaggerated pattern of normal reflex tone.

Patients may demonstrate paralysis or weakness of both contralateral limbs, usually the arm being more severely involved than the leg, although when the anterior cerebral artery is occluded, the contralateral lower limb alone may be affected.

There is often dysfunction of the trunk muscles but, as these are innervated bilaterally (Dardier, 1980) total contralateral paralysis does not occur; however, any decrease in respiratory muscle function will lead to fatigue following physical effort.

There may be poor head control, unilateral facial weakness, hypotonus of oral musculature apparent in facial asymmetry, and perhaps drooling. Orofacial weakness may cause difficulties in expression, speech (dysarthria), mastication, and swallowing (dysphagia), and is seen particularly following brain stem damage.

If only the cortico-spinal tract is damaged the result may be a simple motor paresis with a reasonable change of recovery. In many cases, however, there are diffuse motor deficits, which are compounded by sensory loss and impaired higher cortical skills.

(b) *Impaired balance*. The major determinants for normal balance are vision, proprioception, and labyrinthine (vestibular) function, and at least two of these systems need to function adequately to maintain balance. Parietal damage resulting in impaired visuospatial skills may also impair equilibrium (Mossman, 1976).

Impairment may cause difficulties in assuming and maintaining a vertical posture, and automatic adjustments to changes of position and antigravity movement. Transient vertigo may also be apparent.

Patients with impaired balance may demonstrate an asymmetrical posture at rest, leaning or falling to the hemiplegic side during mobility practice, and fail to use normal protective reactions when their centre of gravity is displaced.

(c) *Apraxia*: defined as the inability to carry out purposeful movement when normal co-ordinated movement is possible and unaffected by lack of comprehension or motivation. It has been proposed that the left hemisphere has a special role in controlling movement, and that the parietal lobes are responsible for directing movements

towards behavioral goals (Kolb & Whishaw, 1980).

Impairment of the left parietal lobe may result in an apraxia where patients are unable to adjust movement of their own body parts, whilst impairment of the right parietal lobe may result in an inability to adjust the position of external objects (Walsh, 1978; Kimura, 1980). Lesions of either frontal lobes may result in apraxia in which sequencing movement is a major difficulty. Lesions of cortical connections may also produce apraxic behaviour (Kolb & Whishaw, 1980).

Patients experiencing difficulty in praxis or motor planning may demonstrate an inability to carry out a verbal request (often a simple task such as combing hair) although they have been seen to do the task automatically; they may perseverate in purposeless movement, be unable to complete a required sequence of acts, be unable to copy gesture, drawings, or simple spatial constructional tasks.

(d) *Incontinence*. There may be bladder or bowel incontinence due to flaccid distention of bladder with overflow incontinence (Mossman, 1976), or an inability to inhibit the reflex expulsion of waste because of neurological damage. Prolonged incontinence often follows bilateral damage. Incontinence may be a symptom of a communication disorder, and may also be due to disruption of normal routine and diet, lack of awareness of body function, or emotional disorder (Mossman, 1976).

2. Somatosensory dysfunction

Somatosensory dysfunction includes both disorders of sensation and perception. Sensation refers to activity from the peripheral sensory receptors, the afferent sensory tracts, and the appropriate primary sensory cortex; perception refers to activity occurring in secondary and tertiary sensory association areas of the cortex, which integrate other information such as memory, context and experience (Kolb & Whishaw, 1980).

It is sometimes difficult to differentiate between the two, sensation when impaired distorting information from self and the environment, and perception when impaired causing dysfunction in understanding and interpreting information from self and the environment.

There is frequently sensory loss together with motor dysfunction. It seldom occurs in isolation and certainly compounds the loss of functional activity.

(a) *Impaired proprioception*. Proprioception is defined as sensory awareness of the position of body parts. Impairment affects anti-gravity and postural mechanisms, including cortical and subcortical adjustments of tone and position.

Patients with proprioceptive dysfunction may demonstrate an asymmetrical posture, have difficulties maintaining balance, appear to forget affected body parts, be unable to describe the position or movement of limbs, and be susceptible to joint damage.

(b) *Impaired tactile sensation*. Tactile sensation is defined as localization and discrimination of cutaneous stimuli including light touch, fine localization, two point discrimination, and discrimination of shape, size, texture, temperature, and pain.

Impairment affects motor activity as sensory feedback is limited; it also affects functional perception as information needed for interpretation and integration is incomplete. Patients with impairment or loss of tactile sensation may demonstrate a lack of awareness of body parts simply because people tend to forget what they cannot feel. They may also be susceptible to damage of affected body parts, particularly to skin breakdown.

On specific clinical tests they will be unable to localize or discriminate accurately when vision is occluded. Damage may occur at either cortical or subcortical levels.

(c) *Astereognosis*. Stereognosis is defined as recognition of common objects by touch, normally almost spontaneous in adults (Carr & Shepherd, 1980).

Impairment affects functional use of the affected hand whenever vision is occluded, so that tasks such as finding keys or coins in a pocket, or a glass on a bedside table when it is dark, may be difficult. Tracts carrying stereognosis information are those of the posterior columns with proprioception and vibration sense.

Stereognosis requires integration of various modalities such as discrimination of shape, size, weight, texture, temperature, joint position sense, fine touch and spatial conceptualization in order to interpret the identity of the object. Patients with impaired tactile and spatial perception may appear to have bilateral difficulty in recognising objects by touch. Astereognosis is not clinically observable without specific tasks.

(d) *Asomatognosia*. Somatognosia is defined as the knowledge and awareness of one's own body and its condition. Loss most commonly results from a right parietal lobe lesion.

Impairment of body awareness will affect motor performance, postural reactions, and the understanding of and response to sensory stimuli from the affected side. It may vary from mild neglect to absolute denial and confabulation, and Critchley (1953) has listed nine categories of this disorder. When asomatognosia is present recovery is slow and difficult.

Patients with loss of body awareness may demonstrate neglect of body parts (contralateral neglect), or denial of parts and dysfunction (anasognosia); they may have asymmetrical posture, poor balance, visual inattention to the affected side, and may be susceptible to damage to affected body parts and make bizarre statements about limbs found in unexpected places. Theories about why contralateral neglect occurs include the thought that as parietal lobe lesions disturb sensory integration, spatial aspects are misperceived locationally and are ignored (Denny-Brown & Chambers, 1958), or that it results from a defect in attention to stimuli, (Critchley, 1953; Heilman & Watson, 1977). The inability to localize and name body parts usually results from lesions of the left parietal lobe and is known as autopagnosia.

3. Visual dysfunction

(a) *Homonymous hemianopia*: defined as loss of vision in one half of the visual field (the temporal half of one eye and the nasal half of the other), following lesions of the optic tract, the lateral geniculate nucleus of the thalamus, or the visual cortex in posterior cerebral artery occlusion. Should the lesion be partial, quadrantic hemianopia results. Loss of vision and hemiplegia occur on the same side (Fig. 2.16).

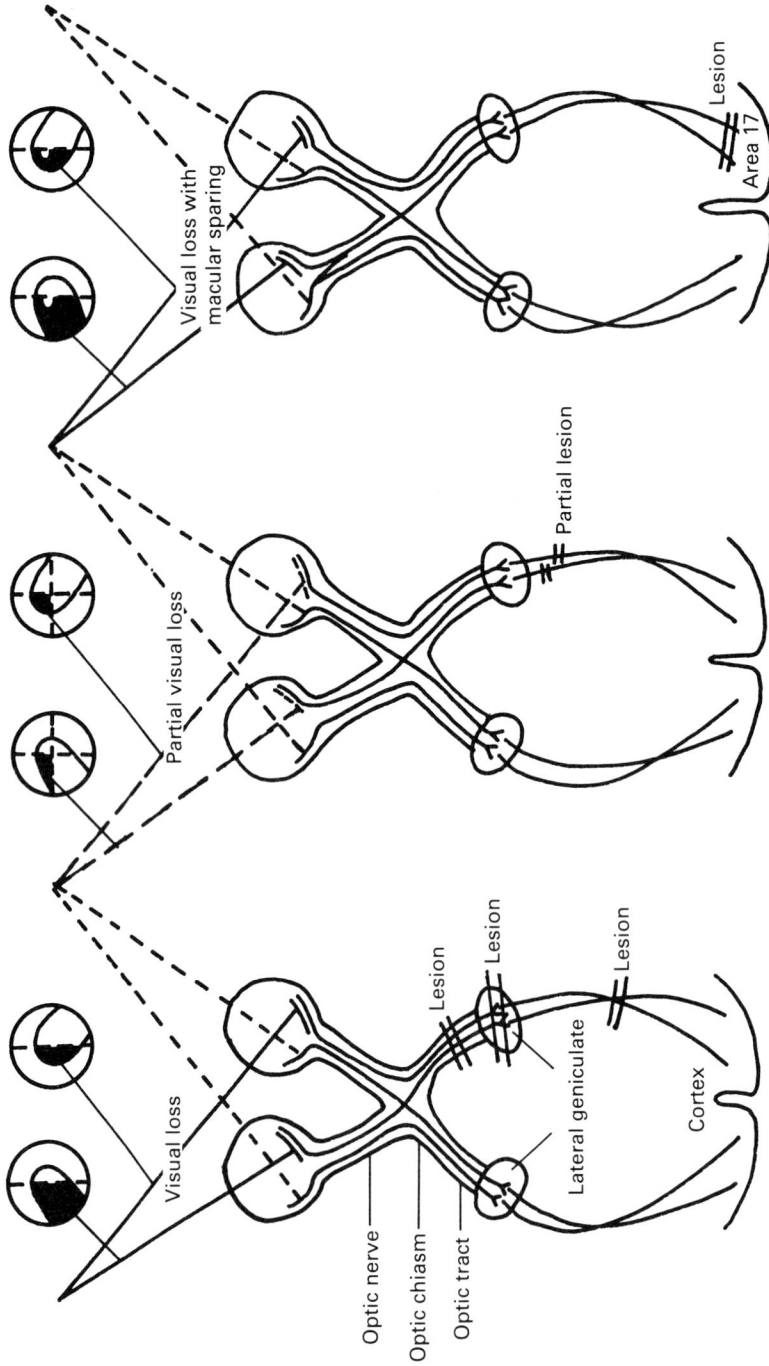

Fig. 2.16 Common visual disorders resulting from lesions to the visual system (Kolb & Whishaw, 1980).

Impairment of the visual fields will decrease the patient's awareness of the environment and affect the performance of motor tasks.

Patients with homonymous hemianopia of either side may demonstrate a lack of response to people, objects, or the environment on the affected side, lack of appreciation of the need to scan or turn their head to the affected side unless prompted or taught to do so, and may bump into objects or be startled by their sudden appearance (Pedretti, 1981). They may also be unaware of their visual deficits. Patients with left visual field loss tend to appear more functionally disadvantaged by the loss, as the visual disorder may be complicated by contralateral neglect.

(b) *Visual inattention*: defined as the lack of response to stimuli on the affected side when simultaneous stimuli are applied to both sides and there is no actual visual field defect.

Injury to either hemisphere may cause impaired visual exploration of the contralateral field (De Renzi et al, 1970; Walsh, 1978). Impairment usually occurs with other sensory dysfunction such as proprioceptive loss and asomatognosia.

Patients may demonstrate difficulty in scanning and shifting their gaze, particularly towards their affected side, and in responding to the environment on that side. In clinical testing patients will be able to see a visual stimulus placed on the side contralateral to the lesion, but fail to perceive it when there are simultaneous bilateral stimuli.

(c) *Visual agnosias*: defined as disorders of recognition of visual stimuli, usually following a lesion of the visual association areas. They appear less common than agnosias of a visuo-spatial nature which follow parietal and frontal lobe damage.

(d) *Visuo-spatial agnosias*: defined as difficulty in understanding the relationship between objects, and between self and objects.

Impairment causes problems in conceptualizing and using extra and intrapersonal space, appreciating distances and directionality between objects, in accurately perceiving vertical and horizontal, in discriminating objects from background, and in appreciating object constancy when orientation is changed.

Patients may demonstrate impairment of visuo-spatial perception by losing their way in a familiar environment, being unable to trace a route on a map, being unable to pick out objects from a cluttered environment or to recognise the same objects when placed differently, being unable to copy drawings or simple construction, and may have difficulty in many functional (spatial) tasks such dressing and reading a newspaper.

4. Auditory dysfunction

When there is a unilateral lesion affecting the primary auditory cortex deafness does not result; rather, on the side contralateral to the lesion, sound is diminished. When lesions occur in the left secondary area there may be difficulties bilaterally in differentiating simultaneous speech sounds (auditory figure ground) and in phonemic hearing. When lesions occur in the right secondary auditory area analysis of music, particularly tonal and timbre memory, may be impaired. There may also be difficulty in locating the source of sounds (Kolb & Whishaw, 1980).

The most common auditory agnosia is amusia which can include the inability to discriminate tonal difference or to recall or recognise a melody. Agnosia for sounds may also occur, and this is characterised by not understanding, or confusing, non-verbal sounds.

5. Language dysfunction

The major language disorder of middle cerebral artery stroke is dysphasia or aphasia.

(a) *Dys/aphasia* may be defined as a multimodality impairment in the capacity to interpret and formulate meaningful language (Sells, 1983). Language involves complex interaction between verbal memory, automatic motor skills, symbolic associations, syntactic ability and sensory integration. Primary language areas are located in the left hemisphere and include those known as Brocas and Wernickes' areas and also parts of the association areas, particularly of the temporal lobe. Other language function takes place in association areas of the right hemisphere and the posterior thalamus and basal ganglia (Kolb & Whishaw, 1980).

Impairment may be varied from cases where subtle use of language is altered, to total loss of functional speech, and can include auditory and visual (reading) comprehension, and verbal and written expression.

Patients with dysphasia may demonstrate difficulties in participating in conversation, perhaps displaying an apparent lack of attention or inappropriate input; they may also have difficulties in word finding, in constructing sentences, in using appropriate words, in reading and in writing and in appreciating abstract aspects of language such as humour. They may have no functional language but display automatic or serial speech and writing. They may also appear emotional, expressing frustration, anger, or inappropriate laughter or tears.

(b) *Dyspraxia* in language function may be defined as an impairment of voluntary ability to use the speech mechanisms. It most frequently co-exists with dysphasia (Sells, 1983). Patients may demonstrate impairment by having difficulties with oral or articulatory movements on command, or in imitation, but may be able to use automatic and serial speech and singing.

(c) *Dysarthria*: is defined as imperfect articulation due to disorders of motor control. Patients frequently demonstrate asymmetry of facial expression, with drooping mouth, drooling, and extended tongue.

6. Cognitive dysfunction

Difficulties with planning, concentration, abstract reasoning, judgment and foresight, and impairment of verbal fluency may occur. These are thought to be due to lesions of the anterior frontal lobe.

Patients with impairment may demonstrate impulsive behaviour or anxiety, and may appear to have limited spontaneous speech, with verbal responses often showing an echolalic quality. They may perform poorly on clinical tests which demand sequential reasoning and problem-solving skills. Short-term (working) memory disorders may occur with parietal lesions, and memory for order of events may be affected by frontal lobe lesions. Impairment may cause difficulties in accurate recall of day to day activities, people and newly learned procedures. A right C.V.A. usually causes more difficulties with visual memory and left C.V.A. with verbal memory. Gross memory disorders are more common, with posterior cerebral artery occlusion affecting the medial temporal lobe and hippocampus (Kolb & Whishaw, 1980).

7. Emotional dysfunction

Depression, denial, anxiety, and fear may occur as a result of the C.V.A.

Patients experiencing emotional disturbance may demonstrate sleeplessness, agitation, irritability, apathy or depression; they may be euphoric or tearful; they may seem dependent on external support and attention demanding. They may try to isolate themselves, resist treatment, and be afraid of physical exertion. Lesions of left or right hemisphere may produce differences in affective behaviour; for example the left hemisphere is thought to analyse the content of sensory stimuli literally, whilst the right analyses its emotional tone. Lesions to the right are generally thought to 'release' talking, whilst lesions to the left reduce talking (Kolb & Whishaw, 1980).

Various studies have been made about differences in affect and social behaviour between patients with right and left vascular lesions (Goldstein, 1939; Gainotti, 1972).

A depressive-catastrophic reaction is described as occurring with left hemisphere lesions, particularly when dysphasia is a factor, and an indifference reaction with right hemisphere lesions particularly in the presence of unilateral neglect.

Researchers report that the catastrophic reaction was most often seen after patients with dysphasia repeatedly failed in communication (Walsh, 1978). Goldstein (1939) found that physical as well as emotional distress symptoms occurred, and that following such a reaction there was a reduction in activity performance with patients failing in tasks previously possible.

Gainotti (1972) lists anxiety reactions, tears, vocative utterances, depressed or sharp renouncements, and refusals to continue the task in hand, as symptoms occurring with left-sided lesions. With right-sided lesions he lists anosognosia, indifference, a tendency to joke, and expressions of hate towards affected body parts.

Bilateral effects usually transient may be observed following a unilateral lesion. They are possibly due to diaschisis apart or remote from the site of lesion, or to a reduction in blood flow and metabolism in both hemispheres (Walsh, 1978).

REFERENCES

Benton A L 1959 Right-left discrimination and finger localization. Harper & Row, New York

Benton A L 1969 Disorders of spatial orientation. In: Vincken P et al (eds) Handbook of clinical neurology Vol 3. North Holland Publishing Co, Amsterdam

Bladin P F 1976 Strokes. In: Stanley G V, Walsh K W (eds) Brain impairment, proceedings of the 1976 Brain Impairment Workshop, the neuropsychology group. University of Melbourne, p 47–52

Blumer D, Benson D F 1975 Personality changes with frontal and temporal lobe lesions. In: Psychiatric aspects of neurological disease. Grune & Stratton, New York

Bobath B 1978 Adult hemiplegia evaluation and treatment. Heinemann Medical Books, London

Brodmann K 1909 Vergleichended Lokalisations lehre der Grosshirnrinde in Prinzipien dargestellt auf Grund des Zellenbaues. J A Barth, Leipzig

Brown J 1972 Aphasia, apraxia and agnosia. Charles Thomas, Springfield, Illinois

Burrow D D 1983 Unpublished lecture notes. Neurology and neurosurgery for O.T. students, Adelaide

Butters N, Brody B A 1968 The role of the left parietal lobe in the mediation of intra and cross modal associations. Cortex 4: 328–343

Carr J, Shepherd R 1980 Physiotherapy in disorders of the brain. Heinemann Medical Books Ltd, London

Critchley M 1953 The parietal lobes. Arnold, London

Dardier E 1980 The early stroke patient. Cassell Ltd, London.

Denny-Brown D, Chambers R A 1958 The parietal lobes and behaviour. Research Publications of the Association for Research into Mental Disease 36: 35–117

De Renzi E, Faglioni P, Scotti G 1970 Hemispheric contribution to exploration of space through the visual and tactile modality. Cortex 6: 191–203

Dorff J E, Mirsky A F, Mishkin M 1965 Effects of unilateral temporal lobe removals in tachistoscopic recognition in the left and right visual fields. Neuropsychologia 3: 39–51

Dorland's Illustrated Medical Dictionary 25th Edition 1974 Saunders, Philadelphia.

Dunphy J E, Way L W 1981 Current surgical diagnosis and treatment, 5th edn. Lange Medical Publications, California

Elliot H 1969 Textbook of neuroanatomy. Lippincott, Philadelphia

Gainotti G 1972 Emotional behaviour and hemispheric side of lesion. Cortex 8: 41–55

Gersten J W 1975 Rehabilitation potential. In: Licht S (ed) Stroke and its rehabilitation. Waverly Press Inc, Baltimore

Geschwind N 1965 Disconnexion syndromes in animals and man. Brain 88: 237–294; 585–644

Goldberg S 1979 Neuroanatomy made ridiculously simple. Medmaster Inc, Miami

Goldstein K 1939 The organism: A holistic approach in biology. Derived from Pathological Data in Man. American Book Co, New York

Guyton A C 1981 Basic human neurophysiology. Saunders, Philadelphia

Hecaen H 1969 Aphasic, apraxic and agnosic syndromes in right and left hemisphere lesions. In: Vincken P, Bruyn G (eds) Handbook of clinical neurology, Vol 4. North Holland Publishing Co, Amsterdam

Hecaen H and Albert M L 1975 Disorders of mental functioning related to frontal lobe pathology. In: Benson D F, Blumer D (eds) Psychiatric aspects of neurological disease. Grune and Stratton, New York

Hecaen H, Albert M L 1978 Human neuropsychology. J Wiley & Sons, New York

Heilman K M, Watson R T 1977 The neglect syndrome. In: Harnard S et al (eds) Lateralization in the nervous system. Academic Press, New York

Jones-Gotman M, Milner B 1977 Design fluency: the invention of nonsense drawings after focal cortical lesions. Neuropsychologia, 15, p 653–674

Kimura D 1980 Neuromotor mechanisms in the evolution of human communication. In: Steklis H D, Raleigh M J (eds) Neurobiology of social communication in primates. Academic Press, New York

Kolb B, Milner B 1981 Performance of complex arm and facial movement after frontal brain lesion. Neuropsychologia 19(4): 491–503

Kolb B, Whishaw I Q 1980 Fundamentals of human neuropsychology. Freeman, San Francisco

Laurence S, Stein D J 1978 Recovery after brain damage and the concept of localization of function. In: Finger S (ed) Recovery from brain damage. Plenum Press, London

Levenson C 1971 Rehabilitation of the stroke hemiplegia patient. In: Krusen F H, Kottke F J, Ellwood P M (eds) Handbook of physical medicine and rehabilitation. Saunders, Philadelphia

Levy L 1975 Examination and diagnosis. In: Licht S (ed) Stroke and its rehabilitation. Waverly Press, Baltimore

Luria A R 1973 The working brain. Penguin, New York

Milner B 1958 Psychological defects produced by temporal lobe excision. Research Publications of the Association for Research in Nervous and Mental Disease 3: 244–257

Milner B 1964 Some effects of frontal lobectomy in man. In: Warren J M, Akert K (eds) The frontal granular cortex and behaviour. McGraw Hill, New York

Milner B 1970 Memory and the medial temporal region of the brain. In: Pribram K H, Broadbent D E (eds) Biological bases of memory. Academic Press, New York

Milner B 1974 Hemispheric specialization: scope and limits. In: Schmitt F O, Worden F G (eds) The neurosciences: third study program. M I T Press, Cambridge, Mass

McKissock W, Payne K W, Walsh L S 1960 An analysis of the results of treatment of ruptured intra cranial aneurysms; a report of 722 consecutive cases. Journal of Neurosurgery 17: 762.

Mossman P L 1976 A problem oriented approach to stroke rehabilitation. Charles Thomas, Springfield, Illinois

Noback C R, Demarest R 1977 The nervous system, introduction and review (2nd ed). McGraw Hill, New York

Pedretti L W 1981 Occupational therapy practice skills for physical dysfunction. C V Mosby Co, St Louis

Perret E 1974 The left frontal lobe of man and the suppression of habitual responses in verbal categorical behaviour. Neuropsychologia 12: 323–330

Piercy M, Hecaen H, Ajuriagueura J 1960 Constructional apraxia associated with unilateral cerebral lesions—left and right cases compared. Brain 83: 225–242

Pincus J H, Tucker G J 1974 Behavioural neurology. Oxford University Press, New York

Rubenstein D, Wayne D 1980 Lecture notes on clinical medicine, 2nd ed. Blackwell Scientific Publications, Oxford

Sells R 1983 Unpublished lecture notes on disorders of language for O.T. students. Adelaide

Semmes J, Weinstein S, Ghent L, Teuber H L 1960 Somatosensory changes after penetrating brain wounds in man. Harvard University Press, Cambridge, Mass

Semmes J, Weinstein S, Ghent L, Teuber H L 1963 Impaired orientation in personal and extra personal space. Brain 86: 747–772

Sparks R, Goodglass H, Nickel B 1970 Ipsilateral versus contralateral extinction in dichotic listening from hemispheric lesions. Cortex 6: 249–260

Taylor L 1979 Psychological assessment of neurosurgical patients. In: Rasmussen T, Marino R (eds) Functional neurosurgery. Raven Press, New York

Teuber H L 1964 The riddle of frontal lobe function. In: Warren et al (eds) The frontal granular cortex and behaviour. McGraw Hill, New York

Twitchell T E 1977 The restoration of motor function following hemiplegia in man. In: Payton O D, Hirt S Newton R A (eds) Scientific bases for neurophysiologic approaches to therapeutic exercise. Davis, Philadelphia

Tyler H R 1969 Disorders of visual scanning with frontal lobe lesions. In: Locke S (ed) Modern neurology. J & A Churchill, London

Vignolo L A 1969 Auditory agnosia. In: Benton A L (ed) Contributions to clinical neuropsychology. Aldine Publishing, Chicago

Walker E A, Blumer D 1975 The localization of sex in the brain. In: Zulch K J et al (eds) Cerebral localization. Springer-Verlag, Berlin

Walsh K W 1978 Neuropsychology, a clinical approach. Churchill Livingstone, Edinburgh

Warrington E K, James M, Kinsbourne M 1966 Drawing disability in relation to laterality of cerebral lesion. Brain 89: 53–82

Warrington E K, Weiskrantz L 1973 An analysis of short-term and long-term memory defects in man. In: Deutsch J A (ed) The physiological basis of memory. Academic Press, New York

Weller R O, Swash M, McLellan D L, Scholtz S L 1983 Clinical Neuropathology. Springer-Verlag, Berlin

RECOMMENDED READING

Gainotti G 1972 Emotional behavior and hemispheric side of lesion. Cortex 8: 41–55

Gersten J W 1975 Rehabilitation potential. In: Licht S (ed) Stroke and its rehabilitation. Waverly Press, Baltimore

Goldberg S 1979 Neuroanatomy made ridiculously simple. Medmaster Inc, Miami

Guyton A C 1981 Basic human neurophysiology. Saunders, Philadelphia

Kolb B, Whishaw I Q 1980 Fundamentals of human neuropsychology. Freeman, San Francisco

Luria A R 1973 The working brain. Penguin, New York

Twitchell T E 1977 The restoration of motor function following hemiplegia in man. In: Payton O D, Hirt S, Newton R A Scientific bases for neurophysiologic approaches to therapeutic exercise. Davis, Philadelphia

3

Evaluation

AN INITIAL APPROACH

The process of evaluation should commence from the initial source of information, usually the referral. All observations, data from formal tests, and discussion with patient, relatives and professional colleagues may be used to increase information available for treatment planning.

Assessment of the absence of function, or the presence of dysfunction and the measurement of its severity, should be ongoing and related to functional ability. Many therapists prefer to make a complete formal assessment before treatment commences, but there may be good reason to suggest that evaluation should be carried out by the occupational therapist as part of the treatment program. The advantage is that the evaluation will reflect more accurately the patient's normal performance, as responses will not be affected by a 'test' situation. The initial approach is therefore important for early identification of problems as well as being a time to establish rapport with the patient.

General considerations

The patient's case notes should be read for data on the nature of dysfunction, and for any personal and social information, which may provide some guidelines for initial communication with the patient. It is useful to observe the patient from a distance before approaching, as this is likely to give indications of disorder. For example, the position of patients may indicate their postural and tonal status, the presence of a visual field disorder, or unilateral neglect. Before approaching it is also useful to assess the environment and the relationship of objects within it to the patient, particularly to the side of dysfunction. For example, the position of the bed in the ward, and its relationship to walls, windows, doors and bedside table, and to other patients, may increase the patient's discomfort and contribute to dysfunction. At this early stage it is essential that in order for patients to feel as comfortable as possible, maximum use is made of the part of the environment they are able to appreciate and control. The major part of the ward, bedside locker and personal treasures should initially be located within the visual field of the unaffected side, as should the most direct access for visitors or staff. Windows on the affected side may encourage rotation for pleasurable rather than necessary reasons. In later stages of treatment, when visual and mobility activities have commenced, the positioning of the patient within the environment should be changed to assist in increasing awareness.

Procedure

The therapist should approach from the sound side so that problems of a sensory or visual nature will not confuse the initial contact. After a brief introduction some indication of future treatment should be given.

If the patient has language problems, speech should be slow and distinct, with care taken to ensure the use of adult tone and language. Sentences should be short and words simple, with meaning emphasised by the use of personal and environment clues.

Patients should be allowed time to respond, should not be prompted, and full attention should be given to their efforts. If the patient becomes frustrated, it sometimes helps to let them know that their problems and frustrations are understood; and it may also help if an alternative way of communicating, such as pointing, is suggested. It is important to check that a referral has been made to the speech pathologist. If the patient does not understand the language of the treatment agency, efforts should be made to locate an interpreter as soon as possible.

The therapist should ask how the patient is feeling both generally and about the hemiplegic side, and should then touch the hemiplegic side and ask the patient to locate the touch. The patient's responses will provide information about sensory-motor impairment, body awareness, sensory inattention, visual scanning and localization, and ability to follow simple communication.

If the patient is lying or sitting asymmetrically, the therapist may need to facilitate a more upright position. Use of manual contact against the unaffected side of the head may be appropriate to assist the patient's symmetry at this stage, as it often

proves an effective facilitator of movement through space, without gross lifting or complex serial instructions being necessary. The patient is asked to push against the therapist's hand until sitting upright, told when sitting straight, and asked to maintain that position (Fig. 3.1). The patient's response will provide information about balance and postural impairment, and body awareness.

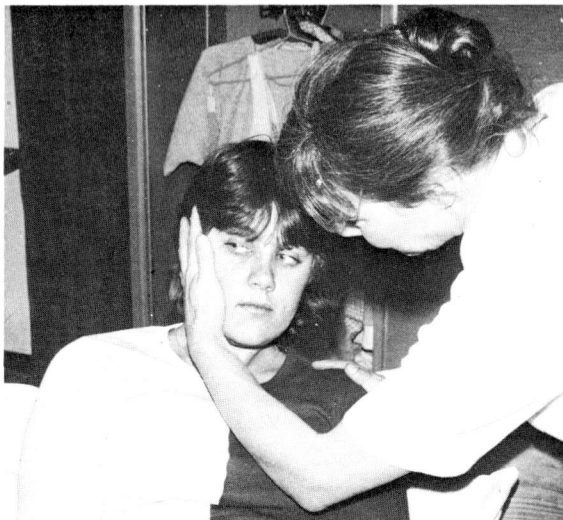

Fig. 3.1 Use of manual contact to the face to facilitate symmetrical sitting.

After establishing eye contact and directing the patient to eye follow, the therapist should move to the hemiplegic side. If eye contact is lost, the therapist should return to the patient's field of vision and try again. The patient's response will provide information about visual impairment of a primary sensory or perceptual nature. It is important not to address patients from the hemiplegic side until they are able to respond to a person in that position. Stimulation of any sort on the side of the dysfunction can cause acute discomfort to patients if they are not able to appreciate the source (Hewson, 1982). When the patient is able to give attention towards the hemiplegic side, discrete sensory stimulation should be used to maintain this gain. The dysfunctional upper limb can be talked about, touched, supported, and positioned in a reflex-inhibiting position, hand shake hold used in Figure 3.2.

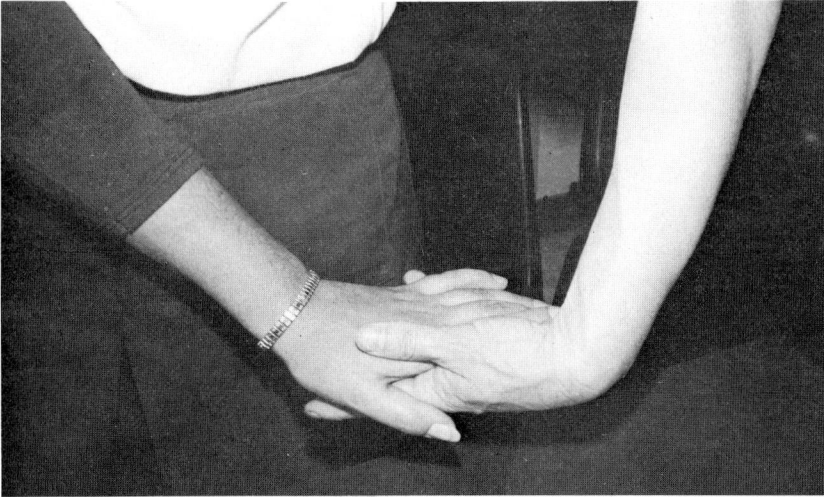

Fig. 3.2 Hand shake hold. This position maintains the wrist and hand in a reflex-inhibiting position. The therapist avoids palmar pressure.

When balance is a continuing problem, an upright position may be maintained with support through the upper limb by the therapist, whilst applying approximation from hand to shoulder. The patient should be encouraged to look at the hemiplegic arm, turn towards and stroke or touch it with the sound hand, whilst the therapist continues to converse slowly, clearly and gently.

Engaging the patient in a small task may extend the therapist's appreciation of impairment and, if chosen wisely, may help in establishing a trusting and therapeutic relationship. An example of a suitable task is to have the patient reach with the sound arm for a personal object, such as a photograph from the bedside table, and pass the object to the therapist on the hemiplegic side, who then discusses it (Fig. 3.3).

The patient's response will provide information about ability to initiate and co-ordinate movement; postural and balance reactions; any reflex activity, such as the occurrence of asymmetric tonic neck reflex (A.T.N.R.) when the patient turns and reaches for the object; ability to visually scan, find and recognise the object and to manipulate it in space; and ability to plan movement, follow simple instruction, and to attend to visual and verbal input from the hemiplegic side. Discussion of the object may also provide information about interests, previous lifestyle, motivation, and affective state; whilst empathy and interest shown by the therapist may encourage the formation of a therapeutic rapport. To end the initial contact and before leaving accurate information about when and where the patient will next be seen should be given.

EVALUATION PROCEDURES

The initial approach technique described will indicate areas of dysfunction which may need formal evaluation. Lengthy assessment is often fatiguing for the patient; may be unreasonable with regard to attention span, particularly early after onset of stroke; takes up valuable treatment time; and in many cases is duplicated by other members of the treatment team. Records of what has already been assessed should be in the patient's notes.

Where possible assessments should be shared by those needing the same information: sensory-motor evaluation with the physiotherapist; perceptual/cognitive/language evaluation with the speech pathologist and neuropsychologist; and social implications with the social worker.

A baseline assessment shared, discussed, and agreed upon by all disciplines may provide inter-team direction and priorities, less confusion for the

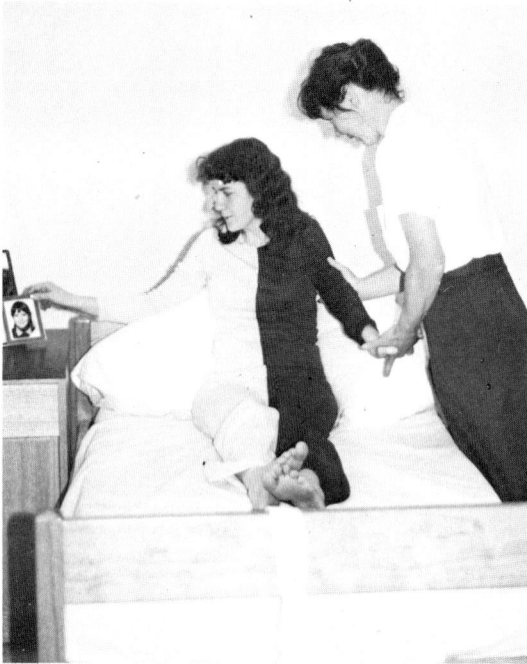
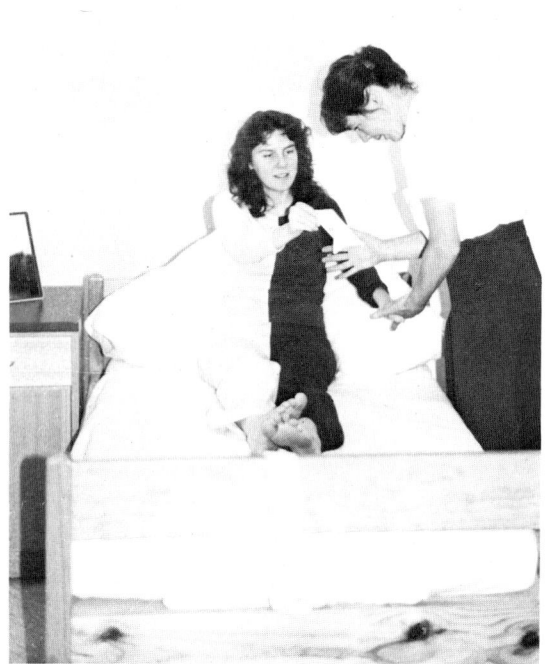

(a)   (b)

Fig. 3.3 Example of a simple task which may be used for initial evaluation.

patient, and, potential for maximal achievement of goals.

The occupational therapist's major contribution should be the functional manifestations of all impairments noted in relation to individual needs. Rusk (1971) indicates that 'the prescription of treatment must be based on the specific functional deficits in the patient'. This is supported by Carr and Shepherd (1982) who hypothesize that effective treatment is based on accurate assessment of functional deficits.

As recovery from stroke is potentially one of constant change, evaluation should be ongoing, proceeding with treatment and recorded regularly. Frequent reassessment is supported by many therapists including Bobath (1978), Brunnstrom (1970), and Carr and Shepherd (1982). Ongoing recording of progress may sharpen the therapist's observation and critical evaluation skills, and indicate the effectiveness of different treatment modalities with individual patients. If recorded effectively and in a standard fashion, it may also provide valuable information for research studies and validation of methodology.

It appears from clinical observation and discussion that occupational therapists are infrequent users of standardized assessments, tending to adapt or change evaluation procedures to what is perceived as necessary for specific agencies and clients. This is supported by a study carried out by Ottenbacher (1980)

In a literature review on the value of neuromuscular assessment in the treatment of hemiplegia, Hayward (1982) suggests that standardized tests should be used whenever possible, so that assessments may be seen as valid and reliable, although none may be considered perfect. She suggests the 'perfect assessment' will probably combine qualitative, quantitative, objective and subjective data to give a total picture of abilities and deficits of a patient's functioning, so that individually specific tailoring may result in more successful treatment.

Most occupational therapists would probably

agree that a perfect evaluation for stroke has not yet been developed, and that its construction is fraught with difficulties. The difficulties are reflected in the many and varied types of assessment forms currently used. The data which is collected on the variety of assessment forms is probably indicative of the chosen priority of treatment regimes used in each agency. Care must be taken that the information collected and recorded on assessment froms is able to be shared effectively with professional colleagues, enabling treatment programs and priorities to be decided.

Some therapists feel that the need to share evaluation material in its collected state (i.e. on a form) with other professionals is unnecessary and a sign of professional immaturity, and that data recorded on occupational therapy forms should be for departmental and research purposes only.

Occupational therapists need to recognise that their understanding of the relationships between different aspects of disorder, rather than being expert in only one area, suggests a responsibility in assimilating an accurate and overall picture of individual patient needs for team appraisal and priority approach planning. To do this an effective method of sharing significant information must be formulated. This may be by reporting briefly to other team members, or by using visually dynamic charts. Table 3.1 which relates impairment to function suggests one method of gaining an overview of dysfunction to clarify priorities of treatment.

This chart (Table 3.1) provides the opportunity to record which aspects of possible disorders interfere with functional achievement. It thus should provide information about how dysfunction may be treated; for example, if bed mobility is impaired intervention to improve it may differ, depending on whether the cause arises from disorders of muscular tone, visual inattention, or contralateral neglect. It should also indicate which aspects of a patient's disorder are causing the greatest number of functional problems, thus establishing possible priorities for treatment.

The patient's strengths should also be obvious, allowing therapists to include some activities in the patient's day for positive achievement, uninhibited by emphasis on improvement of dysfunction. A patient's residual abilities and strengths may also be used either to facilitate improvement or as part of an adaptive approach to impaired function.

More detailed departmental charts will be needed to record specific information about particular aspects or degrees of impairment.

1. Voluntary movement and tone

Changes to muscle tone may be assessed by evaluating muscle resistance to passive movement. When there is flaccidity or decreased tone, the limb feels heavy, and passive movement is free of the tension of stretch sensitivity present in normal muscles (Trombly & Scott, 1977). The patient will be unable to prevent the passive movement or to maintain a posture if support is withdrawn (Bobath, 1978). When there is spasticity or increased tone this will be manifest by resistance to passive movement, when the movement opposes the pattern of spasticity.

Bobath (1978) indicates that passive movement used to evaluate changes in tone should oppose the patient's patterns of spasticity, and that if the passive movement follows the direction of pull of the increased muscle tone, 'exaggerated and uncontrolled assistance' may be felt. Brunnstrom (1970) suggests that in the presence of spasticity, movement patterns rather than individual joint movements be tested and that patterns chosen should be based on the typical recovery stages of hemiplegia. She further indicates that tone will vary according to the gross positioning of the patient, the position of the head in relation to the trunk, and the position of limbs in relation to each other.

Increased tone may be recorded as:
(a) *Mild* if resistance or contraction of the muscles occurs when it is in its lengthened position
(b) *Moderate* if resistance or contraction occurs in its middle range of movement
(c) *Severe* if resistance or contraction occurs in its shortened range, thus limiting range of movement substantially (Trombly & Scott, 1977).

Tone may also be affected by other variables such as the patient's affective state, rapport and familiarity with the evaluator, and the physical environment. The variables which affect muscular

Table 3.1 Visual display, relating stroke impairment to functional performance

	Bed mobility	Transfers	Mobility	Dressing	Personal hygiene	Eating	Meal preparation	Housework	Personal relationships	Personal responsibilities	Social skills	Marketing	Leisure activities	Work activs.	Other
↓ Motor skills															
Tonal change															
Abnormal reflexes															
↓ Dexterity															
↓ Endurance															
Apraxia															
Incontinence															
↓ Proprioception															
↓ Tactile sensation															
Astereognosis															
Asomatognosia															
Visual field defects and inattention															
Visuo-spatial agnosia															
Auditory disorders															
Communication disorders															
↓ Memory															
↓ Attention															
↓ Cognition															
Altered affect/lability															
Other impairment															
Other impairment															

(a)

(b)

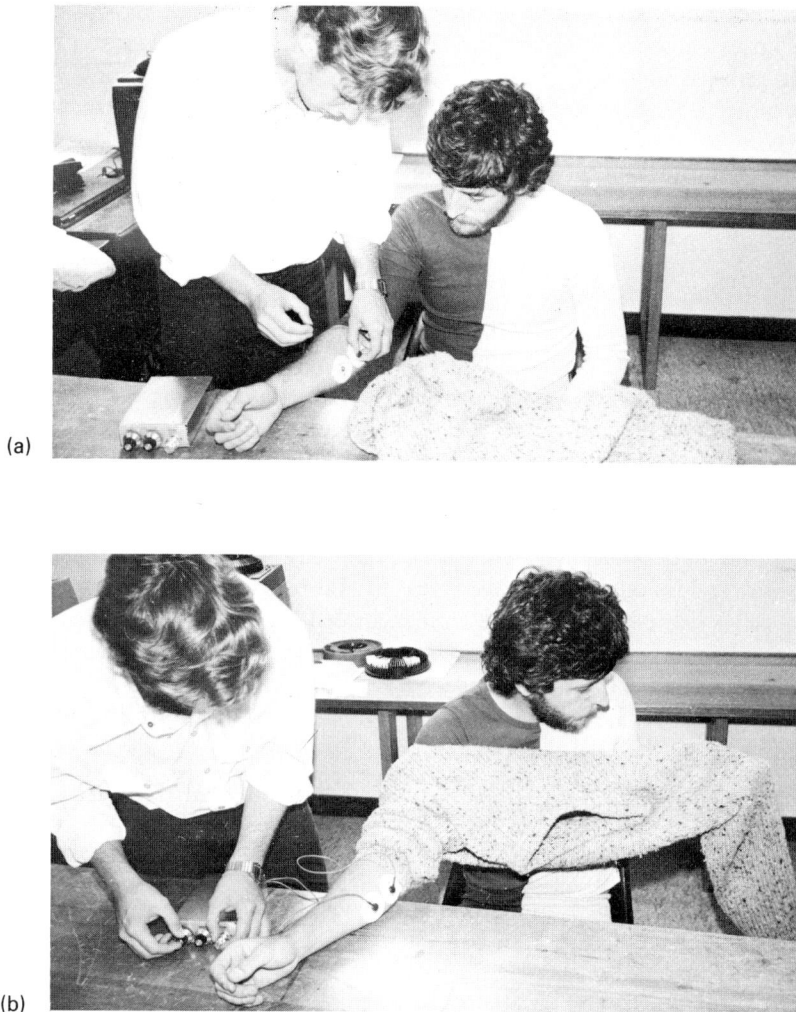

Fig. 3.4 A portable biofeedback machine being used to evaluate tonal changes during dressing activity.

tone are of particular significance to the occupational therapist, who needs to identify the changes that occur when functional activity is performed, so that modification of techniques according to cause can occur if undersirable increases of tone present during evaluation and treatment programs.

During early activities such as bed mobility, self-care, and dressing, therapists should observe, feel and be sensitive to tonal change, should feel the strength of observed changes, and should attempt to modify any that are undesirable. The use of E.M.G. or biofeedback during activity may also provide information about the effects on muscle tone (Fig. 3.4).

2. Reflex activity

Assessment of primitive reflex activity or involuntary stereotyped responses to a particular stimulus is by observation of the response to the given stimulus. If a reflex response occurs the reflex is recorded as positive, and if not, as negative (Trombly & Scott, 1977).

The primitive reflexes which may be observed include the tonic neck reflexes, the tonic labyrinthine reflexes, the tonic lumbar reflexes (Brunnstrom, 1970), and placing reaction.

To test for asymmetrical tonic neck reflex, the head is turned 90° to one side. This causes the limbs on the side to which the face is turned to extend, and the limbs on the side away from the face to flex if the reflex is present.

To test for symmetrical tonic neck reflex, the head is flexed, chin to chest, which causes the upper limbs to flex, and lower limbs to extend if the reflex is present. If no movement occurs an increase of tone may be felt (Trombly & Scott, 1977).

To test for tonic labyrinthine reflexes, when the patient lies in supine the limbs extend, in prone they flex if the reflex is present (Myers, 1982).

To test for tonic lumbar reflexes, rotation of the upper trunk in relation to the pelvis causes increased flexor tone in the upper limb and increased extensor tone in the lower limb on the side to which the trunk is rotated, and increased extensor tone in the upper limb and increased flexor tone in the lower limb on the side away from rotation if the reflex is present (Brunnstrom, 1970).

To test for placing reaction the toes are placed to touch the front of a step. This causes the foot to be lifted and placed on the step if the reflex is present.

Reflex activity may be observed during activities of daily living, for example, when turning the head to find objects to the side, when flexing and extending the head to put on clothing, when assisting the patient to change position in bed, or when taking a patient up steps.

Involuntary stereotyped responses in hemiplegic limbs may be observed when resisting movement of sound limbs, or when patients expend great effort during activity. They may also be observed when voluntary movement at one joint elicits contraction of all muscles linked in basic limb synergies (Brunnstrom, 1970).

Observation of the presence of such reflex activity during functional activity should be watched for and recorded. Some therapists feel that abnormal reflexes should be inhibited at all times, others that reflex activity may be used to promote voluntary movement.

3. Balance

Assessment of balance and postural patterns may be by observation of the patient's unconscious positioning at rest, reaction to movement, and the displacement of the centre of gravity. The therapist may ask the patient to lean or rotate to the hemiplegic side, thus demanding an automatic postural adjustment. This may be done in sitting, standing, or kneeling, and as part of an activity process.

Awareness of balance responses during functional activity is important so that situations or specific parts of an activity which cause greater or lesser difficulty with postural adjustments are noted, thus allowing the therapist to aim treatment directly at problem areas. For example, balance may be affected by a mattress which 'gives' during movement in bed, vision being occluded by clothing or shower water during self-care tasks, and emotional reactions.

Protective extension of the hemiplegic arm is tested by holding the patient's sound hand so that the arm is extended and externally rotated, and pushing the patient off balance towards the hemiplegic side (Bobath, 1978).

4. Manipulative skill

Assessment of fine co-ordination and manipulative skills calls firstly for observation of stability and control of the lower limbs and trunk, and the normal sequence and timing of movement of the upper limbs to flex, and lower limbs to extend if the hands will be affected by impairment of trunk and limb movement. Secondly, the co-ordination of discrete muscle action involved in a manipulative activity should be observed.

Measurements should be taken of the voluntary range of movement at each joint including pronation, supination, flexion, extension, abduction, adduction, and opposition. Any unsolicited effect such as associated reactions or abnormal movement should be watched for and controlled. This should be followed by a functional assessment of grasp/release activities. Brunnstrom (1970) suggests that evaluation should include testing:

mass grasp, mass extension, hook grasp, lateral prehension, palmar prehension, cylindrical grasp, spherical grasp, catch, and throw.

Individual thumb and finger movements should be observed during unilateral and bilateral skilled activity, such as buttoning and unbuttoning, tying shoe-laces, writing to dictation, or any dexterous activity of significance to individual patients. Particular note should be taken of any slowness in performance, specific imbalance between muscle groups causing clumsiness, fatigue causing deterioration as activity continues, or differences in skill of either hand in bilateral or unilateral activity.

It may be assistive to support the hemiplegic upper limb during initial assessment so that effort required to maintain the upper limb against gravity does not detract from the performance demanded of the muscles of the hand. Differences when the same activity is done without support should be noted.

5. Praxis

Since the initial description of apraxia by Liepman in 1900 several descriptive prefixes have been used to differentiate differences of impairment of praxis. Functionally some types of apraxia are difficult to differentiate from visuospatial disorders, particularly those described as constructional and dressing apraxias. Luria (1966) reports that 'defects in spatial perception were usually combined with defects in spatially organised activity' and that some 'writers have suggested calling this condition "spatial apractognosia".'

Both visuo-spatial and constructional praxis activity seems to be initiated from the parietal/occipital area of the cortex and constructional or spatial praxis may be seen as a motor extension of visuo-spatial relationships and orientation (Luria, 1966). Therefore, tests for constructional praxis will also test visuo-spatial motor skills.

To test for constructional apraxia Siev and Freishtat (1976) suggest two-dimensional design copying, such as geometric figures, a house, a flower, or a clock; three dimensional design copying using matchsticks, or 1 inch blocks, and Benton's three dimensional Constructional Praxis Test (Benton & Fogel, 1962).

Both right and left hemiplegic lesions may cause problems with constructional tasks. Patients with right-sided lesions often have difficulty with visuo-spatial aspects of three dimensional construction, such as locating materials, relating parts to each other and with perspective. They are usually not helped by a model. When drawing they may miss out the left side, draw parts scattered over the page, have difficulty with perspective, overscore lines, and their work may be unrecognisable. Practice does not seem to cause improvement.

Patients with left-sided lesions seem to have problems initiating and planning the necessary sequence of movements, and may demonstrate visuo-spatial disorder if they have visual field impairment. They tend to draw hesitantly, but produce a more accurate copy than those with right lesions. They appear to be helped by a model and may improve with practice (Siev & Freishtat, 1976).

Dressing apraxia appears to be a collective term for difficulties experienced during dressing, caused primarily by visuo-spatial or body awareness impairment. It will be discussed as part of the functional assessment of these disorders. Luria (1966) in describing evaluation of motor apraxia, which appears particularly to affect hands and face, suggests that observation of a patient's performance during complex, purposeful tasks such as fastening buttons or tying a shoe-lace may provide preliminary information on praxic skills. Disturbances, unaccompanied by paresis, may be evident in the side contralateral to the lesion, though may sometimes also be present in a weaker form in the ipsilateral hand. Praxic disturbances are indicated by poor reciprocal co-ordination of the two hands, so that movements of each hand are separate and isolated, both hands perform inappropriate similar action, or the hand contralateral to the lesion lags behind the other. Smooth, rapid movement is often impossible. When paresis prevents bilateral assessment, motor tasks involving three consecutive movements of the sound hand may be used. Practice to learn the sequence and establish a rhythm to the movement should be allowed. Impairment will be evident with loss of the correct sequence, repetition of one or two of the movements, loss of automatic rhythmical movement or perseveration.

Kimura's 'Manual Sequence Box', where

patients are required to push a button with the index finger, pull a handle with all the fingers and press a bar with the thumb, is an example of a sequential movement test for apraxia (Kimura, 1977).

Luria (1966) also suggests, as sensitive indicators of praxic ability, tests of (1) a patient's performance of imaginary acts, such as showing how to pour out and stir tea without the objects being present, (2) requesting actions involving symbolic significance, such as beckoning with a finger or saluting, and (3) requesting familiar oral movements, such as chewing, kissing and blowing without reason, and comparing performance with the natural performance of the action.

Siev and Freishtat (1976) indicate the use of the Goodglass test for apraxia (Goodglass & Kaplan, 1972), for the evaluation of motor, ideomotor and ideational apraxias where impaired response is similar, differentiation being qualitative. The test consists of a series of functional buccal/facial, upper limb, and whole body tasks, similar to those mentioned by Luria, which the patient is asked firstly to perform without materials or visual clues. If impaired, the patient is asked to imitate the therapist's performance of the task. If the patient is still unable to complete the task it should be repeated using real objects (Fig. 3.5).

Therapists may design similar tests, using activities of significance to each patient. The 'Solet' test (Solet, 1974) for apraxia has similar testing items and a scoring mechanism.

6. Endurance

Endurance is the length of time a patient can continue an activity before fatigue, distractibility or changes in affect cause deterioration in performance. Evaluation of endurance consists of measuring the time of effective function in activity, and comparing time differences between activities. Awareness and sensitive observation of early fatigue may be critical in the development of appropriately graded activity and successful programs.

Evaluation should take into account the patient's daily schedule and what has been expected of them prior to occupational therapy. Signs which indicate fatigue may be pallor, rest-

lessness, yawning, sighing, pre-occupation with an impaired limb, lapses of attention, irritability, an increase in lability, slowing down of activity, and the occurrence of mistakes. There may be differences between tasks, perhaps indicative of interest or level of achievement possible. Recording of these observations is important.

7. Continence

Therapists should be aware of any bladder or bowel retraining being undertaken by the nursing staff. Observations may need to be recorded during treatment sessions away from the ward, for accurate assessment of the problem.

Information which may be required includes the amount and time of any food or fluid intake; the amount, type, and time of bladder and bowel output; whether the patient was incontinent or aware of the need to empty bladder or bowel; whether the patient was able to communicate the need; and the equipment and position used, such as use of a urinal rather than standing at a lavatory.

Therapists should be aware of signs of bladder overdistention which may include restlessness, perspiration, chills, flushing or pallor, coldness of the extremities, or headache (O'Brien & Pallett, 1978). Incontinence or anxiety about possible incontinence may affect the performance of mobility, self-care, and social tasks.

8. Proprioception

To assess proprioception, the patient's vision should be occluded by the use of a screen or a request for closed eyes. If bilateral movement is possible, the sound limbs are placed into easily described positions, after each change the patient describing the position, or copying it with the limb on the other side of the body.

If paralysis prevents active movement, the therapist may alternatively position the hemiplegic limbs, and request either imitation by the sound side or description. To reduce tactile input body parts should be held laterally over bony prominences (Trombly & Scott, 1977).

Responses are recorded as accurate, imparied or absent. Testing, as for all evaluation which includes occlusion of vision, should not be drawn

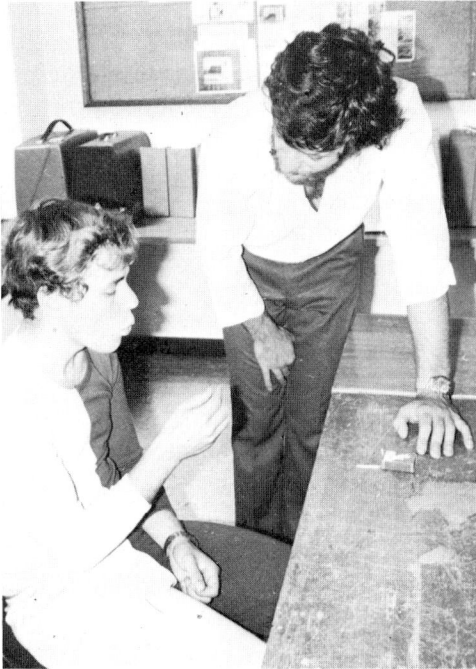
(a)

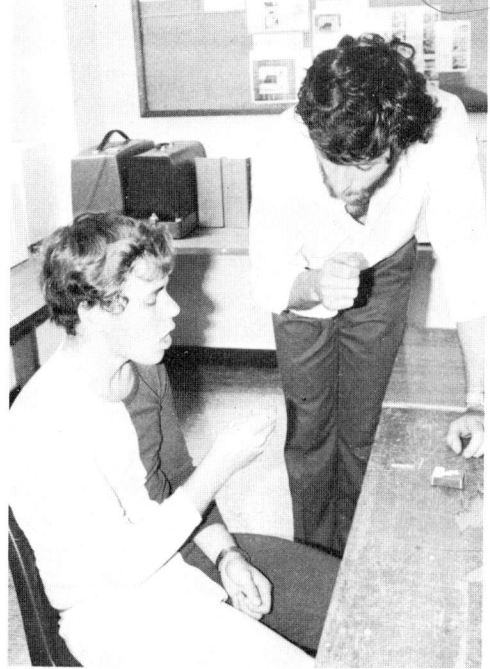
(b)

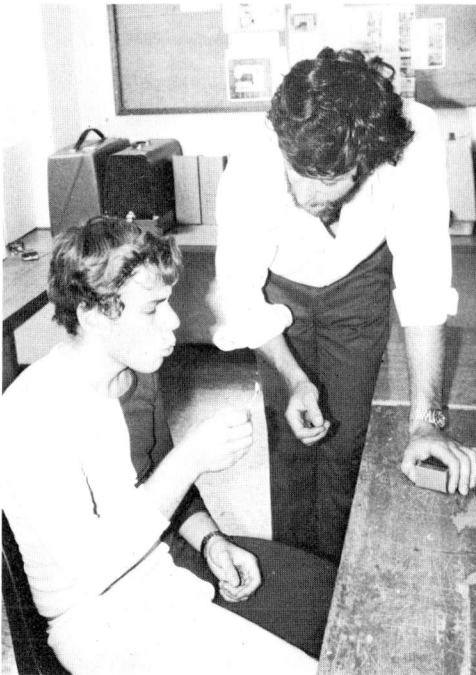
(c)

Fig. 3.5 Testing for apraxia. (a) Therapist asks patient to demonstrate how to blow out a match. (b) Therapist asks patient to copy blowing out a match. (c) Therapist asks patient to blow out a real match.

out as lack of visual stimulation may encourage disorientation or impaired attention.

Functionally, lack of proprioception may be observed by patients neglecting or forgetting body parts, particularly during mobility or self-care tasks, and when reminded being unable to describe the position or find limbs. When made visually aware of their impaired body parts they are able to recognise them as their own unless anasognosia is a complication.

9. Tactile sensation

Formal testing for tactile sensation may be carried out in a manner similar to that described for proprioception, with vision occluded for each part of the assessment, the patient being encouraged to open eyes for instructions between each procedure (Trombly & Scott, 1977). The patient is asked to localise tactile stimuli of:

(a) Light touch, which the therapist applies with a cotton wool ball or soft brush.
(b) Firm pressure, applied by the therapist's finger tips or an aestheasometer.

(c) Sharp or dull touch, applied with either end of a pin. The patient is asked to discriminate whether the stimulus was sharp or blunt.

(d) Two-point touch, applied by the therapist using a two-point aestheasometer (caliper or paper clip). Either a single or double stimuli may be used and the patient indicates whether one or two points are felt. The distance between the two points is reduced to measure how close the two may be before being perceived as one. Two-point discrimination is most refined on finger tips.

(e) Differences in temperature, which the therapist applies using capped test tubes or small film containers filled with warm or cold water, with the request for a 'hot' or 'cold' response.

Stimuli should be applied distal to proximal, in an unpredictable pattern, and with variable times between application. Stimuli should also be applied bilaterally simultaneously to assess whether simultaneous extinction occurs, causing the patient to be aware only of stimuli to the sound side (Trombly & Scott, 1977).

Responses should be recorded as intact, impaired, or absent.

Evaluation of tactile discrimination between size, shape, and texture may be through the patient matching like pairs of chosen stimuli from similar others.

Evaluation of weight discrimination may be through patients grading similar objects according to weight. Functionally, awareness and response to tactile stimulation may be observed when touching the patient on either side during retraining, or by observation of the response to others doing the same. These observations should be recorded so that formal and functional test responses may be compared, as they may differ. This may be particularly significant when tactile inattention decreases the response to tactile stimulation on the hemiplegic side, when bilateral simultaneous tactile stimulation occurs.

10. Stereognosis

Stereognosis may be evaluated by having the patient tactually identify a common object such as a paper clip or tooth brush. Vision should be occluded by either a screen or closed eyes. Patients may either name the object or match the tactually experienced object from an array of others.

Functionally it may be assessed by the patient tactually selecting an object in a pocket, purse, or bag from amongst others, without looking, or observation of difficulty with bilateral tasks when the hands cannot be seen such as manipulating back fastenings on clothing or washing pots under 'sudsy' water.

11. Somatognosia

Understanding and awareness of body gestalt (wholeness) may be apparent in many forms. Impairment may cause difficulties in naming and localizing body parts; inattention and neglect of one side of the body, usually the left, and visual field defects or inattention on the same side; and anosognosia, the denial of defect and illness, to the point of delusion which may be rationalised with confabulation (Critchley, 1965; Walsh, 1978; Kolb and Whishaw, 1980).

The most effective evaluation is of a functional nature:

(a) Observation of posture and movement. Patients with asomatognosia may sit, stand, or lie in an asymmetrical position, with head turned away from the hemiplegic side continuously.

(b) Verbal and tactile stimulation of the hemiplegic side without having first attracted visual attention. Patients may not respond at all, may do so as if the therapist is positioned on the sound side, or may make total body movements (including moving the chair in which seated) before responding to the therapist who, by reason of the patient's actions, is then on the sound side.

(c) Asking and listening to the patient talk about the affected side. Lack of concern, failure to locate or recognise a limb as their own, rationalization or denial of dysfunction, or bizarre statements such as 'finding an arm in a dressing gown pocket' may be considered evidence of disturbance of body awareness.

(d) Observation of the patient in self-care tasks such as dressing, showering, hair combing, or eating will allow identification of the problem when the patient fails to include all or part of the hemiplegic side. This may be obvious as a gross disturbance when, for example, the patient fails to dress the hemiplegic side, tries to put both legs in one half of trousers, or fails to complete the activity despite prompting and instruction; or a minor disturbance such as the hemiplegic shoulder not being soaped in the shower.

Other assessment measures may include the assembly of a 'jig-saw mannequin', drawing a figure, or around the outline of a figure in a magazine. Most patients with a disorder of this nature have been found clinically, on these tasks, to fail to position limbs or head appropriately, to miss out parts, particularly the upper limb, or distal parts of the upper and lower limbs on the same side as dysfunction, or to be very slow in execution of the task, often verbalizing and rationalizing the task method. Right/left discrimination, and naming and localizing body parts, may be tested by asking the patient to touch one part of the body with another, such as 'Touch your right ear with your left hand', or to identify body parts the therapist touches on themselves or on the patient.

Finger agnosia, first described by Gerstmann in 1924 (Kolb & Whishaw, 1980) and considered by him to be part of a syndrome including acalculia, agraphia, and right/left discrimination, may be evaluated by asking the patient to state the number of fingers between two fingers touched simultaneously (Kinsbourne & Warrington, 1962). It may also be tested by asking the patient to identify by touch (on self or therapist), naming, indicating on a chart, or imitating, fingers moved or touched by the therapist (Siev & Freishtat, 1976).

Functionally, it may be observed that patients are hesitant or have decreased dexterity in activity which demands co-ordination between individual fingers, such as typing or piano playing (Siev & Freishtat, 1976.)

12. Vision

As reported earlier the most common visual field defect in stroke is homonymous hemianopia or quadrantopia, with the impaired field of vision being on the side contralateral to the lesion and ipsilateral to the hemiplegia. Visual inattention

may appear functionally similar, but patients are able to appreciate stimuli on the affected side when presented unilaterally, and will be able to respond when reminded to look to the hemiplegic side.

Visual field defects are usually tested by asking the patient to maintain gaze on a fixed point straight ahead, and to report the appearance of stimuli in either periphery or in both (Luria, 1966). Therapists often use two pencils or wiggle fingers on both hands. However, if there is inattention and the patient is able to see only one stimulus at a time (which will be the stimulus on the sound side), incorrect assessment may be made.

Luria (1966) suggests that the degree to which the patient realises and compensates for field defects should also be considered. It is commonly assumed that those with left-sided lesions and right field defects are able to compensate for visual loss by scanning, and that those with right-sided lesions and left field defects are often unaware or unable to scan without training, because anosognosia may be a complication. Luria suggests that tasks such as reading large print or counting cards set out in front of the patient, be used to clarify visual defects, those patients with impairment failing to include material on the hemiplegic side. Clinically, it has not always been found that those with right-sided hemianopia automatically compensate and they should be tested thoroughly. A study by Diller and Weinberg (1977) suggests that those with right-sided hemianopia tend to work slowly and methodically on such activities as visual cancellation tasks, achieving greater success than those with left-sided hemianopia, who tend to be erratic in eye movement and method of performance. Activities that do not allow a slow methodical approach may reveal more evidence of visual field difficulties for patients with left-sided lesions.

Trombly and Scott (1977) suggest as another method of evaluation that a patient be asked whilst looking straight ahead, to bisect equally, by marking, a drawn line. The line is placed centrally to the patient. Those with left or right hemianopia will bisect the line to the right or left of centre.

Evidence of visual defects may be seen in many functional activities, such as failure to find objects placed to the hemiplegic side, difficulties in reading letters or newspapers because part of each line cannot be seen, failure to eat food on one side of a plate, difficulty in finding rooms to the affected side, or bumping into doorways. Sometimes deficits are difficult to determine, particularly those of a milder nature, because of the visual system's ability to complete a visual image from memory of previous experience. This completion phenomenom may be tested by the inclusion of unexpected additions to the visual stimuli or the environment being used for testing. Deficits are sometimes not found until patients are tested for their driving licence.

Visual perception of depth may also be impaired. To evaluate, objects may be hand held or placed at eye level at differing distances from the patient, who is asked to identify the closest object. The objects may then be moved by the therapist who asks the patient to indicate when they are parallel (Trombly & Scott, 1977).

13. Visuo-spatial gnosia

There are many aspects of visuo-spatial disorders that can be individually evaluated, and many specific table tasks have been devised for this purpose, such as design copying, block construction as described for constructional apraxia, negotiating of two and three dimensional mazes, completion of form boards, matching or copying felt pictures, and figure ground puzzles.

Siev and Freishtat (1976) describe several therapist designed tests and also suggest using the Frostig published subtests (Frostig, 1966) for figure ground, form constancy, position in space and spatial relations; the Ayres published subtests (Ayres, 1972) for figure ground, position in space and space visualization; and the Bender Visual Motor Gestalt Test (Pascal & Suttell, 1951), for spatial relations. They also recommend functional tests such as finding and picking out objects (figure ground), identification of similar objects in different orientations (form constancy) and finding the way from place to place (topographical orientation). Pure measurement of specifically named dysfunctions is difficult because of considerable overlap between them, and because integration of various skills is required for the patient to demonstrate intact ability. There is also concern that such

measurement may not give an accurate indication of functional deficits, but is rather a measure of splinter skills.

To consider and evaluate functional deficits caused by visuo-spatial impairment, they may be dichotomized into those of a two or three dimensional nature.

Two dimensional visuo-spatial tasks are those requiring:

(i) recognition, discrimination, and understanding of pictorial and symbolic representations (including words and numbers) in two dimensional form, such as in a book or magazine, on a billboard or poster, on a map, or on television, and
(ii) being able to represent understandable and complete two dimensional material, appropriate to previously held expertise, for such activities as drawing a map, plans or patterns, completing puzzles or carrying out artistic avocational or work skills.

Evaluation should therefore include:
(a) Asking the patient to discuss, point to, or draw around two dimensional material which is appropriate to social and personal needs, and which is graded in complexity of colour, content and specific spatial requirements. Evaluation tools may well be newspapers, magazines, short videotape television programs, and the city street directory.
(b) Asking the patient to draw a map or house plan, and to copy or complete drawings or puzzles graded to suit previously held interests and pursuits (Fig. 3.6).

Three dimensional visuo-spatial tasks are those requiring:

(i) recognition, discrimination and understanding of the environment in which the patient lives, of the functional significance of spatial relationships between people and objects, and being able to move about appropriately and safely. This includes such tasks as finding one's way about, recognising objects which may impede safe mobility (such as a child's toy on a patterned carpet), being able to discriminate like

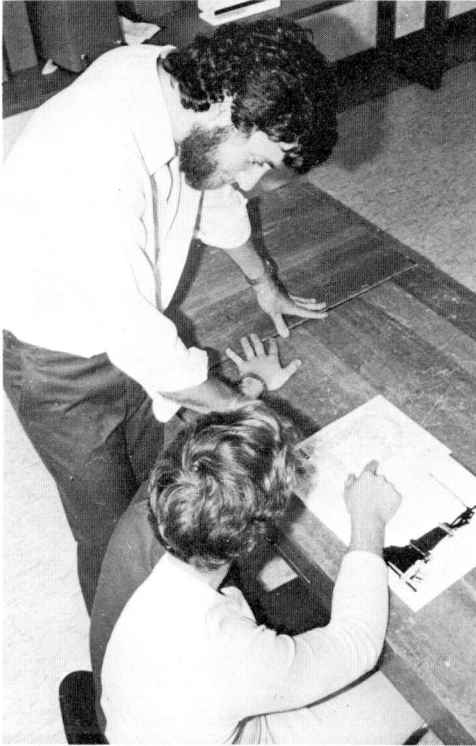

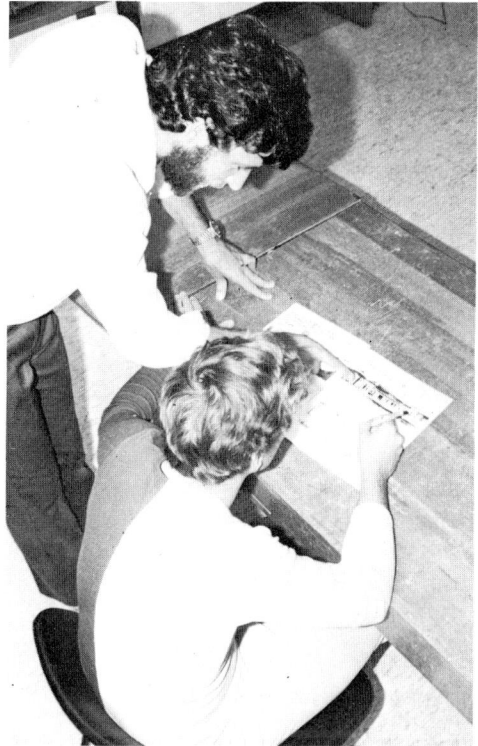

(a)   (b)

Fig. 3.6 Testing for 2-dimensional visuo-spatial impairment. (a) Finding a route on a map. (b) Completing a drawing.

objects in different orientations (such as matching cutlery and crockery), or being able to negotiate to a desired location through a crowd of people and,

(ii) being able to spatially manipulate and construct three dimensional objects to intra or extra personal plans, appropriate to previously held expertise. This includes such tasks as handling clothing so it may be donned efficiently, pouring water into a glass, stacking crockery, building a 'Leggo' space tower according to directions, or constructing a pre-fabricated garden shed.

Evaluation should therefore include:

(a) Asking the patient to show the way to the bathroom or to the occupational therapy department, making sure that mobility training includes negotiation of objects and people (graded to increase difficulty) and discrimination and selection of items from amongst others.

(b) Observation of the patient in self-care tasks such as dressing which require spatial manipulation of objects of a basic and personal nature, and constructional activities involving manipulation of objects to a plan.

Any evaluation should take into account levels of skill prior to the stroke as deficits may not be obvious if all people are taken as capable of the same skills. For example, someone with highly developed two and three dimensional visuo-spatial skills, such as an architect, may have deficits interfering only with his higher level skills and so may not be seen to have any deficits if these are not taken into account.

In Table 3.1, vocational, leisure, family and social skills headings are used to indicate previous levels of function so that assessment takes such factors into consideration.

14. Hearing

Auditory deficits and agnosia are usually evaluated

fully by the speech pathologist. However, patients with specific difficulties in locating, differentiating or recognising sounds may experience functional difficulties which the occupational therapist may need to assess: for example, recognising the noise of a boiling kettle in the kitchen or hearing an approaching car when crossing a road. Evaluation of such specific deficits may be by commercial or individually made tapes of sounds, particularly those relating to safety factors. As the quality of the tapes and the hearing of sounds out of context sometimes makes identification difficult, therapists should test the tape on unimpaired others before using it to evaluate a patient's performance.

For patients with specific auditory needs such as a musician, tests for the appreciation of timbre and tone may be indicated, and referral to a neuropsychologist is recommended, for testing with the 'Seashore Measures of Musical Talents' test, for example.

15. Communication

Based on the speech pathologist's evaluation and recommendations for the most effective methods of communication with each patient, the occupational therapist should further evaluate the effectiveness of verbal approaches, both written and spoken, and approaches using demonstration, mime and sensory cues for functional results and individual achievement during retraining. Any approaches found to be effective or non-effective should be shared with the treatment team.

16. Memory

Neuropsychologists have several standardised procedures available to test disorders of memory, probably the most widely used one being the Wechsler Memory Scale. Referral for this type of assessment is recommended. How deficits in memory functionally affect the patient's day-to-day activities should also be assessed.

Memory traces are formed for all sensory and motor experience including visual, auditory, tactile and kinesthetic, and assessment should consider whether some aspects of memory appear intact when others show impairment. This may be of benefit when establishing adaptive cueing systems for residual deficits.

Memory traces have been found (Hebb, 1961) to build up by cumulative learning of either a conscious or unconscious nature, so assessment of memory should be continuous during repetitive retraining procedures. Even if the patient is unable to recall verbally motor or sensory experiences of the previous day, an increase in speed, assurance, dexterity, or accuracy of performance may indicate motor or sensory memory traces are being formed (Kolb & Whishaw, 1980).

Functional assessment may be carried out by demanding verbal, visual, auditory, tactile or kinesthetic recall for day-to-day activities and events to the maximum extent of the time and amount patients can achieve, and by observing any improvement when stimuli are repeated regularly.

17. Attention

Defects in attention may be functionally evaluated by observation of ability to focus attention at will, evidence of distractability or uninhibited response to happenings around, and whether the duration of effective attention span allows task achievement. Intact attention is necessary for both concentration and conceptual tracking (Lezak, 1976).

Attention defects may be global or specific to visual or verbal modalities, and evaluation procedures should endeavour to find if there are differences between attention modalities to assist choice of methods for either retraining or adaptive approaches.

Well-known verbal tests are:

(a) Forward and backward digit span tests, where the patient repeats a sequence of numbers either exactly as heard, or backwards, immediately after they have been read aloud. The number of digits forwards are graded from three to nine numbers, with the average adult score being six, and most elderly people at least four. The number of digits backwards are graded from two to eight numbers with the average adult score being five and most elderly people at least three. Usually each section is discontinued when the patient is unable to repeat two number sequences of the same length (Lezak, 1976).

(b) Serial subtraction tasks such as subtracting seven from a hundred, from ninety-three etc.; or three from fifty, from forty-seven etc.; or counting backwards from twenty to nought. In the serial seven tests, in a normal population a few errors are common, but very defective performances and pauses of more than five seconds between responses may be indicative of defects in attention (Smith, 1967).

Attention to visual stimuli may be assessed by any activity demanding looking and concentrating for task completion, such as picture matching, simple to complex jig-saws and table games such as noughts and crosses, concentration, and draughts.

Visual cancellation tasks may also be used for assessing attention and concentration. These consist of rows of numbers, letters, pictures or shapes, and the patient is instructed to cross out all examples of a designated target, such as all the 'Cs' or all the triangles. Other skills are also necessary for visual cancellation tasks, such as visual scanning. In a study by Weinberg et al, (1972) it was even demonstrated that scanning eye movements accompany the performance of such conceptual tracking tasks as 'digits backwards'.

More complex dysfunction in attention involving double or multiple conceptual tracking (Lezak, 1976), may need assessment, particularly for some patients' vocational needs. Multiple tracking may demand the patient remembering one thing whilst doing another, or that several stimuli need to be attended to sequentially or alternatively. These skills should be evaluated functionally with appropriate activity for individual patients' social or work demands.

18. Cognition

Assessment of cognitive dysfunction, including such things as abstract reasoning, planning, judgment, and foresight, may be by observing the patient's responses to conversation and instructions, noting such details as ability to follow or question verbal input, to associate verbal and environmental happenings appropriately, to control impulsive behaviour so that effective activity is possible, and whether learning from direct or indirect teaching is possible or difficult.

Evaluation may be complicated by patients having communication or perceptual problems, and should make use of skills likely to be intact. For example, if a patient is experiencing problems with verbal processing, assessment tasks should emphasize visuo-spatial processes.

Video and table games are often useful tools for measuring reasoning and planning skill, and should be graded according to each patient's level of functioning and social requirements. Care should be taken that they are age appropriate.

Evaluation using such tasks does not need a standardized or pre-organized manner of presentation. Patients should be given plenty of time to plan moves and may be prompted or cued if necessary, as performance requiring such assistance is probably indicative of problems, particularly if practice does not improve performance. It should be noted whether the patient learns immediately from therapist intervention, if the learning is carried over to later in the game, or to other tasks, and if the patient can concentrate.

The use of ongoing creative or recreational activity may combine assessment and retraining of cognitive deficits in a non-threatening form.

Patients likely to return to work or family responsibilities and domestic duties, need ongoing assessment of work specific cognitive abilities, using real tasks of significance to each individual, which gradually the patient should be expected to co-ordinate into a complex daily program. If difficulties are experienced the therapist should carefully re-analyse factors in the situation, so that emphasis and practice may be aimed at problem areas. Luria (1966) suggests that in investigating intellectual processes the patient's understanding, ideas and problem-solving ability should be considered, and recommends the use of thematic pictures and/or texts, both of a single and sequential nature, which demand subject analysis and identification of essential elements for interpretation of the theme or story. Close observation to evaluate how the patient goes about the task is essential, for such behaviour as: impulsive and overconfident judgment about the subject after a brief glance; whether conclusions are based on individual details, separate parts or the whole context; whether perseveration or self-correction occurs; whether the emotional tone of the context is perceived; and cause and effect relationships can be appraised.

To evaluate concept formation verbal and/or spatial tasks may be used involving:

(i) comparison and differentiation, such as indicating the odd word or picture in a series, or object in a drawer,

(ii) logical relationships and classifications, such as putting objects with those of a similar nature, and

(iii) analogies, or the carrying over of concepts of relationship from one given task to another, such as finding the word to complete a pair with the same relationship to each other as in an example previously given, e.g. 'meal—food', 'garden—? (plants)'.

Care must be taken to choose activities so that communication or visuo-spatial perceptual disorders are not interpreted as intellectual dysfunction. Particular attention should be given to whether the patient can use and appreciate abstract as well as concrete concepts.

Evaluation of problem-solving skills which involves the setting of goals, planning strategies for solutions, and restricting and inhibiting digressions which prevent the continuance of planned strategy, Luria (1966) suggests may be by use of simple to complex arithmetical problems. Occupational therapists have the advantage of being able to use any appropriate and individually chosen activity such as making a basket, playing lawn bowls, meal planning, or bathing the baby using only one hand, to evaluate problem solving skills and cognitive responses.

19. Affect and lability

Evaluation and research into affective disorders following stroke are poorly documented, and form observations of current assessment forms, would seem to be afterthoughts rather than significant factors requiring attention.

Depression, thought to be most often associated with left hemisphere lesions, and indifference, associated with right hemisphere lesions, and labile behaviour may be inhibitory to relationships and to retraining programs. Specific data needs to be recorded, analysed and published to increase understanding and awareness of symptoms associated with them, so that their effect may be reduced in the future.

Observation should be made of patients' behaviour when they are at rest without people around, when they are with others who are personally important to them, and when they are with hospital personnel, as well as observing the patient at work during retraining.

Data which may be important to record includes the manner, type and amount of verbal and non-verbal responses, motivation, drive, energy, aggression, anxiety, fatigue levels, disturbances of sleep, and the level of pre-occupation with or indifference to impairment.

N.B. In some places administration of published psychological tests may only be by registered psychologists. Therapists should check if tests have restricted usage.

ACTIVITIES OF DAILY LIVING (A.D.L.)

Most occupational therapy departments use A.D.L. assessment forms to record patients' personal and home care skills. These are usually detailed check lists of common functional activities, which are used at various stages throughout rehabilitation. They should reflect the cultures of the people which each agency serves. If assessment is carried out in the rehabilitation setting, the equipment, materials and layout of the environment should closely resemble those of individual patients. If this is not possible assessment will be most useful if done in the home. Habit and familiar patterns of activity are likely to cause different responses to those resulting from activity carried out in strange and unfamiliar surroundings.

Most forms do not provide space to record why tasks cannot be done, but simply whether they can be done independently, with help, or not at all. If this type of assessment were expanded to include reasons for difficulty or dependence in tasks, all the information required by the occupational therapist to retrain patients may be provided. If assessment is academic and removed from functional activity, the information gained has to be transferred and related to patients' life needs, to be useful to the occupational therapist.

A.D.L. indices, which have been developed mainly for research purposes to study the effects of rehabilitation programs, are usually much briefer than A.D.L. assessment commonly used by occupational therapists, and may be used in conjuction with them.

PROGRAM PLANNING

Program planning should be based on the outcome of evaluation following discussion with others in the treatment team. Occupational therapists need to be receptive and adaptive to issues of importance to other disciplines, so that common goals and priorities may be agreed upon. Both short- and long-term treatment procedures should be planned for each problem to suit likely discharge arrangements.

The treatment team may be asked to assess patients for inclusion in long-term rehabilitation, and thus obtain early indication of discharge plans. If this procedure is not followed, therapists should read patient records daily to check whether discharge plans have been made, or discuss the possibilities with the Medical Officer. Selection of patients for rehabilitation programs is dependent upon the policy of each agency regarding the purpose and length of admissions, the role the agency serves in the community, and the type of treatment program offered. If the patient is likely to benefit more from programs offered elsewhere, transfer should be recommended. If, however, no more suitable treatment agency is available, programs should be extended to meet diverse patient needs.

Decision making about the future, taken on behalf of patients by treatment personnel and relatives, does not always appear to consider sufficiently individual patient preferences or possible potential should they participate in long-term rehabilitation. There is sometimes conflict between patients and relatives about the future, possibly as a result of concern for the patient's safety or worry about extra burdens which may be placed on willing or unwilling family members, and sometimes for less altruistic reasons. There is also sometimes conflict between treatment personnel about patient suitability for rehabilitation.

If patients are to be discharged early to dependent care, immediate programs to facilitate maximum functional ability and mobility prior to discharge should be implemented, particularly if rehabilitation facilities are not available at the discharge location.

If patients are accepted for long-term rehabilitation, the therapist should discuss programs with them, at a level appropriate to their understanding and affective state, so that what the patients perceive as major priorities may be considered in program planning. This is an important issue which should be implemented despite difficulties caused by impairment in language, perception, cognition, or the level of acceptance of the stroke. When the treatment is directed towards patient goals, motivation, participation and success are more likely. An early understanding of relationships of importance to the patient, such as those with spouse, children, grandchildren, friends or family pets, may assist in developing a meaningful therapeutic program. A knowledge of the patient's cultural background, role in the community, and daily or regular pursuits is similarly important; for example, whether the patient reads the newspaper; watches television; spends hours in the garden, kitchen or pub; brings work home from the office or plays golf at every available opportunity; and whether work, social, leisure or home activities are primarily important.

Such understanding may enable the patient and therapist to view long-term goals in specific terms which may assist in selecting tasks to meet short-term goals. For any program to be maximally effective a realistic time should be spent in treatment. In some hospitals a 'time audit' may reveal that although patients appear busy because of ward schedules, they may only receive one hour of actual treatment five days out of seven. Such limited programs are inefficient in use of expensive hospital facilities and patient expectations, and may retard recovery.

Promoting a reasonable program, within a daily and weekly time frame, which allows for patient work, rest and leisure in an ordered way is a valuable and often overlooked aspect of therapy. A daily program varying in the nature of the demands made on each patient may be used to promote and stimulate alertness, cognitive abilities, and sensory motor skills, to lessen introspection through purposeful activity which is enjoyable, and promote natural fatigue at the end of the day.

The total rehabilitation team may need to consider how best to implement a co-ordinated daily program within the framework of each agency's routine. Mutual co-operation and agreement upon the importance of the total treatment package, rather than individual units within it, should assist adaptability between staff, to meet individual needs as they arise.

REFERENCES

Ayres J A 1972 Southern California sensory integrative tests. Western Psychological Services, Los Angeles

Benton A L, Fogel M L 1962 Three dimensional constructional praxis, a clinical test. Archives of Neurology 7: 347–354

Bobath B 1978 Adult hemiplegia evaluation and treatment, 2nd edn. William Heinemann Medical Books Ltd, London

Brunnstrom S 1970 Movement therapy in hemiplegia: a neurophysiological approach. Harper and Row, New York

Carr J, Shepherd R 1982 A motor relearning programme for stroke. Heinemann Medical Books Ltd, London

Critchley M 1965 The parietal lobes. Hafner Publishing, New York

Diller L, Weinberg J 1977 Hemi-inattention in rehabilitation: the evolution of a rational remediation program. Advances in Neurology 18: 63–82

Frostig M 1966 Developmental test of visual perception. Consulting Psychologists Press, Palo Alto, California

Goodglass H, Kaplan E 1972 The assessment of aphasia and related disorders. Lea & Febiger, Philadelphia

Hayward D 1982 A literature review of the value of neuromuscular assessment in the treatment of hemiplegia. Australian Occupational Therapy Journal 29.3: 103–107

Hebb D O 1961 Distinctive features of learning in the higher animal. In: Delasfresnaye J F (ed) Brain mechanisms and learning. Blackwell, London

Hewson L 1982 When half is whole. Dove Communications, Blackburn, Victoria

Kimura D 1977 Acquisition of a motor skill after left hemisphere damage. Brain 100: 527–542

Kinsbourne M, Warrington E K 1962 A study of finger agnosia. Brain 85: 47–66

Kolb B, Whishaw I Q 1980 Fundamentals of human neuropsychology. W H Freeman, San Fransisco

Lezak M D 1976 Neuropsychological assessment. Oxford University Press, New York

Luria A R 1966 Higher cortical functions in man. Basic Books, New York

Myers B J 1982 P.N.F. Assisting to postures and application in occupational therapy activities, a developmental approach as taught by Voss. Unit II Video, Rehabilitation Institute of Chicago, Illinois

O'Brien M T, Pallett P J 1978 Total care of the stroke patient. Little Brown & Co, Boston

Ottenbacher K 1980 Cerebrovascular accident, some characteristics of occupational therapy evaluation forms. American Journal of Occupational Therapy 34.1: 268–271

Pascal G K, Suttell B 1951 The Bender gestalt test—its quantification and validity for adults. Grune and Stratton, New York

Rusk H 1971 Rehabilitation medicine, 3rd edn. Mosby, St Louis

Siev E, Frieshtat B 1976 Perceptual dysfunction in the adult stroke patient, a manual for evaluation and treatment. Charles B Slack Inc, U.S.A.

Smith A 1967 The serial sevens subtraction test. Archives of Neurology 17: 78–80

Solet J M 1974 Solet test for apraxia. Thesis, Boston University

Trombly C, Scott A D 1977 Occupational therapy for physical dysfunction. Williams and Wilkins, Baltimore

Walsh K W 1978 Neuropsychology, a clinical approach. Churchill Livingstone, Edinburgh

Weinberg J, Diller L, Gerstmann L, Schulman P 1972 Digit span in right and left hemiplegics. Journal of Clinical Psychology 28: 361

RECOMMENDED READING

Bobath B 1978 Adult hemiplegia evaluation and treatment, 2nd edn. William Heinemann Medical Books Ltd, London, ch 2

Brunnstrom S 1970 Movement therapy in hemiplegia: a neurophysiological approach. Harper and Row, New York

Luria A R 1966 Higher cortical functions in man. Basic Books, New York

Siev E, Frieshtat B 1976 Perceptual dysfunction in the adult stroke patient, manual for evaluation and treatment. Charles B Slack Inc, U.S.A.

4

Treatment modalities; principles and techniques

PURPOSEFUL ACTIVITY

The individually motivating, somatic, extrasomatic, and integrative nature of activity is a prime indicator for its potential as a rehabilitative modality. It may also be seen as a direct method of treatment, as without the achievement of volitional activity, any rehabilitative techniques are of little value.

People measure themselves in their society by the achievement of activities applauded by that society; they express what they are by what they do. Inability caused by the symptoms resulting from stroke, in survival, self and society rewarding activities, is likely to provoke anxiety, depression, and damage self-concepts.

The promotion and maintenance of achievement for each patient from the earliest days after stroke, should be a priority of the occupational therapist.

1. Factors affecting choice

The activity must be of significance to the individual, as attention to its achievement is likely to promote memory of the processes involved, and facilitate repetition and retention of them. Factors which may influence activity choices are:

(a) Home commitments

The sudden nature of stroke often means that patients are prevented from carrying out immediate or ongoing responsibilities and from making alternative arrangements. Particularly when others have been dependent on the patient, anxiety, preoccupation, or concern about other than recovery is possible. Occupational therapists should make it their concern to discover such responsibilities and commitments, as it may be possible to include

57

caring activities within the treatment program. For example:

- An elderly spouse may participate daily with the patient in A.D.L. and recreational activities;
- A young mother may include caring for a baby or infant in treatment sessions;
- A brief visit to water a carefully nurtured garden may be possible;
- A pet cage-bird may be cared for in the day room of a rehabilitation ward;
- And pet visits may be possible during visiting time, patients being assisted to continue in a caring role.

The value of including families in treatment is being recognised, and occupational therapists should take a major role in promoting practical participation.

The importance of animals in therapy has recently received much attention, but situations where this occurs tend to be isolated and fairly structured. To an elderly person living alone, a pet may have been a constant and close companion for years, and some shared time during rehabilitation may be motivating and emotionally satisfying to

the patient. Neurophysiological and neuropsychological treatment techniques may be incorporated into caring sessions (Fig. 4.1).

(b) Relevance to daily life

Repetition and practice of activities of daily living improves patients' abilities in these tasks. Approaches may incorporate neurophysiological and neuropsychological treatment, rather than only teaching compensatory methods.

Many patients find it difficult to relate exercise to function, or to understand and accept perceptual cognitive impairment, so that the inclusion of daily living tasks often makes treatment more acceptable to them. The tasks are seen as necessary to independence and do not have a 'childlike' connotation that some other activities may have.

(c) Cultural differences

Making sure that treatment medium is of significance to each patient, and pertinent to life style, is made more difficult when the patient's cultural

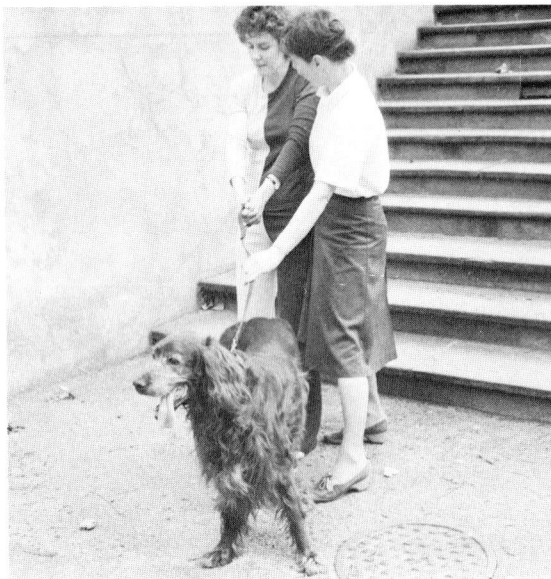

(a)

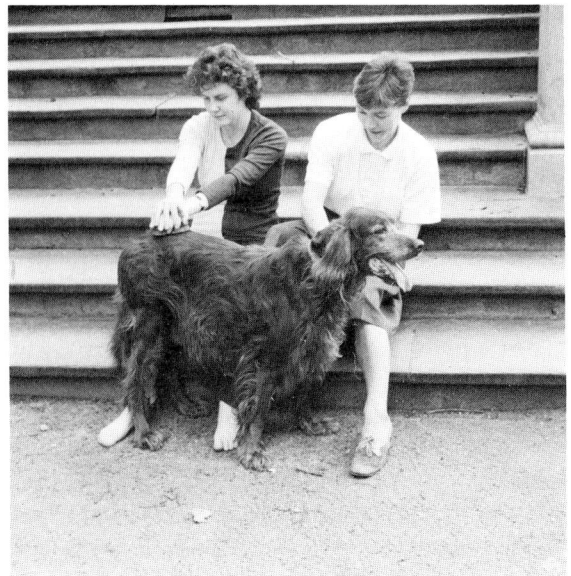

(b)

Fig. 4.1 Incorporating neurophysiological approaches into pet care. (a) Balance and mobility retraining, holding lead with bilateral clasp grip. Therapist assists with support and control of lead. (b) Bilateral upper limb extension in rhythmic, repetitive movement.

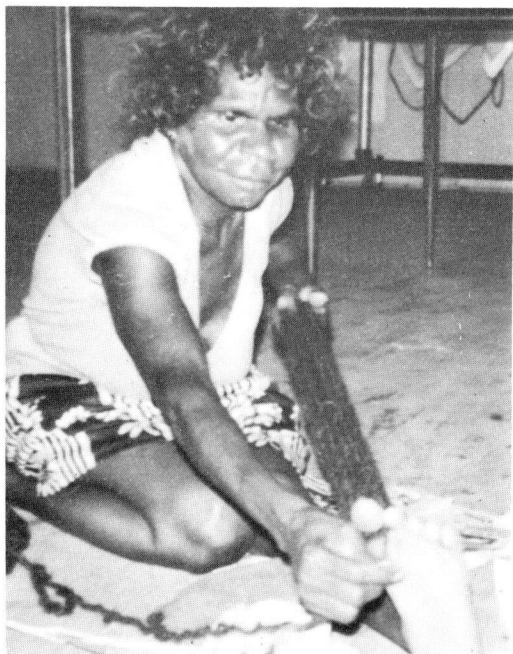
(a)

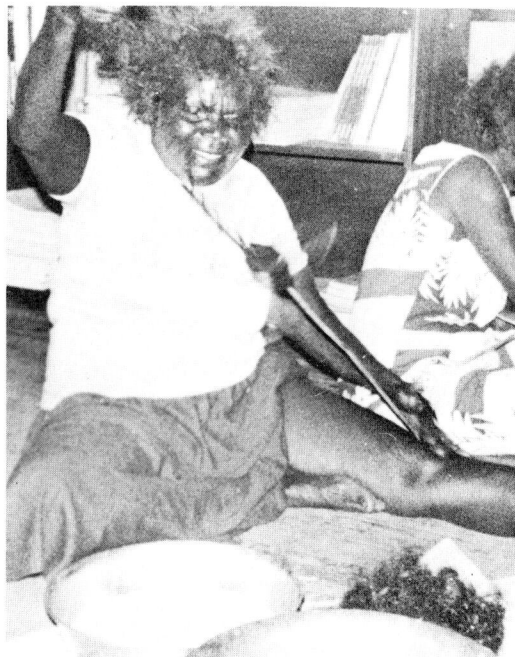
(b)

Fig. 4.2 Treatment medium relevant to patients' culture and lifestyle. Australian aboriginal spinning and weaving skills shared in group treatment.

and social situation differs from that of the treatment agency. This may be true of persons of different ethnic backgrounds living locally, or for those specifically referred for treatment from remote areas, where rehabilitation is not available. Difficulties are compounded when there are language differences.

Daily living, recreational or specific therapeutic activities should reflect the skills previously used by the patient. Encouraging groups where skills unknown to the others are presented and taught by the patient, may be extremely useful in integrating the patient group and increasing the patient's feelings of self-worth (Fig. 4.2).

Therapists may need to build up a resource reference, to assist with such patients, finding out about local agencies, interpreters and community groups who may provide valuable information, or be included in treatment sessions.

Cultural reaction and custom in reference to the sick role should be explored. Despite rigorous A.D.L. retraining and the ability to be independent, those whose culture indicates that the impaired be dependent and cared for, with families supporting and fulfilling this expectation, are unlikely to use the independence skills learned. In other cultures, those with residual disabilities may only be accepted by their society if the lowered status inferred by impairment is negated in some way, such as the acquisition of equipment different to that usually found in the society.

(d) Recreational activities

Leisure activities that the patient has enjoyed prior to stroke may be of great value in motivating participation and in redeveloping sensory motor and cognitive skills. The use of possible future recreational activities is recommended during all stages of treatment.

It is interesting to note that information regarding recreational ideas and adaptations is much sought after by stroke patients after treatment (Independent Living Centre, Sydney, 1983), which may imply the need for more thorough application during rehabilitation.

Simplification or adaptation of recreational activities may be necessary so that intact neuronal mechanisms may be utilized. This may enable a patient's participation in enjoyable activities, which may not otherwise be possible, and which, because of the highly integrative nature of most activity, still stimulates impaired mechanisms. Assistance can be decreased and complexity increased as patients show improvement.

(e) Vocational activity

This can be used similarly for those for whom it is appropriate.

(f) Interesting adult activities

Interesting adult activities which meet particular therapeutic requirements are indicated for treatment rather than simple, purposeless activities such as moving an object from one place to another which, though meeting short-term goals, may appear childish and of no value to a patient. Careful activity analysis should be carried out to assist therapists in considering how to use each activity.

2. Activity analysis

In order to fully utilize activities which patients need or are interested in doing, therapists should analyse them for neurophysiological (Trombly & Scott, 1977) and neuropsychological factors, for example:

(a) Motor aspects:

- sequence and timing of body, head and limb movement;
- balance and equilibrium;
- whether facilitatory or inhibitory to reflex movement or stereotyped postures;
- developmental level of gross postures and patterns of movement;
- mobility or stability demands on joints;
- nature of hand skills in relation to usual return of function;
- Whether any or all the above can be changed by positioning of patient or activity parts.

(b) Sensory aspects:

- developmental level of sensory components;
- direct sensory input, such as nature of tactile and auditory stimulation;
- indirect sensory input, from the environment;
- visual and auditory demands;
- inherent proprioceptive input.

(c) Perceptual aspects:

- number and complexity of steps;
- attention directed to movement or goals;
- primarily unilateral or bilateral;
- relates to body or extrapersonal space;
- Recognition, selection and manipulation of objects;
- 2 dimensional information requires translation into 3 dimensional terms.

(d) Cognitive aspects:

- number and complexity of steps;
- memory, concentration and conceptual tracking;
- verbal and calculation skills;
- problem solving, adaptability and understanding of cause and effect;

Fordyce (1971) suggests that when analysing vocational or leisure activities they may be classified in 3 ways:

(a) *Symbol centred*, which are those activities concerned with words, numbers, concepts, and ideas.

(b) *Motor manipulative centred*, which are those activities concerned with physical movement and manipulative skills.

(c) *Interpersonal centred*, which are those activities concerned with people, and participation in social and organizational ventures.

Classification of a patient's previous activities in such a way, may lead to a better understanding of therapeutic activities which may be motivating, and of those which may be of little use.

Carr and Shepherd (1982) emphasize the importance of activity analysis in identifying the essential components, or key elements of activity, so that repetitive practice of those which the patient finds difficult, is possible. These may then be incorporated into total functional activities.

Evaluation will have made the therapist aware of specific impairment which may prevent achievement.

Careful analysis provides information enabling therapists to simplify procedures, so that components too demanding of disordered neuronal mechanisms may be reduced, and achievement becomes possible. It also enables appropriate grading of activities. For example, Farber (1982) suggests that when parts of an activity are too demanding, sub-cortical activity should be utilized to reinforce treatment goals in early stages of treatment, such as instead of asking a patient to turn his head, the patient's attention should be directed to an appropriate visual stimulus, which is moved to facilitate head turning.

TECHNIQUES TO FACILITATE ACTIVITY

Volitional activity demands activation of cortical mechanisms, which can be enhanced by use of peripheral or 'central' stimulation. Harris (1980) suggests that therapists should decide when to use peripheral and/or central input to modify muscle tone or strength of muscle contraction, when considering each patient's motivation, capacity for motor learning, and the circumstances of treatment, based on priorities of functional importance such as self-care, mobility, and manipulative skills.

Techniques which may be used before or during activity to facilitate achievement, and gradually taught to patients so they may self-apply facilitatory procedures, include:
1. Positions and patterns of movement of body parts;
2. Various types of stretching, proprioceptive and cutaneous input;
3. Increased sensory information;
4. Application of principles of learning.

1. Positions and patterns of movement

(a) Developmental sequence

Developmental approaches follow the order of human development, because recovery from stroke is thought to mirror the developmental sequence (Twitchell, 1951), return of function occurring in a cephalocaudal direction, proximal before distal, and gross movement before discrete. It is believed that recapitulation of previously experienced motor learning will make motor re-education easier (Knott & Voss, 1968), and that as normally primitive reflex activity is sequentially controlled, with maturity of balance and postural mechanisms, following the same progression in rehabilitation will facilitate control of movement (Bobath, 1978).

Neuromuscular development progresses through: reflex head extension in prone; positive supporting reflexes in upper limbs, and visuo-motor reflex effects on neck, trunk, and limb muscles; head control in supported sitting; independent sitting; creeping; supported standing; exploratory crawling; positive supporting reflexes in lower limbs; supported walking; independent standing and walking (Wyke, 1975).

The major developmental stages used in re-education of balance and gross mobility progress as appropriate to individual patients through:
(i) Development of head control, using prone and supine positions, and rolling;
(ii) Development of trunkal extensor tone for stability, using maintenance of an upright sitting posture, utilizing visual, tactile and proprioceptive cues;
(iii) Inhibition of abnormal trunkal tone using rotation, with the head leading the movement, so that voluntary changes of position are possible;
(iv) Re-education of equilibrium reactions, and use of limbs to maintain balance when the centre of gravity is altered;
(v) Practice in voluntary control of postural mechanisms with the upper limb free for activity.

Appropriateness is determined by evaluation of postural status, balance reactions, age, other disability, and affective state.

Developmentally, infants start exploratory activities of a simple nature from a wide, stable base, and progress as they become safe to more complex activity, a less stable base, and reduced support. In balance retraining, this progression may be included.

(b) Vestibular stimulation

Therapists favouring a multi-sensory approach stress the importance of the vestibular system in the developmental sequence, and propose that treatment should follow the order of sensory development. The vestibular system which matures early is important in directing the position and movement of the head in space, facilitating extensor tone, and maintaining stable visual perception when movement occurs (Galley & Forster, 1982).

Vestibular stimulation aimed at normalizing impairment, is applied early in treatment by rolling, rocking, and rotational movement, producing an immediate response which lasts only as long as the stimulus (Trombly, 1983).

Farber (1982) tables a summary of the suggested sequence of vestibular stimulation commencing with inversion of the upper trunk, and progressing through anteroposterior movement such as rocking over a ball or bolster, or in 4 point kneeling; side to side movement in prone; 4 point kneeling, kneel stand, and standing; diagonal rocking in crawling, 4 point kneeling, kneel stand, and standing; linear acceleration using equipment such as swings, and rotation.

Some of the positions used may be inappropriate and contraindicated for many stroke patients, and therapists are referred to *Neurorehabilitation—a multi sensory approach* (Farber, 1982) for information.

(c) Reflex inhibiting patterns (R.I.Ps)

Reflex inhibiting patterns of movement are an important component of the neuro-developmental approach pioneered by Bobath (1970), who hypothesises that before attempting to elicit normal voluntary movement, abnormal reflex activity, which has been released from mature central nervous system control following stroke, must be inhibited.

The abnormal reflex activity is manifest in changes of muscle tone causing stereotyped abnormal patterns of spasticity, most commonly, mainly flexor hypertonicity in trunk and upper limb, and extensor hypertonicity in the lower limb. Because of the stereotyped nature of these

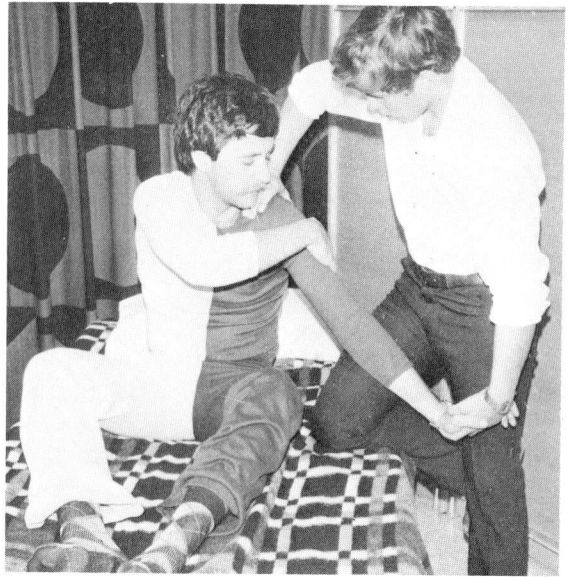

Fig. 4.3 Upper limb reflex-inhibiting pattern; external rotation at the shoulder, elbow extension, wrist extension with supination, and abduction of the thumb.

abnormal patterns it is possible to prescribe positions and patterns of movement which reverse them, and it is these which are known as R.I.Ps.

The main R.I.P. recommended to reverse the abnormal postural pattern of the upper limb and trunk, is extension of the neck and spine, external rotation of arm and shoulder, elbow extension, wrist extension with supination, and abduction of the thumb. An upper limb R.I.P. is shown in Figure 4.3.

The main R.I.P. recommended to reverse both extensor or flexor spasticity in the lower limb is extension, abduction and external rotation at the hip, knee extension, dorsiflexion of the ankle, dorsiflexion of the toes and abduction of the big toe. Also particularly recommended is rotation between the shoulder and pelvic girdles. By changing part of the abnormal patterns, tone may be reduced in the rest of the body.

R.I.Ps should be immediately combined with activation of the patient, that is, the process should be dynamic, the therapist requesting purposeful movement and controlling and preventing any undesirable reaction from occurring.

Because effort, including that produced by the sound side, may provoke associated reactions by a process of irradiation which may increase spasticity, many occupational therapists have been inhibited from using a wide range of activities. Bobath (1978) states 'The occupational therapist should avoid causing effort and stress. It has been mentioned repeatedly that any effort, especially voluntary effort, increases spasticity.' However, Harris (1980), in his discussion of the Bobath approach, suggests 'The strict neuro-developmental therapy adherent loses out on other valuable possibilities by virtue of failing to provide opportunities for learning skills necessary for discrete, functional movements—which could be accomplished through involvement of the patient in motivated volitional activities.'

With both these opinions in mind and to improve the patient's affective state, it seems important to include task achievement and some measure of independence early in treatment without increasing spasticity. R.I.Ps can be successfully integrated into a graded activity program from the earliest days, the therapist monitoring patient responses and adjusting the activity should unwanted tone be elicited.

(d) Synergy modification

Brunnstrom (1970), who advocates following the sequence of recovery as described by Twitchell (1951), hypothesises that during early recovery stages patients should be encouraged to utilize, control, and modify abnormal reflex activity or gross movement synergies, as these always precede the restoration of voluntary movement following stroke, and may be seen as a necessary intermediate stage of recovery.

To elicit basic limb synergies of the hemiplegic side maximum effort of the sound side is demanded. Associated reactions thus elicited by irradiation are usually the same bilaterally in the upper limbs, and opposite in the lower limbs. Interdependence of upper and lower limbs on each side is demonstrated by the same response in each. For example.

(i) Resistance to extension in the sound upper limb elicits an extensor synergy of the hemiplegic upper limb.

(ii) Resistance to extension in the sound lower limb elicits a flexor synergy in the hemiplegic lower limb.

(iii) Resistance to extension of the hemiplegic lower limb facilitates extension of the hemiplegic upper limb.

Irradiation recruits contraction of muscles in gross flexor or extensor synergies (Fig. 4.4). The typical abnormal hemiplegic posture combines elements of both flexor and extensor synergies. By alternating flexor and extensor synergic movement, using them functionally, gradually controlling and refining away from synergy patterns, voluntary movement is facilitated.

When the synergies occur, local muscle tapping and cutaneous stimulation are used to facilitate contraction of individual muscles; for example, stimulation applied over the extensors will be facilitatory to them and inhibitory to the flexors.

The effects of tonic neck and lumbar reactions are utilized in the demand for voluntary movement of limbs, and postural stability and mobility of head and trunk. Souque's phenomena, involuntary extension and separation of the fingers which occurs when the arm is elevated more than 90°, is used during retraining of hand movements. Harris (1980) suggests that the effects of tonic head and neck reflexes are weak, but that the cumulative effect when used with other modalities may be significant.

Patients experience satisfaction from self-initiated movement, which may motivate increased participation in therapy. Because recovery may cease at any of the stages, ongoing application of functional skills encourages the patient to make use of limited movement and to be more aware of the affected side.

(e) Mass movement patterns

Knott and Voss (1968) hypothesize that proprioceptive input enhances motor response and that by resisting mass movement patterns, which are based on normal movements of work and sport, activity in weaker muscles is stimulated by overflow from the stronger muscles involved in maximum effort. The amount of resistance applied does not prevent movement but allows the patient to achieve.

The movement patterns used are of a spiral and diagonal nature, which elongate all muscles and involve all the joints in the moving body part. A

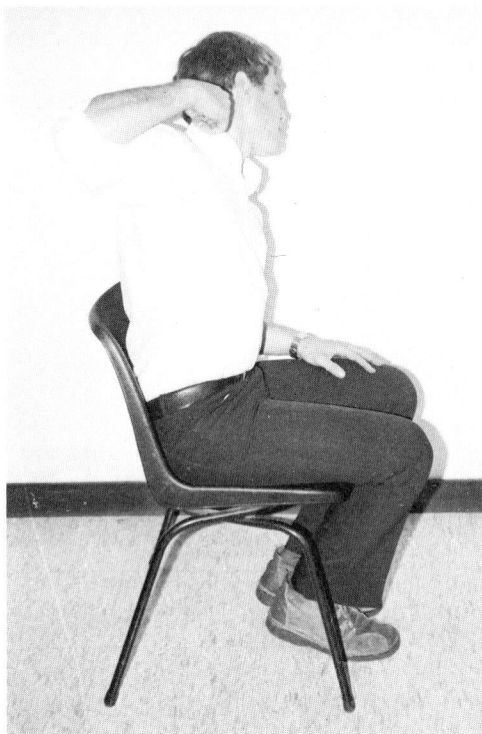

(a)

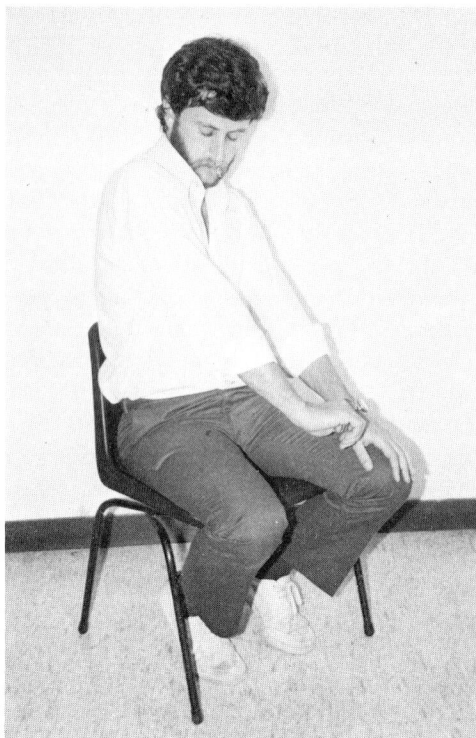

(b)

Fig. 4.4 (a) Flexor synergy of the upper limb — retraction and/or elevation of shoulder girdle, shoulder external rotation and abduction, full range forearm supination and elbow flexion. Wrist and fingers usually flexed. (b) Extensor synergy of upper limb, protraction of shoulder girdle, shoulder internal rotation and adduction, full range forearm pronation and elbow extension. Wrist usually extended and fingers flexed.

full range of patterning is not always useful, and the range and pattern should be selected for individual lack of function (Todd, 1972). A developmental sequence is advocated with developmental postures being described as total patterns.

The spiral diagonal movements for upper limb treatment are shown in Figure 4.5. The terms 'Diagonal 1' and 'Diagonal 2' are used to differentiate between the two upper limb patterns of movement (Trombly, 1983). These movements may be incorporated into occupational therapy activities, and an example is shown in Figure 5.23.

Movement in the desired spiral diagonal tracks may initially be assisted, and other sensory stimuli incorporated as appropriate. The sensory stimuli suggested include normal timing and sequence of movement, manual contact, auditory and visual stimulation and feedback, stretch, joint traction and approximation. These may be facilitatory to

increased awareness of body parts and cross modal matching. Todd (1972), reporting on facilitation of movement as taught at Vallejo, states that: 'All activities of daily living are facilitated by manual guidance or resistance (and all the techniques of P.N.F.), thus enabling quicker learning and eliminating so much frustration for the patient'.

Therapists following this approach believe that the movement patterns assist in the integration of primitive reflex behaviour and support voluntary effort, by restoring balance between flexor and extensor activity. Some authorities have suggested that mass movement patterning may not lead to fine controlled movement and its value may be in the early stages of treatment to elicit return and possible integration of reflex activity. (Mossman, 1976). The movements may also be useful to promote patient awareness of the feel of normal movement.

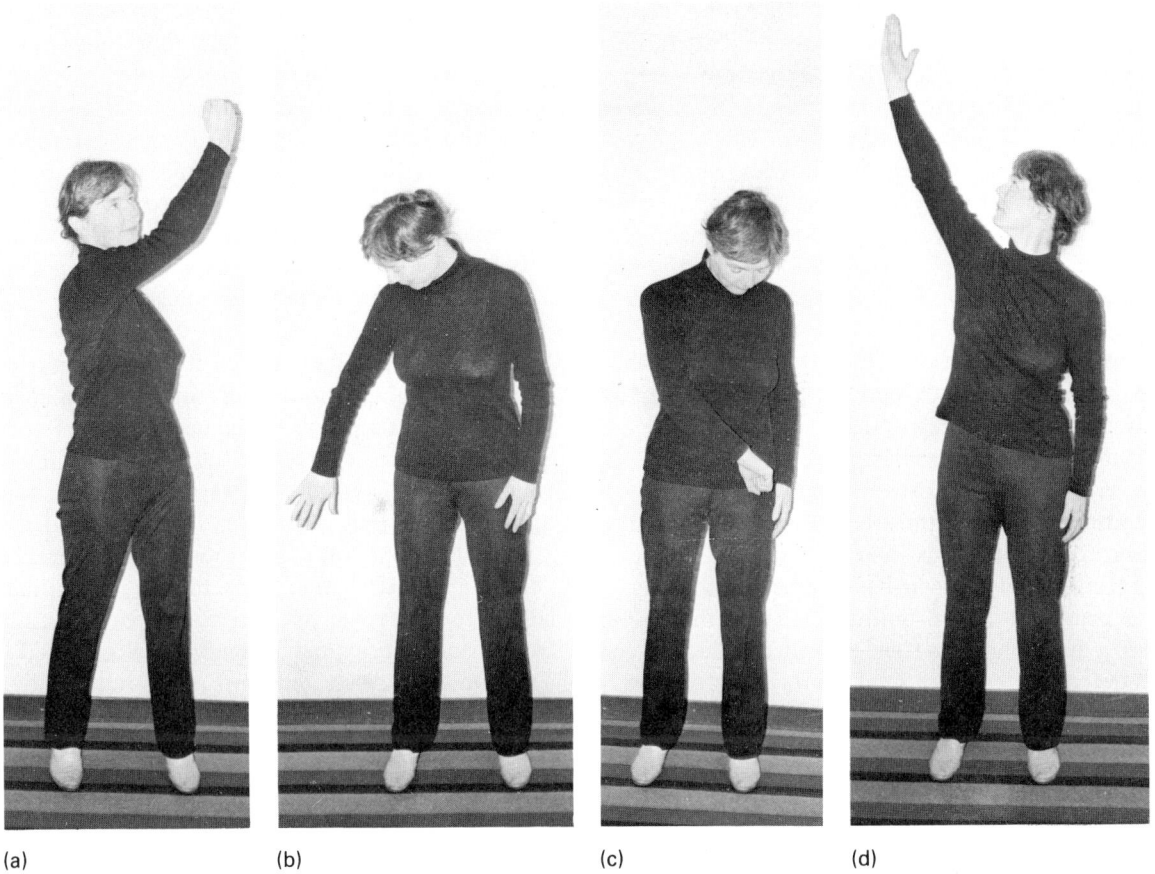

Fig. 4.5 P.N.F. patterns of the upper limb (Trombly, 1983), (a & b) Diagonal 1 pattern. (c & d) Diagonal 2 pattern.

2. Peripheral stimulation

Techniques aimed at modifying peripheral motor neuron excitability may be used by the occupational therapist before or during the use of activity aimed at eliciting a cortical response, as the same motor units may be activated by both central and peripheral nervous systems, increasing the likelihood of effective intervention (Harris, 1980). Peripheral stimulation includes:

(a) Stretch

A quick, light stretch facilitates contraction of the muscles stretched and inhibits the antagonists. The stretch reflex, initiated by mechanical distortion of the stretch receptors within the muscles, occurs when the therapist quickly moves the joint through a full range of movement opposite to the direction of the desired movement.

The afferent fibres arising from the stretch receptors are of large diameter and therefore rapid conductors of impulses. They make monosynaptic, facilitatory connections with the motor neurons, innervating the muscles from which the afferent fibres arise, and polysynaptic, inhibitory connections with motor neurons, innervating the antagonist muscle (Harris, 1980). Quick, light stretch may therefore be used to facilitate contraction of the muscle stretched or relaxation of its antagonists.

The reflex is delicate to elicit and before applying stretch the therapist should feel the tension throughout the limb, ensuring that the muscles to be stretched are at their lengthened range. A quick pressure at this point will elicit the opposite movement (Todd, 1972). At the moment the reflex is elicited, the patient should attempt the opposite movement, so the therapist must prepare and practise the patient using brief verbal command at the point of stretch.

Inhibition of hypertonic muscles can also be obtained by progressive desensitization of stretch receptors by applying very slow and maintained stretch (Trombly & Scott, 1977). The inhibitory effect on hypertonic muscles may be used by immediate activity of weaker muscles, or by maintaining the relaxation achieved in a R.I.P. whilst involving other body parts in purposeful activity. Harris (1980) suggests that slow stretch is the best stimulus to achieve relaxation.

Pressure on muscle insertion also inhibits contraction of the muscle. Pressure must be firm and constant. This may be applied manually during activity, or tool handles may be constructed to provide pressure during their use, thus inhibiting finger flexors. Cone-shaped handles are considered particularly useful for this (Farber, 1982).

(b) Thermal stimulation

Prolonged deep cold which penetrates the muscle mass produces a block on the receptor excitatory process or afferent fibres, temporarily preventing the conduction of impulses, so acting in an inhibitory fashion (Harris, 1980). This inhibitory effect may be achieved in several ways:

(i) Total immersion of part of a limb, e.g. forearm and hand, in icy water. Both origin and insertion of muscle to be relaxed must be immersed for one minute. Some patients find this very unpleasant and it may therefore be contraindicated. However, dipping the limb several times briefly, may be helpful, especially if the therapist participates by sharing in the immersion. This may assist the patient's acceptance of the process and the patient's joints may be eased into anti-reflex positions as they relax.

(ii) Limbs may be wrapped in icy towels. The towels should be of a thick, soft variety for greatest effect and should be kept in icy water all day ready for use. Excess water should be wrung out and the towels applied either directly over the antagonist muscle group or all around the limb. Knott and Voss (1968) recommend approximately three minutes use of the compress, during which time the towel is changed at least once.

(iii) A more convenient method may be the use of commercially available ice packs wrapped over the body part in the same manner as the towels, making sure a protective layer of material is between the ice pack and the skin.

Before using cold, therapists should discuss its use with the patient to promote acceptance and participation.

Thermal stimulation applied to specific areas of the skin to modify tone and stimulate particular muscle contraction was pioneered by Rood. Stroking the skin with an ice block, leads to innervation of the stretch receptors of the muscles underlying the skin stimulated (Harris, 1980).

Application is over the muscle belly or the dermatomal distribution of the muscle to be stimulated, from three to five seconds, stroking firmly from distal to proximal (Trombly & Scott, 1977). The muscle stretch receptors are brought to a heightened state of excitability which makes them more responsive to the quick stretch reflex, which may be applied by the therapist before demanding functional use of the movement elicited.

It has been said that the maximum excitability of the muscle is reached thirty minutes after the thermal stimulation, but the time may vary with individuals even to the maximum response occurring immediately, so therapists should test response time span with each patient (Harris, 1980). Therapists should also check the effect of icing over several hours in case there are any adverse manifestations, and should not apply ice to the posterior trunk, the head, or the neck, as a protective sympathetic nervous system response (vasoconstriction) may result (Trombly, 1983).

Neutral warmth may be used to induce relaxation, thereby facilitating the use of weak muscle contractions without having to overcome strong synergic activity. 33° to 37° Celsius is the recommended temperature (Farber, 1982).

Neutral warmth is less specific than the other modalities mentioned, but skin receptors, especially those of pressure and vibration, have their lowest threshold between 36° and 38° Celsius (Geldard, 1972), so neutral warmth may be used as a preliminary to specific stimulation using these modalities.

It is a pleasant stimulus and may be achieved by the use of a tepid bath or shower in an A.D.L. retraining session if the weather is warm, or by wrapping limbs in warm towels. An alternative to this might be the use of a dacron filled sleeve, similar to an air splint. Wrapping may be used during non-specific treatment times, maintaining the limbs in a R.I.P. and to assist in resisting the establishment of strong spastic patterning. The fact that neutral warmth may be used for specific treatment also indicates the importance of the temperature of the working environment.

(c) Cutaneous stimulation (Trombly, 1983)

Brushing with a battery operated camel hair brush against the direction of hair growth is another of the specific techniques used by Rood. The rationale and technique is as for quick icing, previously described, and the same precautions and contraindications apply.

Tapping and *vibration* are other forms of cutaneous stimulation in common use. They act as a series of sudden muscle stretches, stimulating the underlying muscle, and are applied before and during voluntary movement.

Tapping with the finger tips should be light and initially quite fast, and several bursts may be needed before a response is felt, then tapping may be slowed and the intervals between taps prolonged. If the tapping rhythm is unchanged when a response is elicited, the stimulus loses effectiveness.

Vibration, using a battery-operated vibrator, can be used over the muscle belly or tendons of smaller muscles, or the musculo-tendonous junction of large muscles. Vibration should be applied in short bursts of one to two minutes at five second intervals rather than continuously.

These techniques should not be used on hypertonic muscles or those likely to become hypertonic, but on their antagonists, and it is useful to alternate them with, or use as part of reflex-inhibiting activity.

If undesirable tonal changes occur, inhibitory techniques should be used to promote relaxation. The modulating effects of peripheral stimulation are brief, with maximum response usually occurring very shortly after input, so the timing of

voluntary movement is critical and should be monitored by the therapist for each patient (Harris, 1980).

Manual contacts when assisting the patient to move should also be considered for facilitatory or inhibitory effects (Knott & Voss, 1968). Manual pressure may be over the muscles involved in the movement, used to provide sensory cues, or as a directional guide. Pressure should not be painful or a withdrawal response may be elicited.

Whichever procedure is considered most appropriate to the individual, additional use of other sensory modalities may be included to increase patient awareness, particularly simple verbal instruction, and having the patient watch any movement which is elicited in the limb.

(d) Proprioceptive stimulation

Approximation or joint compression stimulates the joint proprioceptors, facilitates extensor tone and assists stability and co-contraction of muscle around the joint.

It can be applied manually (Fig. 4.6), for example after achieving extension in the upper limb, or whilst leading a limb into functional activity. It may also be used as a training mechanism for weight bearing when hypotonicity causes joints to be very unstable.

Approximation can also be used naturally during weight bearing of both upper or lower limbs. Care should be taken to correctly align joint surfaces before body weight is allowed to apply compression. Added manual compression may be given. If weight is taken for any length of time, through upper limb joints particularly, discomfort or pain may result, so care should be taken to change position frequently.

Johnstone (1978) recommends the use of air pressure splints to increase sensory input, as it produces deep, sustained pressure which bombards the proprioceptors, thereby increasing awareness of that body part. If applied correctly with the limb in a R.I.P. it inhibits muscle spasm and will assist in decreasing tone in the rest of the body. Whilst wearing the splint the patient should be encouraged, and assisted if necessary, to move the limb. When the splint is removed the patient should use the limb in activity so that benefits

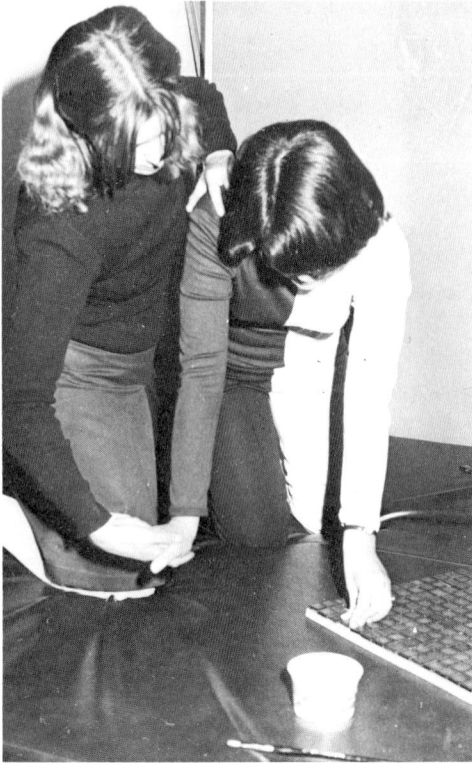

Fig. 4.6 Manual application of upper limb approximation to stimulate joint proprioceptors.

gained from its use are maximized. Air splints should be inflated by human blowing as this will prevent over inflation and constriction. It will also ensure that warm air fills the splint, adding another pleasant, relaxing sensory modality.

3. Increased sensory input

In recent years occupational therapists have been particularly interested in sensory aspects of cortical integration and its effects on functional activity. This interest was stimulated by the work of Rood and Ayres, who stressed the importance of sensory input in the production of motor output.

(a) Sensory engrams and feedback

Harris (1980) and Guyton (1981) report on animal research studies (Mott & Sherrington, 1895), which demonstrate functional impairment resulting

from sensory denervation is far greater than impairment from a lesion in the primary motor cortex.

Harris concludes that tonic postural and phasic motor output become defective without sensory input, that normal postural stability and voluntary movement depend on accurate kinesthetic feedback, and many impairments of balance and movement may be caused by lesions affecting the sensory rather than the motor system.

Guyton indicates that in many activities the motor system acts as a servomechanism, merely following a pattern (engram) located in the sensory system. If the motor system fails to follow the pattern, sensory feedback allows modification of motor activity.

Sensory engrams are memories of different movements recorded from experiences received in the sensory and sensory association areas. Patterns of control of rapid co-ordinated movements, such as writing or piano playing, are probably established within the motor system after frequent practice of the skill, as there is insufficient time for effective sensory feedback during the activity, and this is provided retrospectively to help correct the motor pattern, if necessary, when next used (Guyton, 1981).

The facilitatory effects of peripheral stimulation may be partly due to improvement in sensory rather than motor mechanisms, the provision of extra sensory input from skin, muscle and kinesthetic receptors heightening awareness of a hemiplegic part, and increasing the possibility of the initiation of voluntary movement (Harris, 1980).

Carr and Shepherd (1982) report on the work of Taub (1980) and others, who have demonstrated that animals can learn to use sensory denervated limbs by training and increasing motivation and learning time. They suggest this implies that although sensory feedback may be necessary for the fine tuning and accuracy of movement and at certain stages of motor learning, peripheral information from movement may not be as important as some think, because many motor programs are genetically endowed.

Sensory information is certainly needed when new motor skills are being learnt by 'normal' people. Guyton (1981) suggests that even highly skilled activity is possible, if done extremely slowly so that kinesthetic sensory feedback is able to guide step-by-step movement. Other sensory systems are probably intimately involved during the learning stage, particularly the visual and auditory systems. Guyton points out that the somatic proprioceptive system is faster than the others in recognising motor error, and therefore when the sensory engram depends on visual feedback, activity is usually much slower.

Carr and Shepherd (1982) indicate that emphasis should be placed on visual, verbal and vestibular feedback in the relearning of motor control, rather than proprioceptive input such as resistance, which they suggest has little effect on accuracy of movement if the other inputs are not used. They further state that motor re-education utilizing continuous visual, verbal and manual guidance to increase patients' understanding of their performance of activity, will also improve impairment of sensory perception.

(b) Combining sensory modalities

Cross modal matching between sensory systems may be assisted by combining proprioceptive and tactile modalities with patient awareness via visual monitoring of movement and touch, verbal cues, and encouraging concentration on residual impressions of somato-sensation.

Therapists who follow a sensory integrative approach (Farber, 1982) propose that sensory input is most useful if it follows the sequence of sensory system development, tactile and vestibular inputs being emphasised before visual and auditory inputs. Stimulation should be designed to produce an adaptive response, which is defined by Farber as 'behaviour of a more advanced, organized, flexible, or productive nature than that which occurred before stimulation.'

Graded use of sensory modalities from a single stimulus to complex multi-sensory stimuli is advocated, progression occurring when consistent adaptive responses are achieved at each stage. This enables gradual acquisition of intersensory processing, at association areas of the sensory cortex. Intersensory processing, or cross-modal integration, is necessary for an individual to cope independently within a changing environment.

Indiscriminate use of sensory stimulation is contraindicated because over-bombardment with inhibitory or facilitatory stimuli may cause over-stimulation and confusion (Farber, 1982).

Johnstone (1978) recommends that to obtain a response from sensory stimulation, the input or demand must be increased until a response is gained. As part of that increased demand she advocates the use of air pressure splints, as described previously, to stimulate deep sensation, including proprioception, during procedures to develop normal movement. She also advocates thoughtful and dynamic use of hearing, vision, and touch.

It appears there is general agreement that movement is enhanced or retarded by the effects of sensory stimuli, both of primary sensation and perception, visual, spatial, kinesthetic and auditory modalities being of particular importance in the achievement of goals. By awareness, evaluation and application of sensory modalities during retraining of movement, a more holistic and realistic approach to integration of neurological function is achieved. It is important for the therapist to consider the appropriateness of sensory cues, stimulation or the environment and their effect on the level of achievement.

Patients should watch and follow limb movements, and should be encouraged to touch and talk about their hemiplegic side. Therapists should use attention demanding procedures when appropriate, such as language for specific effect, altering tone, speed and amount of words to facilitate or relax movement; touch and pressure to reinforce the action required and to integrate sensation and movement; and visual stimuli to give purpose to the movement.

(c) Timing of sensory input

Guyton (1981) points out that voluntary activity may not occur until minutes, hours or days after sensory input, depending on cerebral processing, that is analysis, storage, retrieval and integration of sensory and motor memory, and initiation of motor response.

As in everyday life, people often need time to 'sleep on' an idea, so may patients sometimes need time to 'sleep on' response to sensory input. Responses to some specific inputs, such as quick stretch, will be immediate, but repetition of a stimulus from time to time, which has not previously been seen to initiate activity, may be appropriate.

(d) Order of sensory input

The order of sensory inputs used is seen by some therapists as important, the emphasis of combined sensory modalities may also be significant. Patients early after onset of stroke frequently experience disturbed body image, whether or not the lesion directly affects cortical areas responsible for spatial understanding of an extra- or intra-personal nature. As infants develop and mature by initially relating sensory experiences to their own body, before being able to relate them to the environment and to respond appropriately and independently within it, so may the stroke patient need to be made more aware of their own body, before being expected to respond to complex activities of an extrapersonal nature.

Sensory input relating to the body and its needs is suggested as an important initial treatment modality. Occupational therapists may use personal care tasks such as dressing, washing, showering, eating and transferring to increase patient awareness of their body from the earliest possible opportunity, because these activities if used appropriately, will maximise, without bombardment, visual, tactile, kinesthetic and auditory imput. As patients become more aware of their body, particularly of the hemiplegic side, the sensory modalities may be extended to include the immediate, and later an expanded, environment.

(e) Utilizing habitual responses

In making use of sensory input to enhance recovery processes, the importance of habitual responses cannot be overstated. Because of the patterned nature of much volitional activity, to expect patients to respond adaptively to familiar activities, when equipment, circumstances and environment are changed, may be unrealistic. At least during the initial stages of treatment, adapting the situation to simulate the patient's

own, as much as possible, may trigger responses more effectively than any applied sensory stimulation.

(f) Biofeedback

Biofeedback or electronic devices may be used as an alternative or supplementary method of supplying information to patients about activity.

4. Principles of learning

In order to learn, patients need to be motivated, provided with an environment in which learning is possible, given appropriate practice, sensory cueing, and a progressive learning experience.

(a) Motivation

In order to facilitate patient participation in the treatment process they need to appreciate the nature of their impairments, wish to improve them, and see the relevance of proposed approaches and techniques. Occupational therapists should assist the patient to gain an understanding of their dysfunction and to appreciate that particular tasks and methods may be helpful. An empathetic, caring approach based on fact is essential. Therapists should develop their ability to talk about the nature of dysfunction at levels appropriate to each person.

It is invalid to assume that patients will have completed an accurate inventory of impairment, particularly if there is sensory loss, language, praxic, spatial or body awareness disorders. For example, a patient may have contralateral neglect, but because of the nature of the disorder feels 'whole'. Patients may be unable to respond with understanding if the therapist suggests they find their left arm (Hewson, 1982), rather they need to have the arm identified. They require information, at an appropriate level, for understanding about the nature of the impairment, reinforced by repetition and sensory cues. An educational approach may be essential before patients are able to adapt their previous self-image to the reality of the present. Relearning may not be possible if patients do not understand their dysfunction.

Regular repetition of information may be necessary. Discussion should progress to the setting of goals, patient and therapist priorities, and a tentative program structure.

Occupational therapists need to create an environment which allows the patient time to grieve, assimilate, and achieve, to appreciate the present, and accept the future challenge.

(b) A therapeutic environment

Although the creation of a therapeutic environment may not be seen as a specific intervention modality, without it, programs, approaches and particular techniques may be less effective.

It is a place where those participating in treatment are comfortable, relaxed yet stimulated, which promotes individual growth, facilitates relearning, and in most cases results in maximum ability being achieved. It is relevant to the society which it serves, promoting and enhancing skills necessary for quality survival within that society. A well-ventilated, attractively decorated, warm, pleasant area will not in itself create a therapeutic situation. What happens within the environment is what creates it.

A major role of each therapist is that of environmental engineer. To be effective in this role therapists need to develop their personal skills so that they promote support and encouragement between patients, patient–therapist interaction which is mutually beneficial, and inter-team understanding, with acceptance, promotion and/or sharing of treatment objectives.

A therapeutic environment encourages the redevelopment of social skills by use of group activities and sharing of problems and solutions, it allows patients the opportunity to adapt their self-concepts to present reality in an empathetic and uncritical situation, and provides a background to individual goals and sensory-motor improvement.

The maintenance of dignity and self-worth is vitally important, so activity which appears childish, or that patients are unable to control to some degree, are contraindicated. The nature of the tasks used in therapy should be of an adult nature, related to real interests and practical requirements, or, understood by the patient for their therapeutic worth. To treat every patient with individually

specific activity may sometimes appear time consuming and difficult, but by offering remediation with real life goals, treatment will be more useful and motivating than by the use of short-term, non-specific tasks chosen for their physical characteristics only.

Emphasis must be on activities in which the patient will be able to succeed, so therapists must have a good understanding of how to do the activity themselves, and how to teach it clearly and simply to the patient. The approach must be flexible, with the therapist ready to change or adapt should stress or frustration become a problem. This does not imply that difficult tasks should not be attempted, as achievement of seemingly impossible tasks may offer an enormous boost to self-confidence, allowing the patient to feel more in control of life. To ensure success therapists need to evaluate the patient's abilities and potential, give practical assistance with appropriate support and cues during the difficult task, and allow the patient to complete the last component of the activity by themselves, if possible.

Praise and recognition from the therapist or other patients may reinforce patient satisfaction. In a study by Anderson (1967) a significant relationship was found between social interaction and self-esteem, self-esteem increasing with opportunities for interaction.

Patients should be encouraged to talk about or express how they feel if they wish to. If they do not wish to, this should be respected, the therapist's empathy and understanding being shown by a touch on the arm, or by leaving the patient alone for a few moments as appropriate. An over-hearty, jolly manner should be avoided. Success in an activity should be shared and enjoyed, but care should be taken that over emphasis on a small achievement does not appear insincere and inappropriate to the patient.

(c) Activity presentation

The therapist should have adequate understanding and physical skill in the activity and techniques chosen for use, should be prepared with any equipment or materials necessary for success and make sure that the patient has spectacles or hearing aid as required so that communication is enhanced, effort is reduced, and patient safety is ensured.

Depending on the site and extent of lesion, and nature of impairments, presentation of the activity or activity parts, may require either mainly demonstration or mainly words. Either should be clear, simple and adult. Appropriate sensory and environmental cues should be used to reinforce instructions. The activity process should be slowed down so that maximum use of information and feedback from intact sensory mechanisms may be utilized. Either a very simple task should be chosen initially, or the patient asked to do only a small part. Forward or backward chaining, when only the first or last stage of the activity is completed independently and assistance is given with other steps is an example of a method useful for grading tasks. The number of steps the patient performs alone is gradually increased, either at the beginning or end, until independence in the total procedure is possible. Using such techniques, practice in everyday skills may be initiated early.

The therapist should make sure, when patients are trying a task for the first time, that they are relaxed throughout, and do not hold their breaths unnecessarily. This is also true for the therapist, as attitudes are easily transmitted between people.

(d) Practice and repetition

It is generally agreed that practice and repetition are essential for any kind of learning. Patterns or engrams of motor function are developed by conscious repetition of a volitional activity, with sensory feedback correcting undesirable or wrong movement (Kottke, 1975).

Therapists who advocate the use of inhibition of abnormal movement at all times, believe that this may prevent abnormal movement engrams becoming established. Those who utilize progressive modification of abnormal movement, believe that repetitive sensory input during practice may provide feedback, to assist redeveloping sensory and motor engrams to self-modify in the central nervous system.

Hebb (1961) demonstrated cumulative learning of verbal skills occurs unconsciously in a study using recurring digits. Corsi (1972) demonstrated that the same type of learning occurs with spatial skills by using blocks instead of digits. Learning can occur with rehearsal even without memory of the activity, that is, even though a patient may not remember previous performances of a task, their skill in the task can show improvement in subsequent performances. (Milner et al, 1968).

Carr and Shepherd (1982) suggest that important components of practice include goal identification and the relevance of practice, appropriate selection of whole or part of an activity, practice without error, patient participation in task rehearsal or mental practice, and augmented practice.

Trombly (1983) with reference to Sage (1977) suggests that a whole activity should be practised initially, aiming at normal timing, and as ability develops, skill in component parts be emphasized; the environment and equipment be natural to the activity; that practice should make use of regular rest so that fatigue does not diminish performance.

Practice should be assisted with sensory cues, appropriate to patients' observed response to them, and should be graded to build skill on skill, so that relearning develops naturally towards more complex activity without the necessity of patients having to 'unlearn' steps previously taught.

Reinforcement by praise and encouragement on achievement, or some method of recording progress which the patient is able to appreciate, will be conducive to ongoing participation.

(e) Consolidation

When patients are able to continue an activity independently or with only occasional help, the activity should be included in a day long program which is additional to specific individual programs. This extends treatment time which has several important benefits. It enables consolidation of re-acquired skills, facilitating learning of subsequent skills by providing a sound basis for progression. It promotes a more structured use of time, possibly providing the 'work time' component of a normal daily cycle, so assisting natural fatigue and possibly reducing dependence on drugs to induce sleep. It provides the opportunity to participate in reality-based activities shared with others to maintain self-concepts.

SUMMARY OF STEPS IN USE OF REMEDIAL ACTIVITY

1. Discovering and analysing the purposeful activities which will be highly motivating or necessary to an individual.
2. Incorporating specific neurophysiological procedures and increased sensory input into the performance of the chosen activity, whilst utilizing neuropsychological components. Both procedure and activity should evoke a desired response appropriate to the stage of recovery reached.
3. Assisting the patient to understand why a particular sequence and method of retraining is being followed and have them learn to incorporate for themselves, as far as possible, approaches which allow them to succeed, discouraging the use of methods which are seen to produce abnormal response.
4. Grading the task to increase both independence and normal volitional components of activities.
5. Providing opportunity for practice of the activity independently to consolidate learning. For patients who do not reach a stage of complete recovery, retraining in activities necessary for daily functioning has progressed with the sensory motor retraining program, and does not have to be tacked on as an afterthought. If necessary activities are left until recovery of volitional movement plateaus or ceases, patients may not be sufficiently practised when they are discharged.

COMPENSATORY TECHNIQUES

Early training in compensatory methods using residual abilities is an approach followed by some occupational therapists and rejected by others. Those who reject the use of compensatory approaches for daily functional tasks early in rehabilitation, do so in the belief that they will inhibit or prevent the return of more normal motor function.

The few comparative studies of outcome between treatment methods have indicated no significant differences between the results of patients treated with early mobility and adaptive self-care regimes, to those treated with strategies based on neurophysiological mechanisms (Feldman & Lee, 1962; Stern et al, 1970).

There may be benefit in adaptive procedures equal to neurophysiological strategies. It is possible that the emotional and cognitive benefits of a motivating, easily understood approach, which facilitates rapid achievement of a functional nature (particularly for those whose abstract reasoning and attention skills are reduced) stimulates neuronal mechanisms significantly.

When there is massive cortical destruction, or when age or other dysfunction decrease the likelihood of good recovery, and institutional care is proposed, the use of repetitive adaptive techniques to maximize limited ability should be used, as there may be insufficient time in the acute hospital setting to assist such patients to reach maximum potential through use of slower remedial approaches. Any simple procedure that will decrease dependence, will improve future quality of life. Intensive retraining utilizing existing ability for the acquisition of independence in simple tasks, is recommended for their short stay in acute care. This may have the additional benefit of increasing patients' awareness of the environment, stimulating sensory and cognitive functioning and possibly facilitating some continued improvement even if no rehabilitative services are available in the institution to which they are discharged.

REFERENCES

Anderson N H 1967 Effects of institutionalization on self esteem. Journal of Gerontology 32: 313–317
Bobath B 1970 1978 Adult hemiplegia: evaluation and treatment. Heinemann Medical Books Ltd, London
Brunnstrom S 1970 Movement therapy in hemiplegia, a neurophysiological approach. Harper and Row, New York
Carr J, Shepherd R 1982 A motor relearning programme for stroke. Heinemann Medical Books Ltd, London

Corsi P M 1972 Human memory and the medial temporal region of the brain. Unpublished Ph.D thesis, McGill University

Farber S D 1982 Neurorehabilitation, a multisensory approach. Saunders, Philadelphia

Feldman D J, Lee P R, Unterecker J, Lloyd K, Rusk H A, Toole A 1962 A comparison of functionally oriented medical care and formal rehabilitation in the management of patients with hemiplegia due to cerebrovascular disease. Journal of Chronic Disease 15: 297–310

Fordyce W E 1971 Psychological assessment and management. In: Krusen F H, Kottke F J, Ellwood P M (eds) Handbook of physical medicine and rehabilitation, 2nd edn. W B Saunders Company, Philadelphia

Galley P M, Forster A L 1982 Human movement—an introductory text for physiotherapy students. Churchill Livingstone, Edinburgh

Geldard F A 1972 Human senses, 2nd edn. John Wiley, New York

Guyton A C 1981 Basic neurophysiology, 3rd edn. W B Saunders Co, Philadelphia

Harris F A 1980 Facilitation techniques in therapeutic exercise. In: Basmajian J V (ed) Therapeutic exercise, student edition. Williams and Wilkins, Baltimore, ch 3

Hebb D O 1961 Distinctive features of learning in the higher animals. In: Delafresnaye J F (ed) Brain mechanisms and learning. Oxford University Press, London, p 37–46

Hewson L 1982 When half is whole. Dove Communications, Blackburn, Victoria

Johnstone M 1978 Restoration of motor function in the stroke patient, a physiotherapist's approach. Churchill Livingstone, Edinburgh

Knott M, Voss D E 1968 Proprioceptive neuromuscular facilitation, 2nd edn. Harper and Row, New York

Kottke F J 1975 Neurophysiologic therapy for stroke. In: Licht S (ed) Stroke and its rehabilitation. Waverly Press Inc, Baltimore, ch 11

Milner B, Corkin S, Teuber H L 1968 Further analysis of the hippocampal amnesic syndrome: 14 year follow up study of H.M. Neuropsychologia 6: 215–234

Mott F W, Sherrington C S 1895 Experiments upon the influence of sensory nerves upon movement and nutrition of the limb. Proceedings of the Royal Society, London 57: 481

Mossman P L 1976 A problem oriented approach to stroke rehabilitation. Charles C Thomas, Springfield

Sage G H 1977 Introduction to motor behaviour: a neuropsychological approach, 2nd edn. Addison-Wesley, Reading, Mass

Stern P H, McDowell F, Miller J M, Robinson M 1970 Effects of facilitation exercise techniques in stroke rehabilitation. Archives of Physical Medicine and Rehabilitation 51: 526

Taub E 1980 Somatosensory deafferentation research with monkeys: implications for rehabilitation medicine. In: Ince L (ed) Behavioural psychology in rehabilitation medicine: Clinical application. Williams and Wilkins, Baltimore

Todd J 1972 Facilitation of movement as taught at Vallejo. Physiotherapy London 58: 415–419

Trombly C 1983 Occupational therapy for physical dysfunction. Williams and Wilkins, Baltimore

Trombly C, Scott A D 1977 Occupational therapy for physical dysfunction. Williams and Wilkins, Baltimore

Twitchell T E 1951 The restoration of motor functions following hemiplegia in man. Brain 74: 443–480

Wykes B 1975 The neurological basis of movement—a developmental review. In: Holt K S (ed) Movement and child development. Heinemann Medical Books Ltd, London

RECOMMENDED READING

Bobath B 1978 Adult hemiplegia: evaluation and treatment, 2nd edn. Heinemann Medical Books Ltd, London

Brunnstrom S 1970 Movement therapy in hemiplegia, a neurophysiological approach. Harper and Row, New York

Farber S D 1982 Neurorehabilitation; a multisensory approach. Saunders, Philadelphia

Guyton A C 1981 Basic human neurophysiology, 3rd edn. W B Saunders Co, Philadelphia

Harris F A 1980 Facilitation techniques in therapeutic exercise. In: Basmajian J V (ed) Therapeutic exercise, student edition. Williams and Wilkins, Baltimore, ch 3

Johnstone M 1978 Restoration of motor function in the stroke patient, a physiotherapist's approach. Churchill Livingstone, Edinburgh

Knott M, Voss D E 1968 Proprioceptive neuromuscular facilitation, 2nd edn. Harper and Row, New York

Trombly C 1983 Occupational therapy for physical dysfunction. Williams and Wilkins, Baltimore

Approaches to acute rehabilitation

INTRODUCTORY CONSIDERATIONS

IN THE WARD (Ch. 5)

Early treatment which takes place in the ward focuses on the establishment of rapport and communication between therapist and patient, and basic somatosensory re-education using body-related activity. Treatment approaches have not been discussed separately in Chapter 5 but suggestions for several have been included to illustrate that a variety of treatments are possible. Readers are referred to the initial approach discussed in Chapter 3, Evaluation.

IN THE RETRAINING UNIT (Chs. 6–9)

When patients are to attend the occupational therapy department, particularly for the first time, it is important for the therapist to be aware that they are likely to be anxious and uncertain about what is going to happen. Factors which may cause discomfort should be eliminated as far as possible, so that relaxation and acceptance of the situation is promoted.

Consideration should be given to factors such as: the order and timing of patient transport; where and with whom patients are placed; the duration of initial and subsequent treatments; that they are met and greeted pleasantly by name when first they arrive; that they are given adequate and appropriate information about procedures; that personal embarrassment is minimized and that they are individually farewelled, having been given an accurate understanding of when they will be returning.

Information gained from observation of the patient within the ward situation should be used as a basis of planning for the initial treatment session in the department, to ensure that some measure of success important to the individual patient is achieved.

Treatment is separated in the following chapters according to the nature of impairments; however, this is for the purpose of clarity only: treatment for gross mobility and balance, impaired function of the upper limb, higher cortical or affective disorders and social problems needing in most cases to occur concurrently.

5

Treatment in the ward environment

GENERAL CONSIDERATIONS

1. Timing

It is important that all patients be assessed and treated as soon as their condition has stabilized, which for many patients is about 2 days after onset of stroke (Held, 1975; Carr & Shepherd, 1982). In order to ensure that patients do not miss being referred, therapists should check admission sheets daily, consult ward charts regularly, and request a referral if it has been overlooked.

2. Daily program

The patient should be out of bed and leave the restrictions of the ward environment as soon as possible, to commence active treatment. However, it is probable that in many hospitals much of the patient's time will be spent in bed and ward in the early post-stroke period. Treatment programs at all stages should extend positively into the ward to prevent lengthy immobility, detrimental positioning, anxiety, depression, and rehabilitation gains achieved elsewhere being negated.

Because of the importance of patients being aware of, and appreciating their wholeness, before they are able to make maximum use of sensory motor retraining, early emphasis needs to be on increased sensory input used in conjunction with neurophysiological movement techniques. Personal care activities of dressing and hygiene tasks, because of their cutaneous sensory nature, are recommended for this purpose specifically, having the advantage of being motivating, because seen as functional and necessary to each individual. That they may also promote personal independence is a secondary, though important factor, at this stage in treatment.

Some patients may be confined in bed for longer than a few days, because of associated or additional medical problems. Techniques to use with patients in bed have been included.

As discussed earlier the patient's day should, as nearly as possible, resemble a daily cycle of work, recreation, relaxation and rest, so that close to normal physiological and socio-psychological demands are experienced, reducing the danger of increasing dysfunction (of a physical or psychological nature) caused by inactivity. This may be more difficult to organise in an acute ward setting than in a specialised rehabilitation unit but intra-team attempts should be made to create such an environment, and to structure timing of specific treatments, so that the patient's daily program is realistic to their individual needs.

3. Relatives and friends

It may also prove advisable to enlist the co-operation and participation of the patient's relatives and friends. This may lead them to a better understanding of the patient's actual problems, and be conducive to increased patient participation and motivation. Such participation may lead to spontaneous sharing of anxieties when 'on the spot' education programs for both the relatives and patient may be beneficial. These should be geared towards particular worries that are expressed, and specific about practical problems manifesting themselves at the time. They should deal simply with why some behaviour is happening, how to handle it, how not to handle it, and realistic assurance. Simple pictures, drawings and demonstration are often helpful. If there are queries beyond the scope of the therapist, these should be referred to the medical officer.

PREVENTION OF PHYSICAL DISORDERS SECONDARY TO STROKE

Before proceeding to practical suggestions on activities to initiate whilst the patient is bed bound, disorders secondary to stroke must be discussed.

1. Subluxation of the shoulder joint

Subluxation of the hemiplegic shoulder is frequently a complication of prolonged flaccidity but may also become manifest when tone increases.

There are many theories about the cause of subluxation, including stretching of the shoulder capsule and cuff muscles, depression of the lateral aspect of the scapula, malalignment of the humeral head when the angle of the glenoid fossa changes, spasticity of muscles changing the force and angle of joints (Cailliet, 1980), and traction on the already stretched muscles and joint by the weight of the flaccid arm (Carr & Shepherd, 1982).

When flaccid hemiplegia is present, and particularly if it is accompanied by loss of proprioception, the patient will be unaware of pain and position of the upper limb, and unable to move it actively. The shoulder joint, unstable because of decreased muscle tone around it, is susceptible to damage.

Opinions differ about prevention of this problem, some therapists feeling that correct handling and positioning alone will prevent subluxation (Johnstone, 1978); some that passive ranging alleviates the problem; others that it causes it, and feel that early facilitation of active movement is the answer (Carr & Shepherd, 1982); some believe in sling support (Tobis, 1957), and others decry the use of slings (Hind et al, 1967). Such wide divergence of opinion indicates that it is a serious problem and that all measures to ensure it does not occur should be considered.

(a) Handling the flaccid arm

Movement and control of the scapula should be facilitated when extending the arm passively, or assisting the patient to utilize limited voluntary movement (Fig. 5.1). At all times the arm should be supported and the scapula assisted to rotate. Internal rotation and adduction should be avoided (Carr & Shepherd, 1982). The patient should be asked to think about the shoulder as it moves, to increase awareness, and discouraged from pulling on the hemiplegic arm, or passively ranging until the scapula moves in a normal relationship with the upper limb.

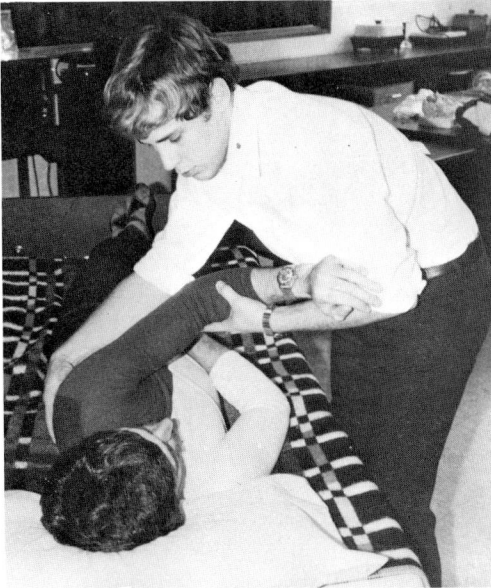

(a)

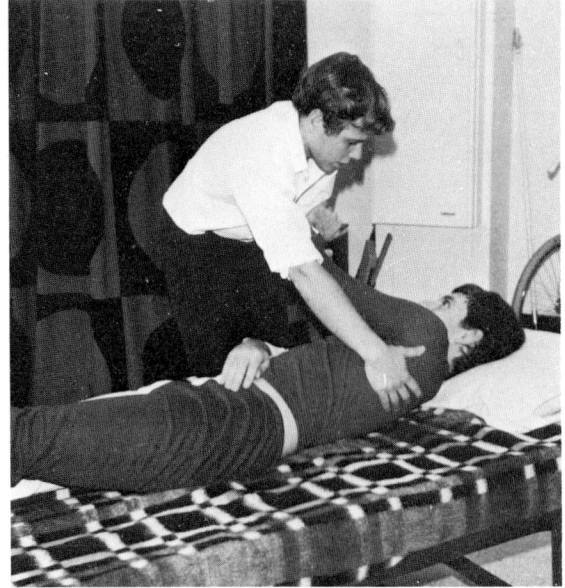

(b)

Fig. 5.1 Assisting rotation of the scapula when re-educating rolling activity. (a) Before assisting the patient to roll, the therapist locates the scapula and supports the forearm. (b) As the patient rolls the therapist extends the supported arm and rotates the scapula.

(b) Positioning

When in bed, seated in a chair or wheelchair, or at a table, the forearm should be supported so that the joints are correctly aligned and the humerus is seated in the glenoid cavity. Pillows, gutter or suspension slings may be used (Fig. 5.2). When sitting, weight bearing through the affected upper limb, the arm abducted and externally rotated, the elbow, wrist and fingers extended, and the thumb abducted is recommended (Cailliet, 1980). This position may require supervision to ensure correct joint alignment (Fig. 5.3).

(c) Facilitation techniques

Cailliet (1980) postulates that every stimulation technique should be tried until voluntary or reflex muscle activity about the shoulder occurs.

When facilitating voluntary movement by mass movement patterns, reflex inhibiting patterns, cutaneous stimulation or any other means, the therapist should ensure a normal anatomical arrangement of the shoulder joint in all positions, and normal sequence and timing of movements (Fig. 5.4).

(d) Support

When the patient is transferring or walking without assistance, some means of support must be applied to prevent traction caused by the weight of the arm, which will increase the degree of subluxation. Various supports and slings currently used are shown below (Fig. 5.5). Concern has been expressed that the conventional hemiplegic sling maintains the arm in a flexed position and fails to support the humeral head in the glenoid cavity. However, if this type of sling is used only at times of greatest susceptibility, such as when transferring or walking independently, and applied before subluxation can occur, to prevent, rather than cure, it will inhibit the occurrence of continuous traction.

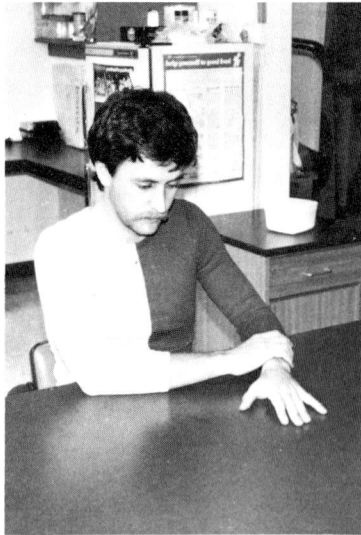
(a)

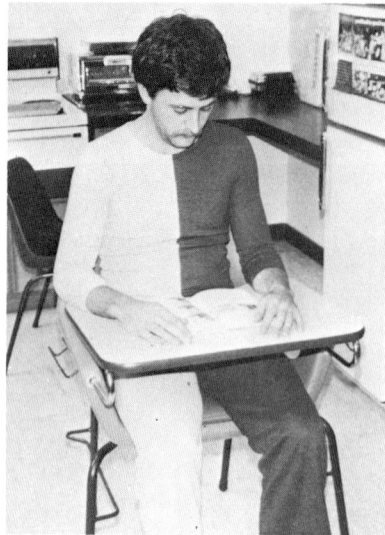
(b)

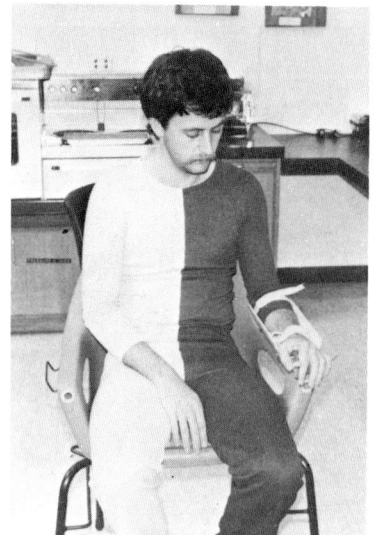
(c)

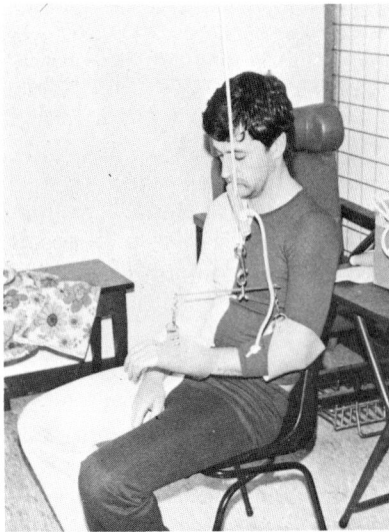
(d)

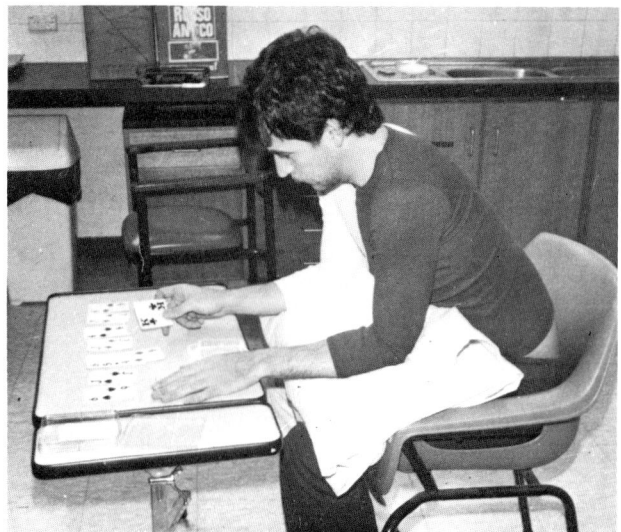
(e)

Fig. 5.2 Forearm support to maintain joint alignment and seating of the humeral head in the glenoid cavity. (a) At a table. (b) Reading using a chair table. (c) With gutter support on chair arm. (d) With overhead sling. (e) Playing cards in elbow support sitting.

Pressure garments for early use and prevention of shoulder joint damage may be worthy of study. A prototype garment, made of lycra, is shown in Figure 5.6, with extra lycra bands following the pull of the shoulder musculature to increase upward movement of the humerus. It is designed to be worn before subluxation occurs, will not hinder movement, may assist with the stability of the elbow in weight bearing tasks, will apply deep pressure which may facilitate proprioceptive response (Johnstone, 1978) and increase awareness of the hemiplegic limb.

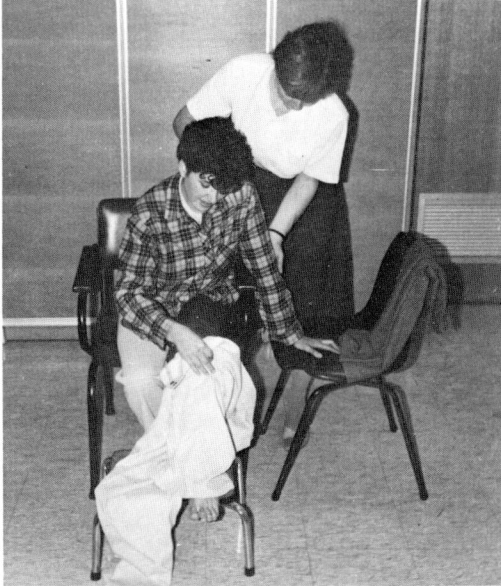

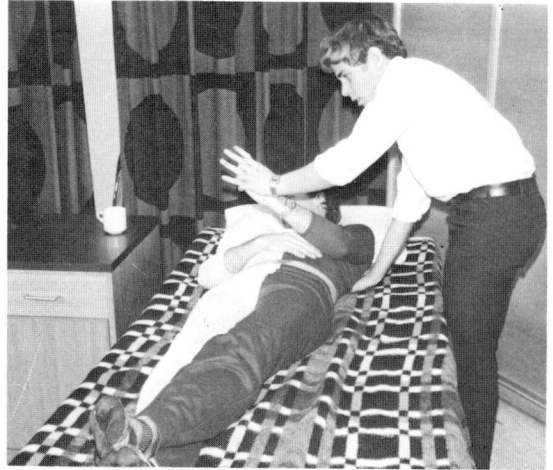

(a)

Fig. 5.3 Weight bearing through affected upper limb — the arm abducted and externally rotated, the elbow, wrist and fingers extended, the thumb abducted. The position is supervised to ensure correct joint alignment.

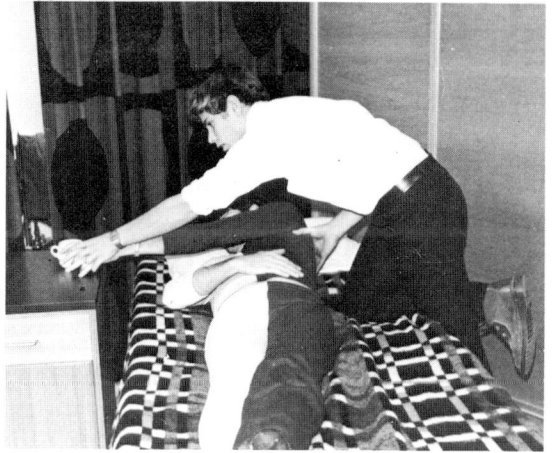

Fig. 5.4 Assisting functional reach whilst maintaining normal anatomical position, sequence, timing of movement.

(b)

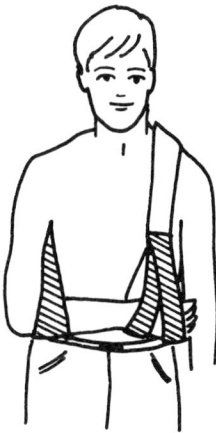

(a)

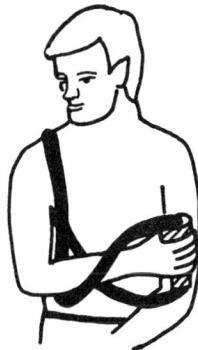

(b)

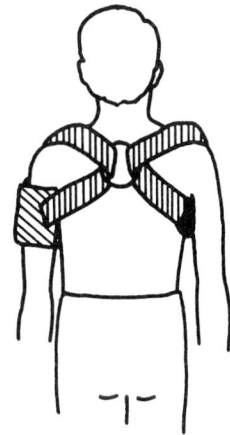

(c)

Fig. 5.5 Examples of slings or supports currently used to discourage shoulder subluxation. (a) Conventional hemiplegic sling, crosses under the hemiplegic arm to the sound shoulder and supports the wrist and hand, separating the thumb from the fingers. (b) Rood sling (Cailliet, 1980). Elastic tubing with cone-shaped hand piece. It is proposed that this stimulates arm extension, radially deviates the wrist, and elevates and derotates the scapula. (c) Cuff and strap support similar to the type recommended by Bobath (1978). Each strap is made of one length of webbing passing through a central back ring to allow freedom of movement. Additional wedge under axilla is fixed with velcro (removable) and webbing is padded under the sound axilla. Design used at Prince Alfred Hospital, Prahan, Victoria.

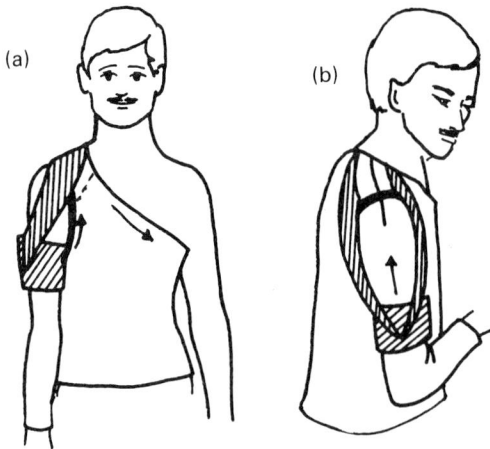

Fig. 5.6 Prototype lycra pressure garment with added lycra bands to increase upward movement of the humerus.

2. Pain and fatigue due to unaccustomed positions

The physical changes associated with stroke can cause muscular and joint pain, discomfort and fatigue because gravity and muscular imbalance of the limbs, trunk and head will cause unaccustomed positions to be assumed.

Sensory changes and emotional factors may increase risks of faulty positions occurring, especially if the patient exhibits contralateral neglect, somatosensory disturbance, visual disorders, fear or depression. Patients may be unable to make the minute adjustments usual for easing and sharing joint and muscular activity, and will therefore be unable to feel comfortable for any length of time; they may feel symmetrical when they are not, and be unaware of their habitual position patterns.

Lorna Hewson (1982) when describing the gross contralateral neglect she experienced following stroke, explains her feeling of wholeness despite complete lack of awareness of her left side, and how her centre of gravity appeared to have moved to the right, to be in the centre of her known body. She was dependent upon others to adjust her position and experienced much discomfort and pain, which she was unable to localize, understand or explain. In retrospect she attributes much of her pain to degeneration of her cervical spine aggravated by her head constantly falling to one side.

Occupational therapists should be responsible, with other staff, for maintaining positions to reduce the development of pain and fatigue, as well as facilitating sensory motor re-education. Figure 5.7 illustrates common abnormal positions patients assume when supine in bed.

Constant vigilance may be required and so it is appropriate that all those working with the patient should share a common concern and purpose in the maintenance of appropriate and comfortable positions.

Some treatment centres advocate the use of bolsters and pillows to assist with propping and

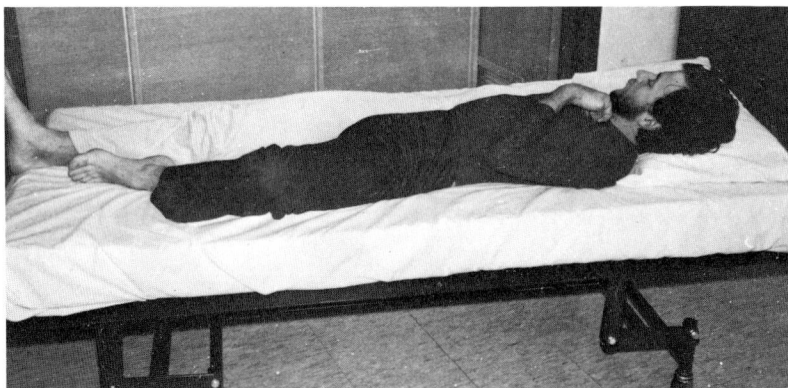

Fig. 5.7 Common abnormal positions assumed due to neurological dysfunction which are contraindicated. Flexion of the upper limb should be avoided. Rotation and retraction of the hip, constant flexion or hyper extension of the knee, and inversion or eversion of the foot should be avoided. Lateral flexion of the neck to the hemiplegic side and rotation of the sound side should be avoided.

positioning, particularly of flaccid body parts, and these may have added value when skin breakdown may result from undesirable pressure.

3. Contractures

In the neglected or untreated hemiplegic, contractures may be expected to occur (Mossman, 1976). The poor positions naturally assumed because of neurological damage and the effects of gravity, if unchecked, are likely to result in the formation of contractures, particularly when strong spasticity is a complication, and limbs are drawn habitually into the same position.

Upper limb contractures are most usually those of flexion in all joints, adduction and internal rotation, and in the lower limb, flexion of the knee and extension of the ankle (Mossman, 1976).

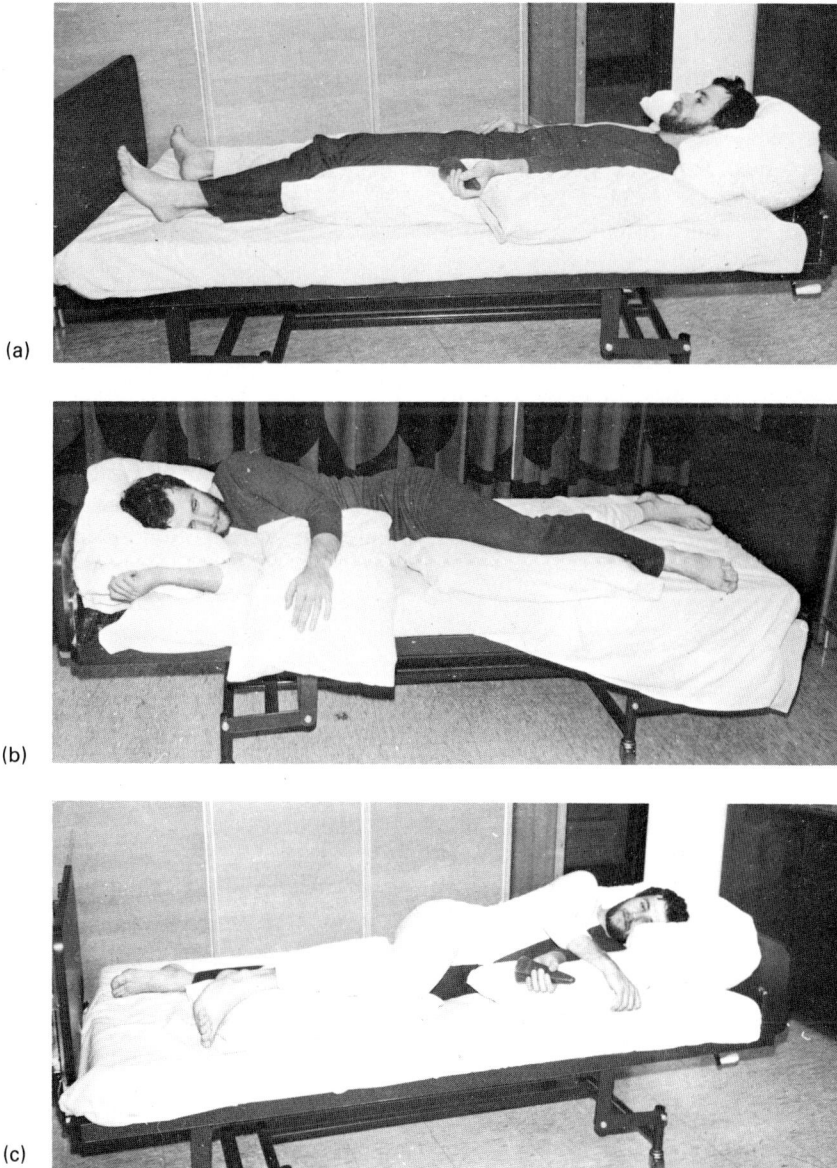

(a)

(b)

(c)

Fig. 5.8 Examples of positions recommended whilst the patient is resting in bed. (a) In supine. (b) Lying on the sound side. (c) Lying on the hemiplegic side.

Early standing and weight-bearing of upper and lower limbs will help prevent the development of contractures, but reflex-inhibiting positions (Bobath, 1978) should be maintained whilst the patient is in bed (Fig. 5.8), and active movement encouraged early (Carr & Shepherd, 1982).

4. Lower limb damage through inappropriate mobilisation

Early weight bearing and standing has many advantages, being assistive to motivation, balance re-education, prevention of contractures, reduction of incontinence and enhancement of normal physiological function; however, if undertaken without due care, may result in joint damage, secondary to neurological deficit. Particularly when limbs are flaccid, joints unstable and unprotected by co-contraction of surrounding musculature, transferring, standing or assisting the patient to move, requires constant monitoring of joint alignment and limb position. In the early stage, foot, ankle, knee and hip may all need support from the therapist. How the therapist moves and stands, so that the patient gains maximum benefit, may differ from therapist to therapist, as different body shapes and sizes alter which body part may be used to best advantage.

ACTIVITY IN BED

Most patients, subject to their condition having stabilized, are encouraged to spend much of each day out of bed, but need to be retrained in bed mobility for independence during evenings, at night time, during rest periods, and for when they return home. Practice in dressing is preferable out of bed, but some patients may require extended bed care, and the sensory stimulation provided by dressing is too valuable in promoting gestalt, to postpone. A few patients find dressing in bed easier and safer.

Many of the movements and positions described in this section may be used when treating patients on a plinth in the retraining unit.

1. Position and mobility

Positioning is important in the facilitation of purposeful activity. In order to position a patient so that activity is maximally therapeutic, the occupational therapist must assist the patient to move as independently as possible, but without undue effort.

As the patient learns to move independently in bed, it is necessary to be aware of problems likely to be evident and those that could develop, either through the natural progression of recovery or through inappropriate or thoughtless intervention.

The specific problems that are interfering with the patient's ability to move about in bed normally, may be: fear of moving, disturbed postural mechanisms, poor head control and balance, disturbed understanding of body parts, altered concept of the objects and space around them, inability to plan movement generally, impairment of range of movement and co-ordination, disturbed proprioceptive and tactile sensation, impaired understanding and judgment, or fatigue.

All members of the retraining team should use similar or complementary techniques, so that the patient does not become confused, and learning is reinforced by repetition.

In order for learning to take place it is important for patients to understand what is being asked of them, and to understand the reason. An occupational therapist should ensure that the reason for moving in bed has a purpose, is goal directed, such as sitting up to eat a meal, to watch television or to talk more comfortably. Both functional gains and sensory-motor re-education should result from the mobility technique taught.

It may be necessary to break the actual instructions for moving into small components, and teach step by step. In such cases the total sequence of movements should be made clear before proceeding with individual steps. To ensure achievement it is recommended that intact neural abilities are utilized initially: for example, if there are spatial disorders or contralateral neglect, use of left hemisphere verbal processing will assist patient understanding; similarly demonstration may be necessary when the speech dominant hemisphere is affected. The use of affected hemisphere skills may be introduced gradually.

2. Moving up in bed (from lying to sitting)

Method (Fig. 5.9)

The sound arm is positioned to allow the patient

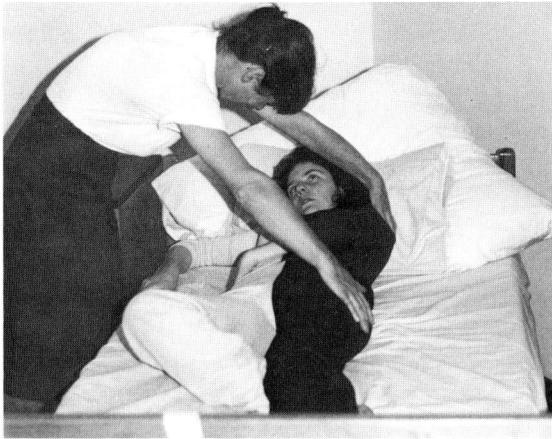

(a)

to push up on it, forward at the shoulder and flexed at the elbow. The sound leg is flexed with the foot under the hemiplegic leg. The hemiplegic arm is brought forward ensuring that the scapula rotates and the therapist, by supporting pelvis and shoulder, assists the patient to roll on to the sound side. The patient is assisted to push up on the sound arm, then to push down on sound arm and foot, and lift up and back. This may be repeated several times until the required position is achieved.

Therapeutic rationale

Because the hemiplegic side is supported and carried by the sound side without over-use, effort is reduced, and early independent movement is possible. The method mirrors the way many elderly people get up in bed or out of bed normally. That is, they roll to one side, push up on one hand and swing their legs out of bed (Carr & Shepherd, 1982). It may therefore assist in the recall of a previously experienced sequence of movement, triggering cognitive, somatosensory and spatial responses. The sequential and ro-

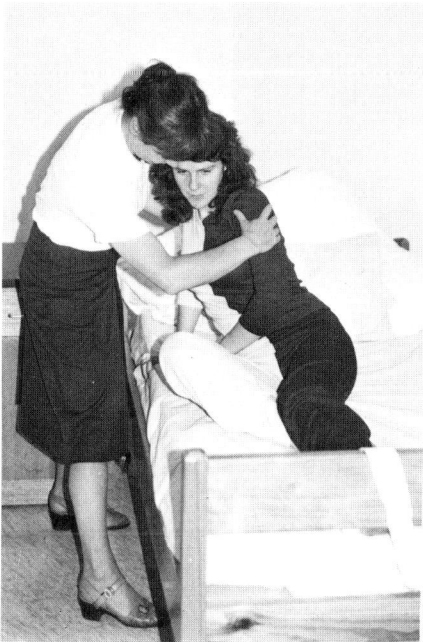

(b)

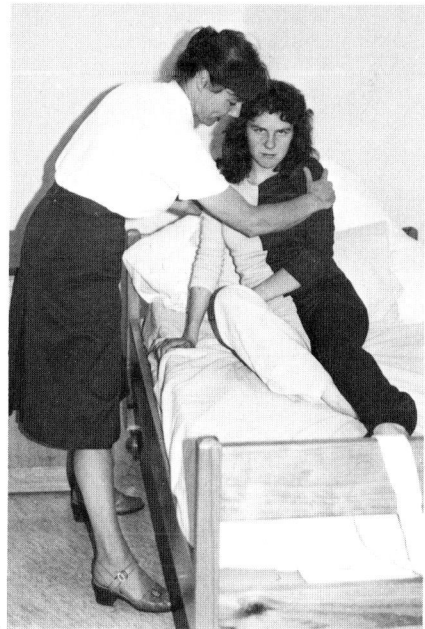

(c)

Fig. 5.9 Assisting the patient to move in bed from lying to sitting.

tational aspects of the movement are those of early motor-development, and may encourage head control, postural, and balance reactions. Early achievement of some measure of independent functioning will help patients to feel some control over their environment.

3. Support sitting

Support and elbow support sitting are used to encourage active controlled neck movement by providing support to the rest of the body and limbs and reducing effort needed to maintain trunk position.

Method: Support sitting (Fig. 5.10)

To encourage neck flexion, pillows or specially constructed wedges support the body totally so

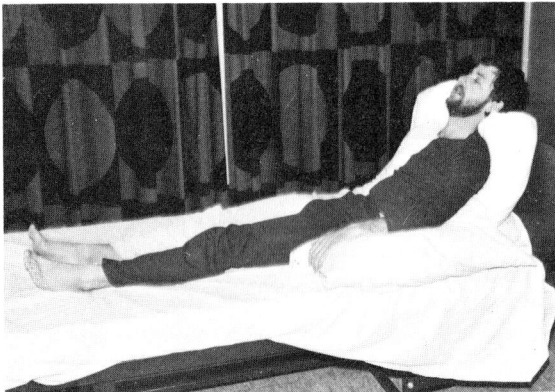

(a)

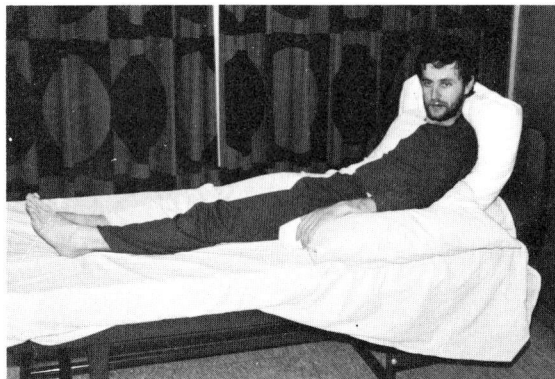

(b)

Fig. 5.10 Support sitting to encourage controlled neck flexion.

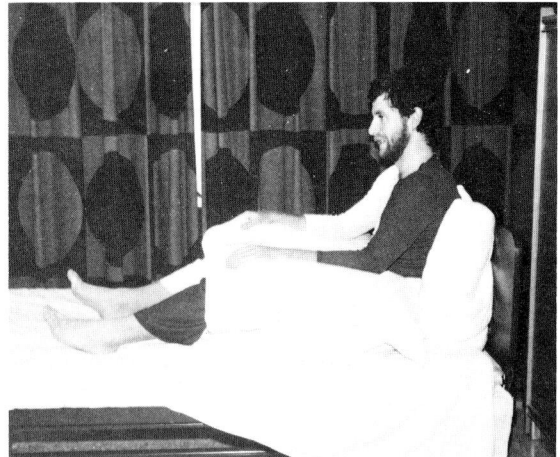

Fig. 5.11 Elbow support sitting to encourage neck extension.

that gravity assists neck extension. Brief activity which demands neck flexion and rotation is used, such as participation in group discussion, games or facial and hair care sessions. Care should be taken to work within the patient's fatigue tolerance.

Method: Elbow support sitting (Fig. 5.11)

To encourage neck extension the patient is encouraged to lean forward, supporting both forearms on pillows or wedges. Additional support may be required under the knees when in bed as the position is more comfortable with the legs flexed. The therapist is advised to stand on the hemiplegic side so that assistance may be given, if necessary, to maintain symmetry and ensure safety. Activity similar to the examples given for support sitting is appropriate.

Therapeutic rationale

- May be used as an alternative to prone lying when age or joint stiffness make it an unsuitable position for individual patients.
- Reduces effort by restricting use of other body parts.
- Encourages early symmetry and balance as head control is a necessary preliminary to normal equilibrium.

- Encourages scanning and awareness of the immediate environment, which may be carried over to times apart from specific treatment—such as talking with visitors.

4. Simple functional activity sitting in bed

Once the patient is sitting up, functional activity may proceed. The task illustrated in Figure 5.12 of hair combing, demonstrates visuo-spatial and body awareness re-education, early balance retraining, and practice in a daily living activity.

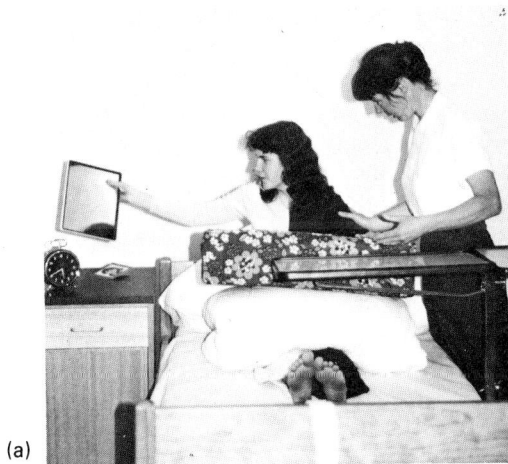

(c)

(a)

(d)

(b)

(e)

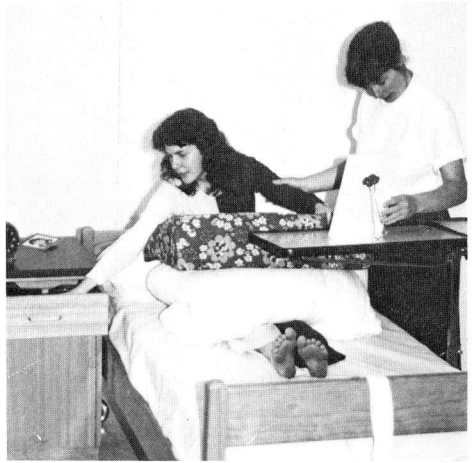

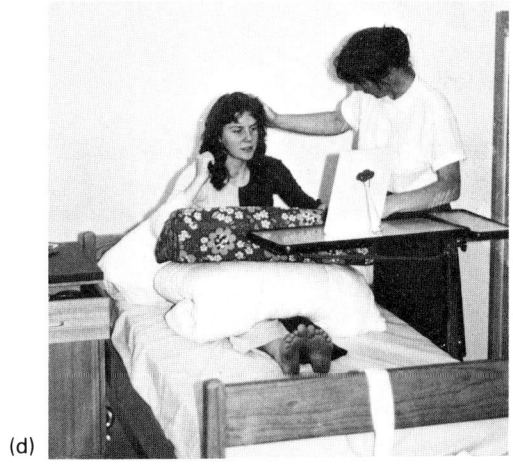

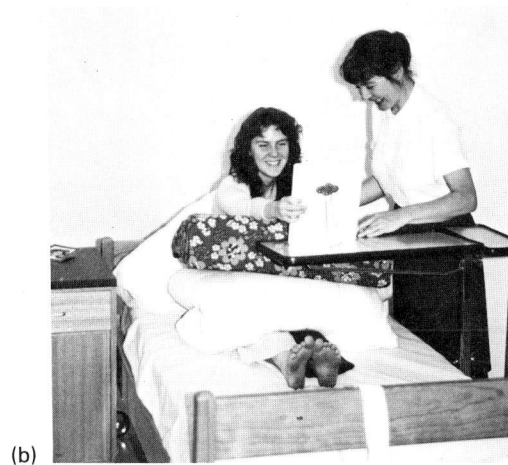

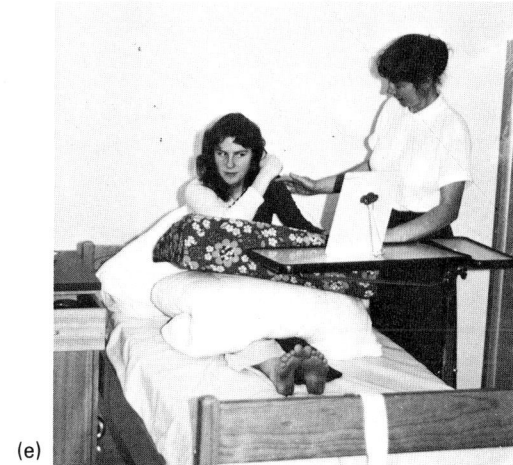

Fig. 5.12 Simple functional activity sitting in bed.

Method

From elbow support sitting which demands head control, the patient is encouraged to rotate and collect objects required for the task. The therapist prompts the activity, helps to maintain balance and the upper limb in a reflex inhibiting position, applies appropriate sensory stimulation and encourages visual scanning, whilst the patient combs her hair, looking in a mirror.

The patient is reminded verbally and tactually of the existence of the hemiplegic side of the body, and is encouraged to take care of it. Use of a mirror often gives patients a clearer picture of themselves as an intact person. Peoples' common experience of their appearance is mirror imaged, and so should not add right/left confusion.

Therapeutic rationale

The activity naturally demands:
- Head control, trunk rotation and alteration of centre of gravity at subcortical level.
- Functional 3-dimensional visuo-spatial skills of object recognition and figure ground in selection of items.
- Praxis through following instructions and manipulating the comb.

Contralateral awareness may be increased by visual, tactual and verbal input and the habitual, previously known nature of the task.

5. Activity in prone lying

Therapists following an ontogenetic sequence in treatment, and finding it appropriate to facilitate head control with activity in prone lying, may do so whilst the patient is in bed. It is a position often naturally assumed to read in bed, and is comfortable for a short while. It should only be used if within patients' physical capacity and fatigue tolerance, and acceptable to them.

Method (Fig. 5.13)

To assist the patient to assume a prone position he should first roll to the sound side and prop on the sound arm, as when sitting up in bed. Instead of moving up the bed he moves his buttocks back-

wards, after taking weight on the sound arm and leg. The therapist places a boomerang pillow between the sound trunk and arm and then assists the patient to rotate and lower the trunk onto the pillow with the sound elbow flexed and weight bearing. Both legs are placed centrally and may be supported at the ankle so that feet are dorsiflexed and knees are slightly flexed.

The patient may be encouraged to read, watch television, or participate in a brief activity, previously organised and positioned to facilitate neck extension and dynamic weight bearing on the hemiplegic arm, as pages are turned, or controls adjusted. Therapists should remain with the patient to ensure joint alignment. As this position can be fatiguing it should be assumed for only short periods, perhaps several times each day. Assuming a prone-lying position encourages mobility, control of balance, awareness of bilaterality, and provides proprioceptive input. Prone lying may be inappropriate for some patients due to other disorder, such as a cardiac or arthritic malfunction.

Both reading and television viewing may be extremely important activities to consider, as they may be a significant aspect of patients' lives, providing companionship or social comment when these are limited from other sources. The ability to continue with these pursuits may have been jeopardized by the stroke, particularly if there are visual field defects, language, perceptual or cognitive impairment and decreased concentration, particularly early after onset of stroke.

Short-term treatment procedures may appropriately include use of television or books. However, programs and reading material should be chosen with care, as patients may be distressed if unable to follow or appreciate personal favourites.

Selection criteria includes the length being in the patients' attention span, appealing yet simple content, and the structure enabling therapists to prompt and cue appropriately. Material may be graded in complexity as improvement occurs.

Therapeutic rationale

- Prone lying is an early stage of the developmental sequence when head control is practised prior to more complex balance skills. Rotation

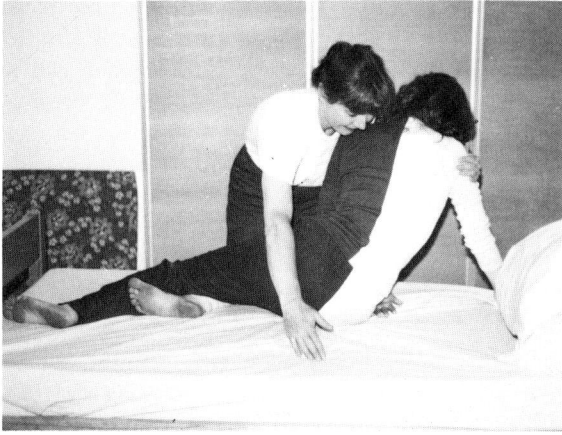

(a)

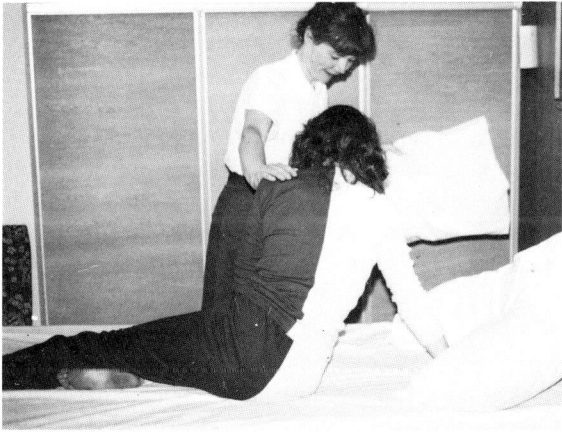

(b)

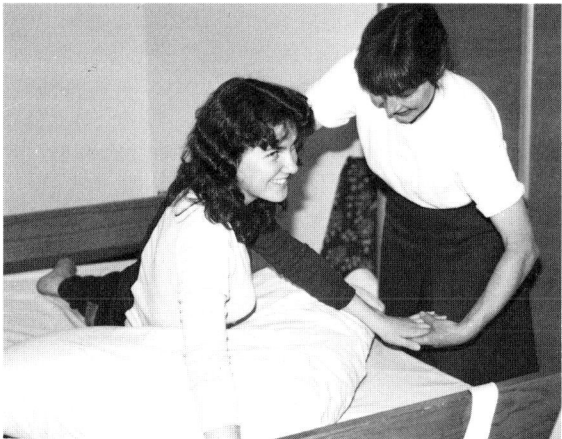

(c)

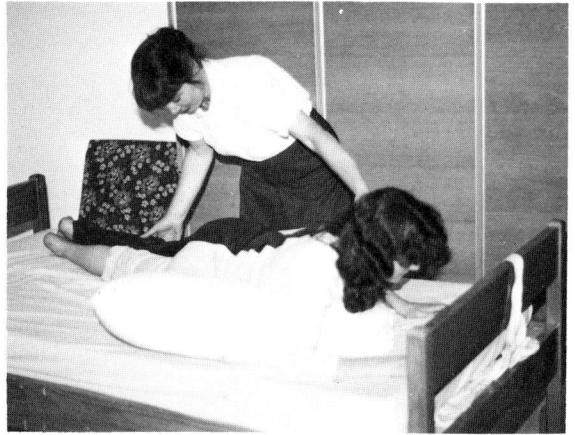

(d)

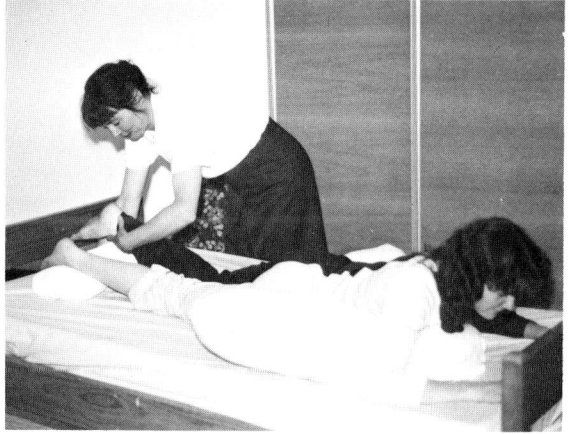

(e)

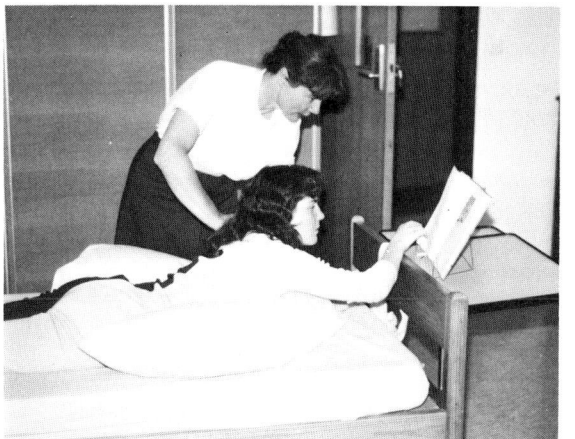

(f)

Fig. 5.13 Assisting the patient to move in bed from supine to prone lying for simple activity.

and mobility are encouraged as the patient moves from lying or sitting into a prone position.

- Weight bearing on the hemiplegic arm provides proprioceptive input.
- Use of television and reading, especially if they are activities followed in the patients' everyday life, may provide relaxation from the stress of the present. Although as therapeutic activities they make only limited physical demands, this may be useful, especially early in treatment, when fatigue is a factor to be considered. They can be selected and graded for visuo-spatial, auditory and verbal input, as well as timing of attention and memory, and may prove valuable tools in assessment, and as a ward activity.

6. Dressing in bed

General considerations

Clothes are an external expression of self, chosen because the colour, texture or style is appealing to the individual, who feels comfortable and appropriate wearing them. Even the most stunning garment may be discarded after one wearing if the wearer does not feel comfortable or appropriate to the social situation. It is therefore important to have patients choose what they wish to wear. The garments they choose may reinforce their self-image and give them confidence to tackle the rehabilitation program.

Clothes have cultural and climatic significance, so an understanding of garments worn by patients in their normal environment should be sought as soon as possible. To teach patients dressing skills unknown to, and of no significance to them, is likely to confuse them and complicate rehabilitation unnecessarily.

There is usually only limited storage space available in treatment agencies, so the number of garments a patient may have is limited. This implies that the occupational therapist should, within the patient's choice and, probably, in consultation with the relatives, advise on what may be appropriate for retraining purposes, at different stages of treatment. For example, knit garments which stretch and give are easier to put on when movement is limited, and yet are not loose and do not conceal body shape, a consideration when regular reference to body parts may be a component of treatment. Similarly it may be wise to suggest slacks rather than skirts to ladies with contralateral neglect (Hewson, 1982), so that they may see their legs individually, and experience cutaneous sensory stimulation to the limb each time they dress or undress. Early concerns are likely to be flaccid hemiplegia, proprioceptive and tactile sensory loss, impaired postural sense, disturbed body and spatial awareness, and impaired communication skills. Dressing may be used as a treatment for these disorders, particularly useful early after onset of stroke, because it relates intimately with body parts, and may be used to supply sensory input, body and limb movement, yet be seen as a useful and necessary activity. Activity to promote body awareness is essential to sensory motor retraining.

As patients are encouraged to sit out of bed as soon as their medical condition has stabilized, it is much more comfortable for them to do so wearing day clothes. To be able to dress independently gives an enormous psychological boost, and practice towards this goal may be commenced whilst pursuing other treatment objectives. In the early stages of treatment if perceptual-motor disorders interfere with dressing, attempts should be made to overcome difficulties by breaking the activity into small components, utilizing intact hemisphere skills, and gradually increasing emphasis on difficult parts of the task. Organisation of clothing and procedures are important, plus repetition of input to reinforce learning and rebuild memory traces.

Compensatory methods of dressing may be considered later when residual deficits are more clearly defined. Other considerations may include whether the dressing method of choice is for a garment put on over the head or front fastening, or whether the patient is capable of understanding and learning more than one procedure. Suitability for physical therapy activities is another consideration, and discussion of what the patient may be doing in treatment may affect their selection of clothes.

Method 1: (overhead garment)

The garment chosen for demonstration is a simple, sleeveless slip (Fig. 5.14). Patients should select what they wish to wear, and the item of clothing should be presented to the sound side, with concise instruction and/or demonstration of how to proceed. Visual clues to assist manipulation of the garment should be pointed out. The slip is placed, front down, on the patient's legs and the therapist instructs the patient to gather up the back towards the arm hole on the opposite side. Meanwhile the hemiplegic arm is extended in a reflex inhibiting pattern, and approximation is applied between the shoulder and hand, held in a hand-shake hold.

The therapist assists the hand into the armhole, instructing the patient to think about the movement and to keep looking at the hemiplegic hand and arm. The hand is released as the patient passes the armhole over it, and held again as the garment is slid up to the shoulder. The hemiplegic arm is maintained in extension and controlled by the therapist assisting in the maintenance of balance as the patient puts the slip over the head and inserts the sound arm into the second armhole. The garment is straightened, with attention directed particularly to the shoulder of the hemiplegic side. A full length mirror should be placed to the sound side and the patient is directed to adjust the garment as they look in the mirror. At this stage in treatment it is important for patients to see their total body, and a mirror so placed will enable those with visual field deficits to appreciate a whole image, although not all patients will be able, or want, to make use of a mirror. The patient is assisted to transfer weight to the hemiplegic side, lifting the sound side slightly so that the slip may be pulled down, with the therapist either supporting the patient by a hand on the sound hip, with the hemiplegic arm maintained in a reflex inhibiting position, the therapist's body or leg controlling the elbow movement, or by placing the patient's hemiplegic hand on the bed and supporting the elbow as weight is borne through the limb. The therapist's other arm may provide pressure against the trunk to maintain balance. It may help for the sound leg to be placed under the

hemiplegic leg, helping to raise it slightly. The slip may then be pulled down over the sound leg. The patient is supported as weight is transferred to the sound buttock, and the slip is pulled down straight.

Method 2: (overleg garment) (Fig. 5.15)

The trousers are placed on the patient's legs, front upwards with the top nearest the patient's trunk. Whilst the therapist supports the patient's hemiplegic side, and arm and hand in extension, the patient gathers up, with the sound hand, the opposite trouser leg, from the top. The therapist encourages the patient to lean forward and place the gathered leg over the hemiplegic foot, which is supported by the sound leg.

The patient takes weight through the sound buttock, and pulls the pants well up over the buttock affected. The therapist maintains the arm and hand in extension, and supports the patient as weight is transferred to the hemiplegic side. The patient then inserts the sound foot into the remaining leg of the pants and pulls them up to the waist.

Therapeutic rationale

- Proprioceptive stimulation applied through manual approximation and weight bearing increases co-contraction and stability of weight bearing joints, and awareness of the hemiplegic limb.
- Cutaneous stimulation through manual contact, touch, texture, and manipulation of the garment increases awareness and helps integrate a total body concept.
- Practice in spatial manipulation through handling the garment and following instructions promotes visuo-spatial skills and eye hand co-ordination.
- Simple, controlled, practice in balance, head control, pelvic control and weight bearing, is promoted during purposeful activity. Effort is reduced by appropriate support from the therapist.
- Self-esteem may be enhanced through achievement of a necessary self-care task, seen as an understandable step towards recovery.

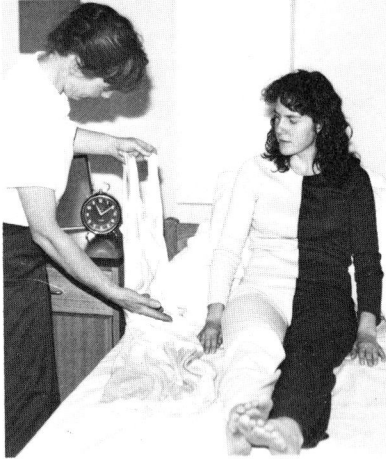

(a)

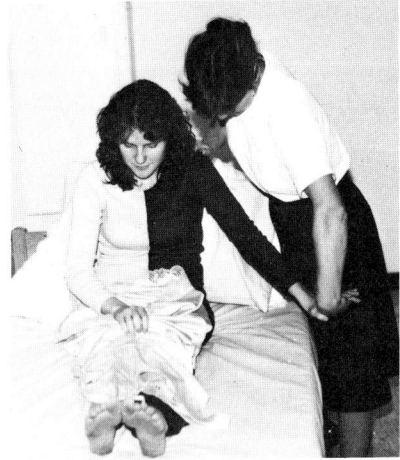

(b)

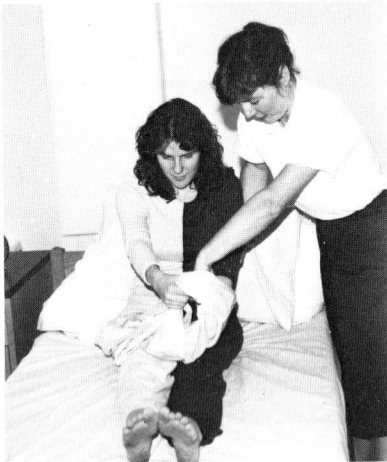

(c)

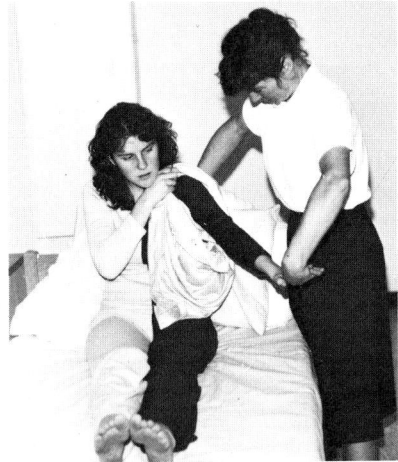

(d)

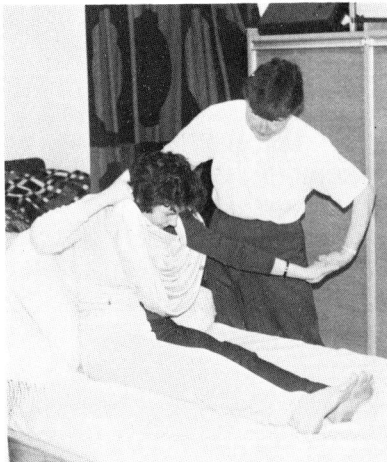

(e)

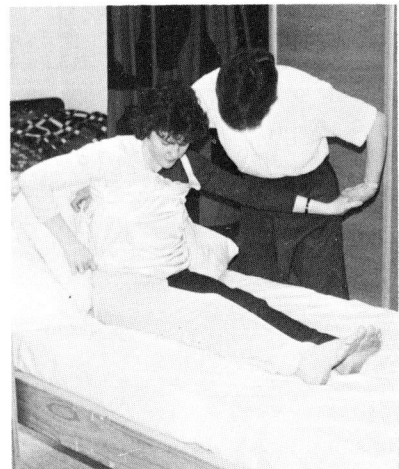

(f)

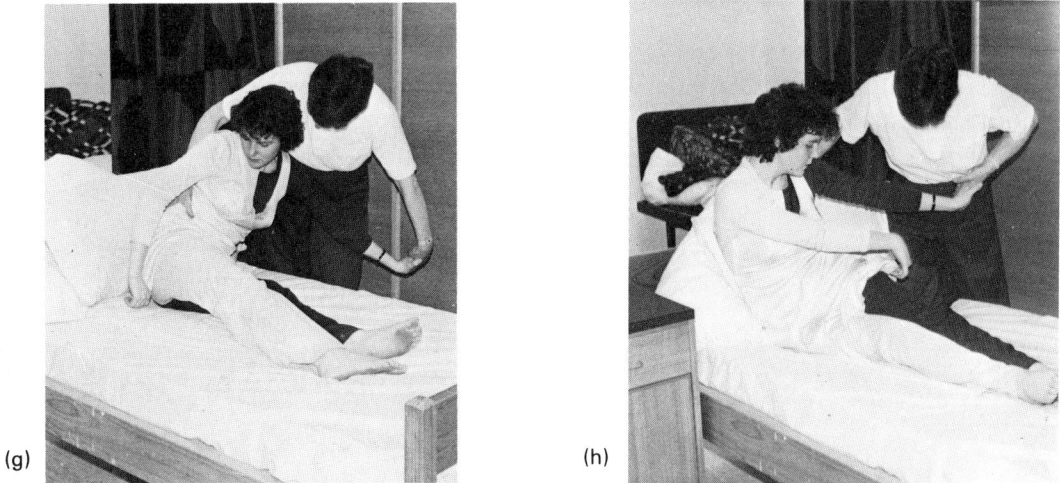

(g)   (h)

Fig. 5.14 Putting on a simple overhead garment whilst in bed. (a) Presented to the sound side initially. (b) Garment, face down, is gathered by sound hand, hemiplegic upper limb in R.I.P. (c) Hemiplegic arm assisted through armhole. (d) Garment is slid up to the shoulder. (e) Patient puts garment over head. (f) Patient puts sound arm through armhole and straightens the garment. (g) Assisted to transfer weight to hemiplegic side so that garment may be pulled down over sound buttock. (h) Weight transferred to sound side so that garment is pulled down over hemiplegic side.

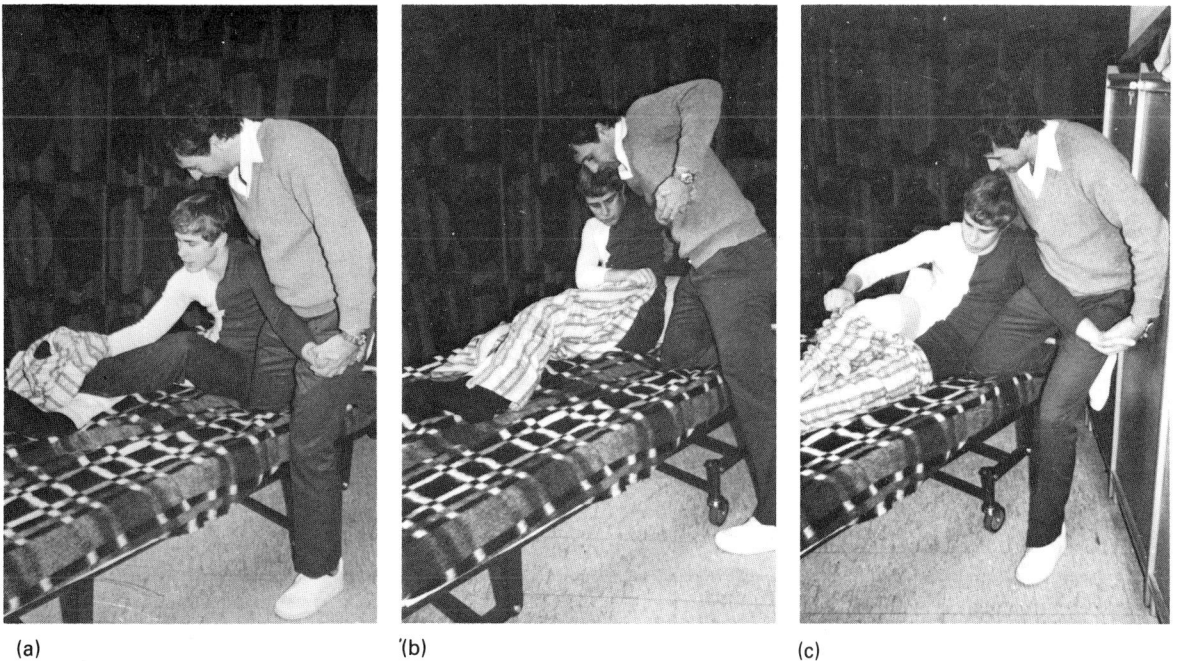

(a)   '(b)   (c)

Fig. 5.15 Putting on an overleg garment whilst in bed. (a) Patient leans forward and places garment over hemiplegic foot, therapist supporting balance and reflex inhibiting postures. (b) Assisted hip hitching to sound side. (c) Assisted hip hitching to hemiplegic side.

7. Bridging

Bridging is normally used to adjust clothing or position when in bed. It is a useful exercise for stroke patients as it may enable them to move up or down the bed symmetrically, pull clothes over buttocks if night wear is uncomfortable or if dressing in bed, lift hips when nursing staff are positioning a bed pan, or reduce undesirable pressure on prominences when lying supine. It also encourages patient awareness and control of the pelvic girdle.

Method

The patient lies supine with both arms extended symmetrically on the bed, and is asked, assisted if necessary, to flex both legs, bringing knees together, facing upwards or slightly to the sound side. The patient is then asked to lift both hips off the bed, and hold the position for a few moments. If assistance is required, the therapist, on the hemiplegic side, helps support the knees in a flexed position and the upward movement of the hemiplegic hip as the patient voluntarily tries to lift both (Fig. 5.16). Two people may be necessary, one on each side, for heavy patients with a poor understanding of what is required (Johnstone, 1978).

Therapeutic rationale

Use of trunk and proximal musculature in early retraining follows developmental principles and the usual pattern of recovery.

It may be seen as an early procedure towards the re-establishment of pelvic control, which is essential for the development of normal walking patterns. It encourages awareness of the hemiplegic side of the body.

MOVING TO SIT ON THE SIDE OF THE BED

Method 1

The easiest and safest method for the patient to move from sitting up in bed to sitting on the side, is to take weight through the sound arm and hand, support and lift the hemiplegic leg with the sound leg, and swing both over the edge of the bed. The therapist assists balance and initially the swing of the legs, from a central position, ready to move to the hemiplegic side as soon as the legs complete the movement (Fig. 5.17). With very little practice the activity may be completed with minimal effort (Carr & Shepherd, 1982) and, being a relatively safe procedure with the weight on the sound side, will reduce risk of tension causing unwanted,

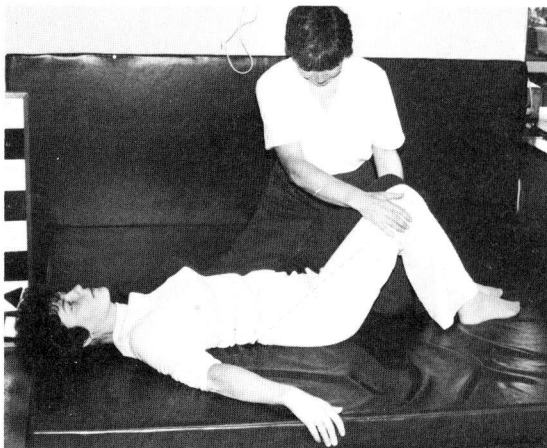
(a)

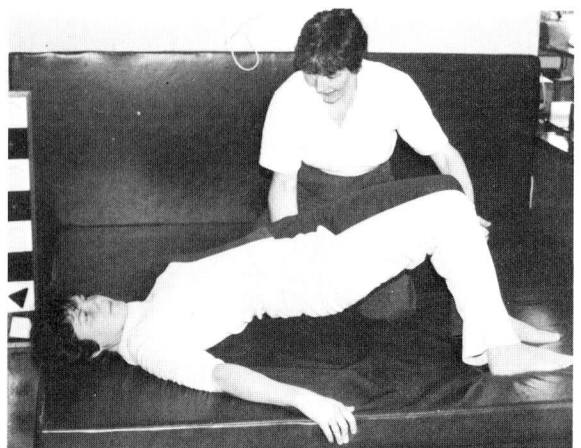
(b)

Fig. 5.16 Assisted bridging — shown on a plinth, but may be carried out whilst patient is in bed, the therapist standing on the hemiplegic side.

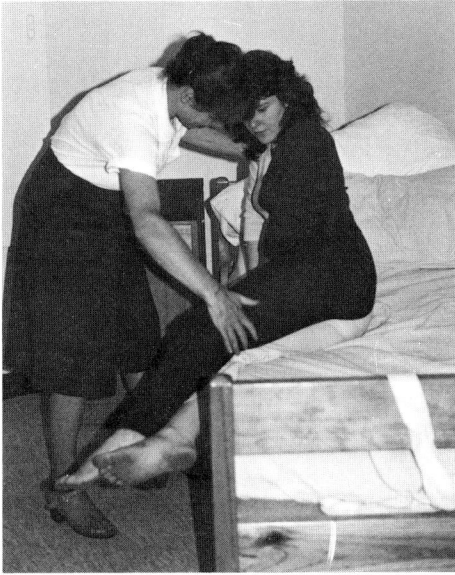

Fig. 5.17 Assisting the patient to swing legs out of bed taking weight through the sound side.

abnormal movement of the hemiplegic side. Once seated on the edge of the bed the therapist may encourage symmetrical sitting.

Method 2

Some therapists believe that this activity with all others should concentrate on use of the hemiplegic side, minimising any activity of the sound side. This procedure makes it initially harder for the patient to achieve (Bobath, 1978), is less safe and should be taught sequentially step by step so that the patient feels secure at each stage (Johnstone, 1978) before progressing to the next.

The procedure is very similar to that already described, except the patient rolls to the hemiplegic side rather than the sound side, is assisted to take weight through the hemiplegic arm, pushes up with assistance into sitting, and swings the legs out of bed (Fig. 5.18). Hands may be clasped during all or part of the procedure, unless the sound arm is needed to facilitate the upward movement of the trunk (Bobath, 1978).

Clasping hands, as demonstrated in Figure 5.19, is considered useful for several reasons. It helps to maintain the patient's awareness of the affected side, and as the hemiplegic side will move with the

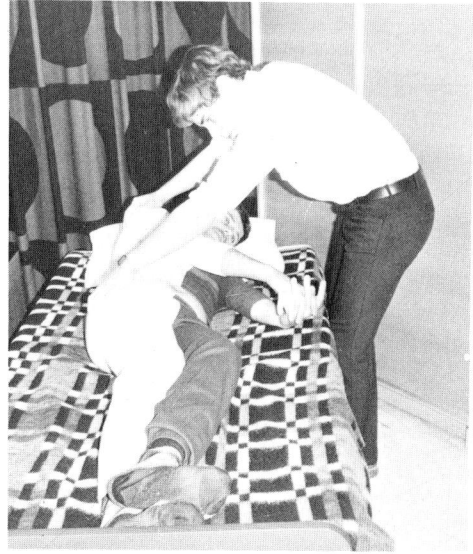

(a)

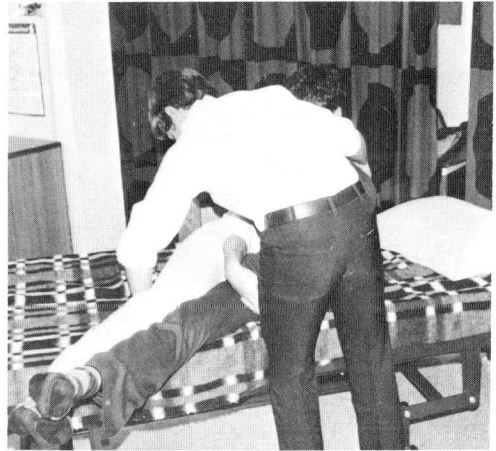

(b)

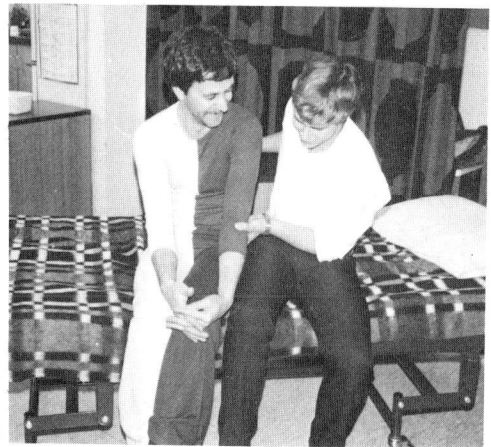

(c)

Fig. 5.18 Assisting the patient to sit on the side of the bed taking weight through the hemiplegic side.

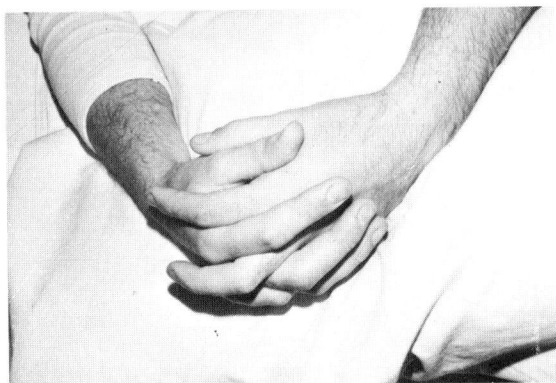

Fig. 5.19 Clasped hands recommended to encourage extension and abduction of fingers and thumb to inhibit flexor spasticity.

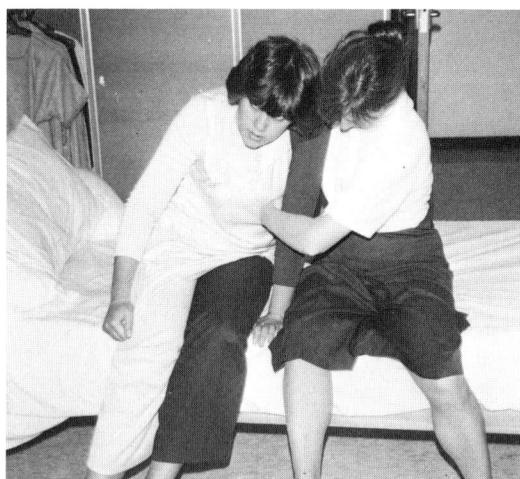

(a)

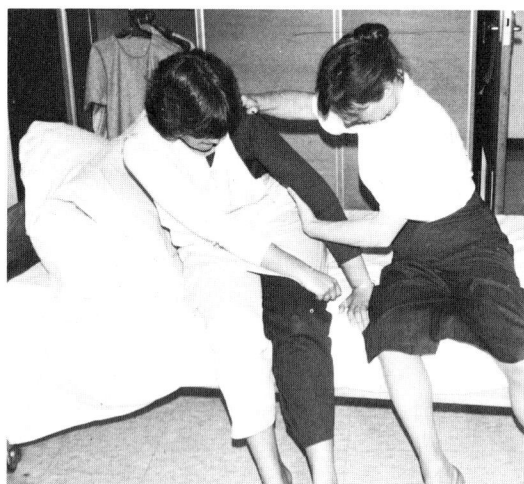

(b)

Fig. 5.20 Clothing adjustment sitting on the side of the bed. (a) Hip hitching to the hemiplegic side. (b) Hip hitching to the sound side.

sound one, gives some kinesthetic sensory input. It may be useful in reducing upper limb flexor spasticity, encouraging abduction of the fingers and thumb, and helping to supinate the forearm (Bobath, 1978). It may be appropriate to suggest the patient clasps hands when resting between tasks, or to adapt tasks to include this action. When hands held in this way prevent the normal execution of activity, it should be discouraged.

1. Dressing

Practice moving to sit on the side of the bed may be incorporated into dressing retraining; for example, clothing adjustment over the buttocks taking place on the side of the bed as an alternative to on the bed.

Method

The patient rocks to the hemiplegic side to pull the garment down on the sound side, with the therapist providing support to the trunk and weight-bearing arm and using shoulder pressure to maintain the patient's affected shoulder in a forward position. The therapist then supports the patient, maintaining upper limb extension as weight is taken on the sound side, allowing the garment to be pulled down over the hemiplegic leg (Fig. 5.20).

The task may alternatively incorporate standing to facilitate garment adjustment. The therapist provides support from the hemiplegic side, maintaining the arm in a reflex inhibiting pattern with

shoulder pressure and hand shake grasp, stabilising the knee and inhibiting forward foot movement if necessary, as in Figure 5.21. The therapist's other hand is placed on the patient's sound hip.

This position provides absolute safety for the patient, as the hemiplegic side, if necessary, can be totally supported by the therapist who is able to control weight bearing and symmetry in even very heavy and dysfunctional patients. Rotation can also be safely demanded and assisted, and normal sequence and timing of movement are not

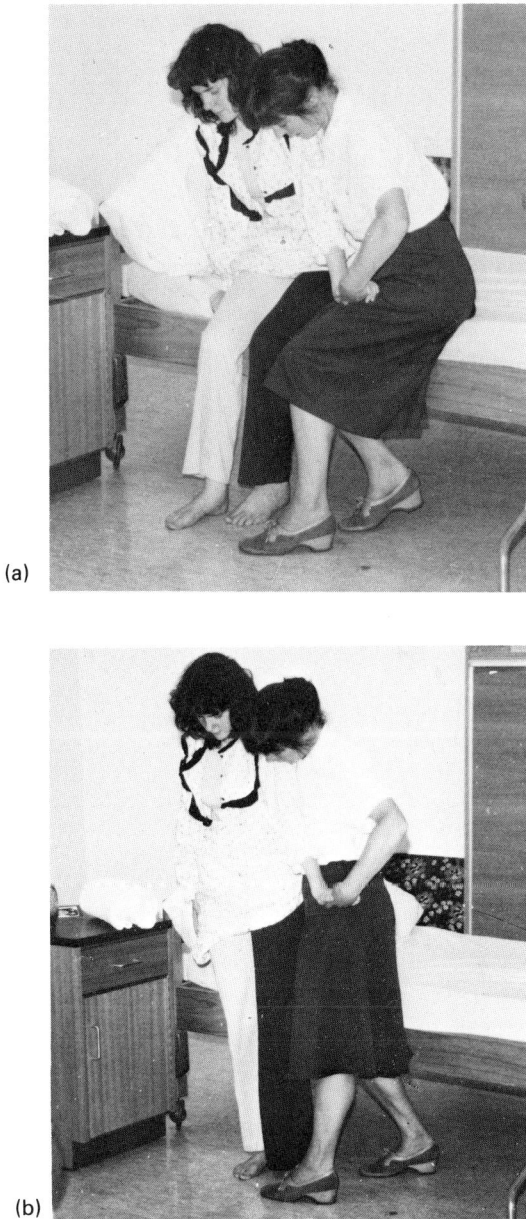

(a)

(b)

Fig. 5.21 Assisted standing from the side of the bed to adjust clothing.

2. Mass movement patterning and dressing

When sitting on the side of the bed it is possible to include mass movement patterning in dressing activities. The spiral diagonal upper limb D2 pattern (Knott & Voss, 1968; Trombly, 1983) may be used in putting on a T-shirt.

Method

The therapist initially guides the movement, and attempts to facilitate some voluntary muscle activity by manual contact, verbal command, and quick light stretch at the point of direction change. The patient watches the movement as the therapist moves or assists the limb several times in the pattern before it is used in donning the garment. The extended arm is pronated from a supinated position, down and in, and supinated from pronation, outward and up, as illustrated in Figure 5.22. The grip shown in close up in Figure 5.23a is an alternative to those used in texts describing P.N.F. movements, and is useful when the therapist wishes to control or assist movement from the extensor surface, whilst encouraging the fingers to maintain extension and abduction.

The garment may be put on in the sequence demonstrated in Figure 5.23, initially arm, then head, followed by the sound arm, or, as in Figure 5.24, both hands put into the sleeves first, then the garment is slid to the shoulder of the hemiplegic arm and put over the head, before the sound arm pushes through the sleeve to complete the activity.

Therapeutic rationale

Various sensory modalities are inherent in this technique, which may stimulate awareness of a neglected side and some muscle activity. The sensory modalities are tactile, visual, verbal and kinesthetic. These are co-ordinated in an integrated procedure to stimulate voluntary movement by the repetitive rhythmic activity and the application of quick light stretch as described.

Those with poor verbal skills may also find the rhythm and repetition conducive to learning. Any unwanted, abnormal synergic action can be felt and inhibited by the therapist, who remains in constant touch with the hemiplegic arm, and demands the prescribed movement.

inhibited by the therapist's body in front of the patient, nor is the patient's view of the world or a mirror obstructed. The therapist does not intrude into the patient's 'personal' space, allowing them to feel more comfortable, and less dependent. Verbal and manual input are maximized on the hemiplegic side.

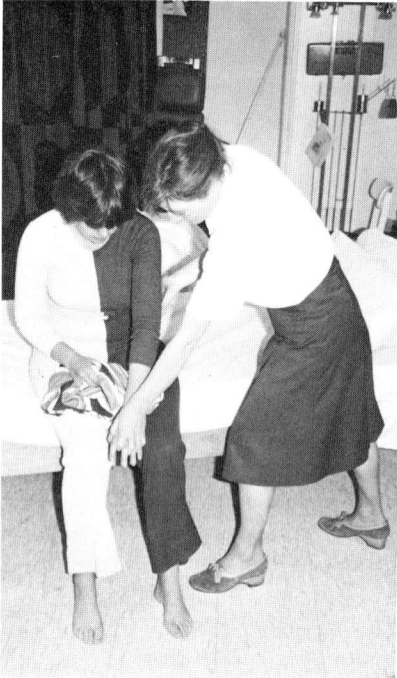
(a)

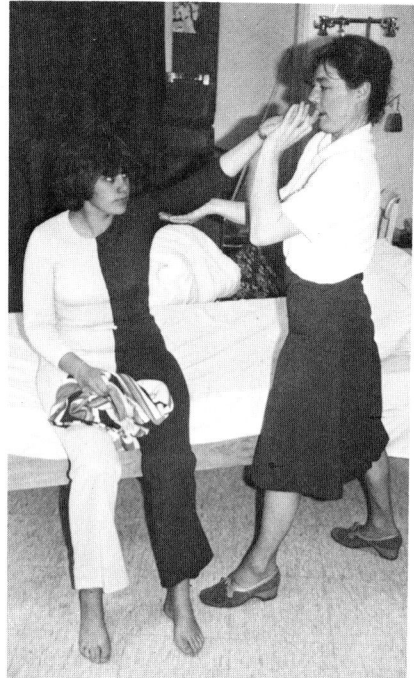
(b)

Fig. 5.22 P.N.F. upper limb pattern 'Diagonal 2' used prior to dressing. (a) Guiding the movement from 'down and in' to (b) 'Up and out', with the patient directed to watch the movement, garment ready to put on.

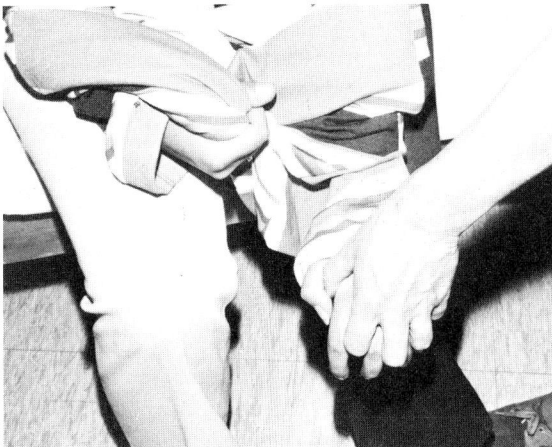
(a)

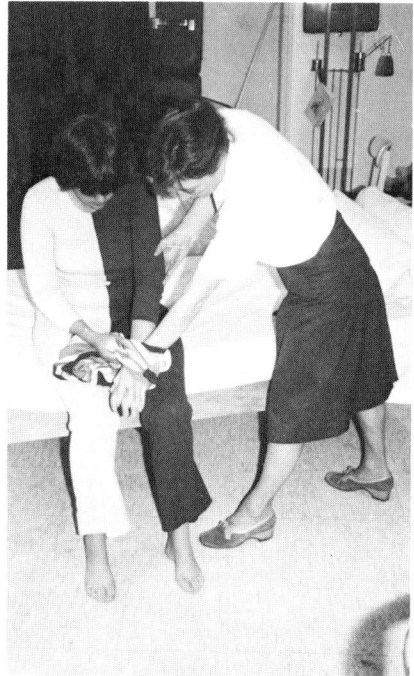
(b)

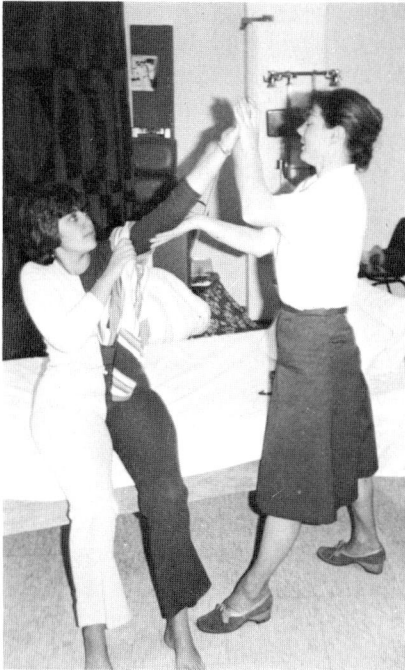

(c)

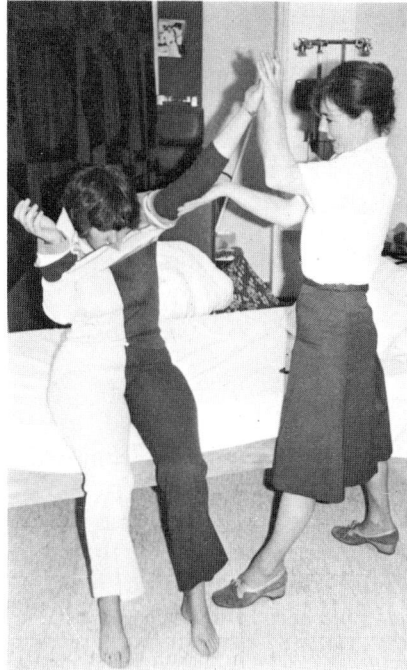

(d)

Fig. 5.23 P.N.F. upper limb pattern 'Diagonal 2' used in dressing. (a) Alternative abductor grip. (b) 'Down and in' movement guides movement through garment arm hole. (c) 'Up and out' movement, garment is slid to the shoulder. (d) Therapist maintains extended hemiplegic upper limb whilst the patient puts the garment overhead and sound arm.

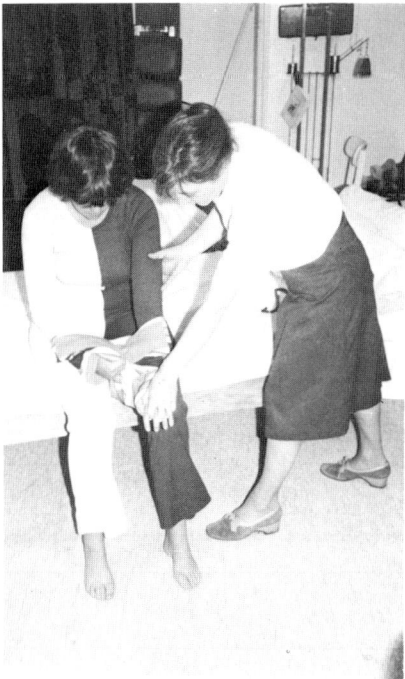

(a)

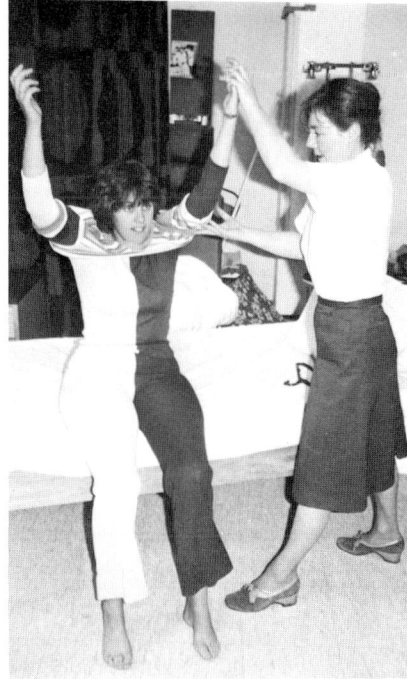

(b)

Fig. 5.24 Using Bilateral P.N.F. Diagonal 2 pattern to dress. (a) 'Down and in' both hands through garment armholes. (b) 'Up and out' as garment is slid up arms and placed over head with the sound hand.

BED TO CHAIR

There are various techniques of transfer advocated. Two of them will be described. Both carry over learning from early bed mobility training, which will decrease confusion and assist the patient to learn. Repetition builds up memory traces (Hebb, 1961), so that utilizing the same patterns of movement in different tasks facilitates learning.

Method 1 (Fig. 5.26)

The therapist assists from the hemiplegic side to control balance, decrease the patient's fear of falling to that side and to maximise tactile, proprioceptive and verbal stimulation. Normal sequence and timing of movement with the head leading, is made easier because vision and movement are not inhibited by the therapist's body.

Before standing, the feet are positioned flat on the floor, and the therapist may apply some approximation through the hemiplegic knee whilst explaining to the patient the procedure about to be followed (Fig. 5.25). The proprioceptive input provided by the approximation may promote increased patient control of the foot.

The feet may then need to be moved slightly under the patient so that the knees are flexed at about 70°. Symmetrical movement is facilitated by the patient pushing up on the sound arm and hand, and the therapist giving support to the hemiplegic limb held in a reflex-inhibiting position.

In the initial trials, weight may be encouraged toward the sound side during upward movement as the patient may feel safer and more in control. Symmetry is resumed in standing when postural adjustment is less complex. Being able to move from an asymmetrical to a symmetrical position is a necessary skill, which should be included rather than avoided in therapeutic situations.

When an upright position is achieved the patient should be encouraged to relax, lift the head, which will encourage lower limb and trunk extension, and gently transfer weight from side to side.

A chair is positioned in front of the patient rather than to the side. This tends to slow down the procedure, making the steps more deliberate, so that practice of controlled movement is emphasised—this is especially useful when judgment of timing is disordered. Forward transfer is also often a necessary basic skill transfer on to a toilet.

The patient is instructed to lean forward and place the sound hand on the arm of the chair facing, whilst the therapist continues to control balance and safety between the hand on the sound hip and body support of the hemiplegic side. The patient is then instructed to turn both feet towards the therapist, transfer the hand to the other chair arm, and move both feet until facing the bed. The patient may then be encouraged once more to stand straight, with head up, before gently lowering into the chair.

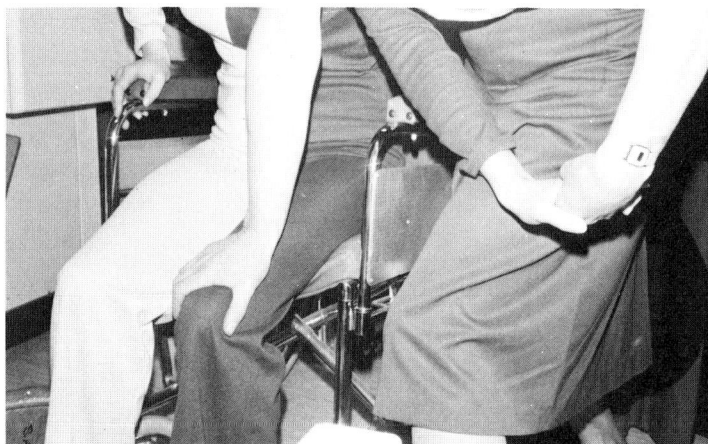

Fig. 5.25 Approximation applied through the knee before asking the patient to stand.

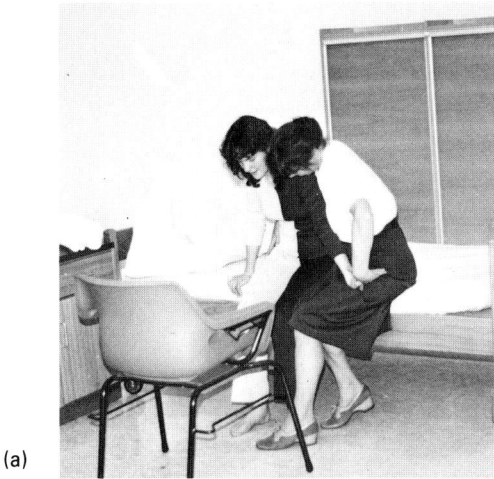

(a)

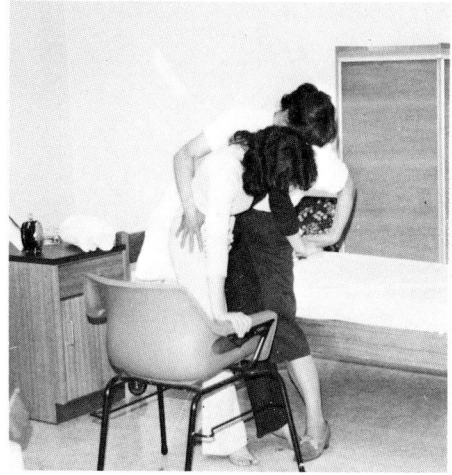

(b)

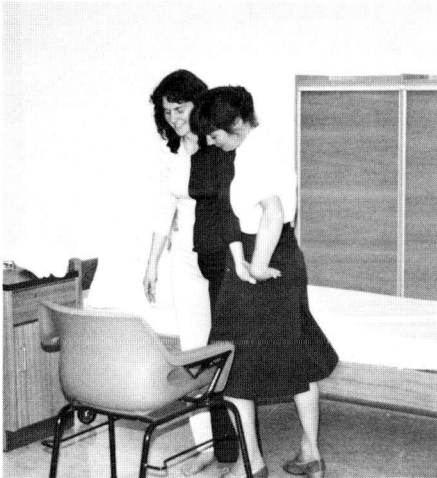

(c)

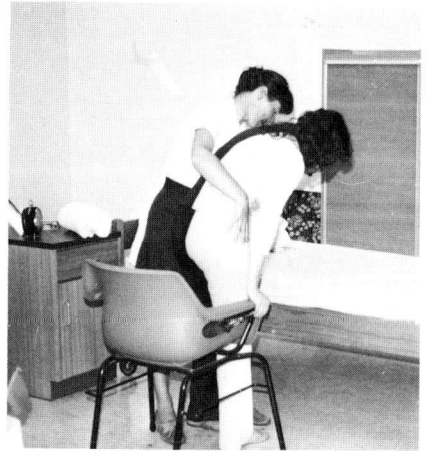

(d)

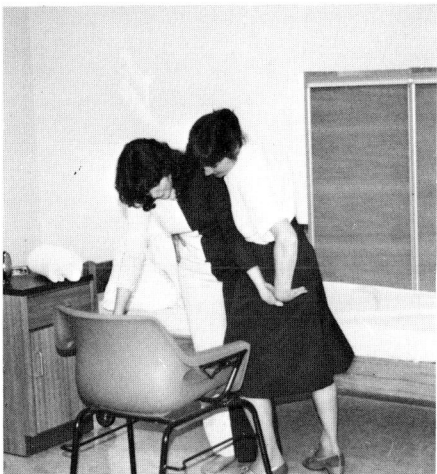

(e)

Fig. 5.26 Bed to chair transfer, method 1. (a) The therapist assists from hemiplegic side, upper limb held in R.I.P. (b) Symmetrical standing, weight transference encouraged. (c) The patient places hand on chair arm facing. (d) The patient turns feet, and places hand on other chair arm. (e) The patient turns back to chair, lowers slowly to sitting.

The type of chair used is important. It must be of standard height to allow feet to be placed firmly on the floor, have good back and arm supports and be stable when weight is placed through one arm. The chair shown in Figure 5.26 was specially designed for geriatric use and includes these features, despite its somewhat fragile, modern appearance.

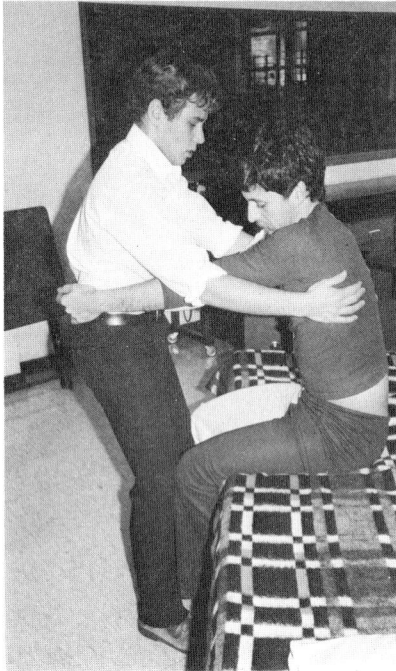

(a)

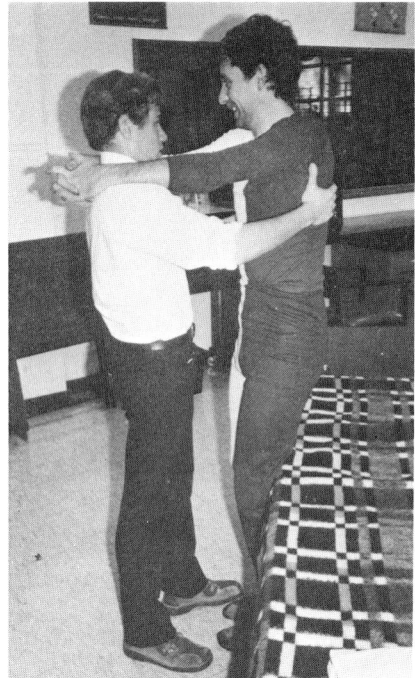

(b)

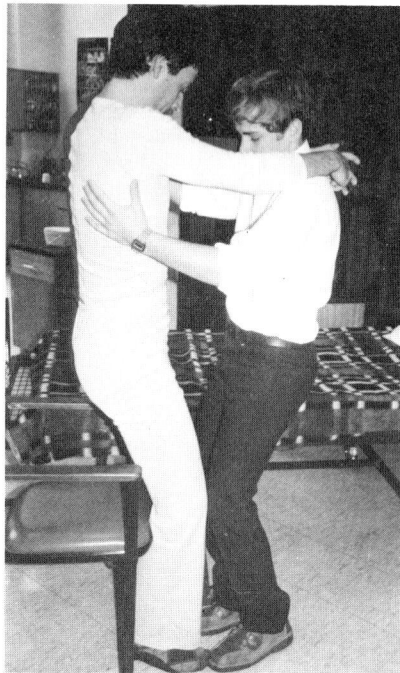

(c)

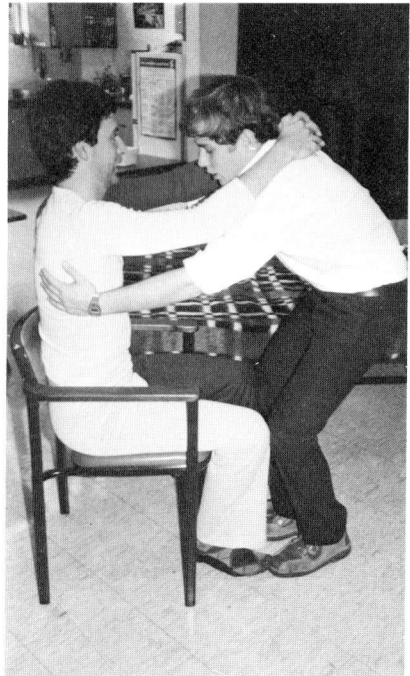

(d)

Fig. 5.27 Bed to chair transfer, method 2. (a) The therapist assists from the front of the patient supporting scapula, upper limb and maintaining symmetry. (b) The patient is instructed to lean forward and stand. (c) The patient turns 90 so back is to chair. (d) The therapist assists gentle lowering to sitting in chair.

This method is recommended for patients who are scheduled for rapid discharge to long-term institutions. Emphasis on taking weight on the sound side for safety, will enable them to be as independent as possible in their transfers, despite limited potential (McIntyre & Mort, 1973). The possibility of damage to unstable joints is reduced, as are feelings of uselessness which patients may experience if they are unable to assist in their own mobility. Treatment for these patients should include constant practice and repetition of simple bed, transfer, and personal care tasks.

Method 2 (Fig. 5.27)

The therapist stands in front of the patient, bends at the knees, instructs and assists the patient to move to the edge of the bed and lean forward and put the sound arm either over the therapist's shoulder or around the trunk. The hemiplegic arm is guided from the shoulder to mirror the movement of the sound limb, and supported to maintain the position. As the therapist straightens up the patient is instructed to lean forward at the hips and stand. When upright the patient may clasp hands behind the therapist's neck. The patient should be assisted to move both feet around 90° so the back of both knees touch the seat of the chair, and instructed to slowly lower into it (Bobath, 1978). A front approach is felt to encourage symmetry.

SITTING IN THE WARD

1. Environmental considerations

The patient may spend many hours sitting in a chair in the ward, which suggests that considerable attention should be given to the type of chair and where it is situated, how the patient sits, and what he does whilst sitting. The chair should encourage symmetrical balanced sitting, be comfortable, safe and suitable for ease of transfer.

The environment in which the patient sits should be stimulating and interesting without overloading dysfunctional neuronal circuits, and should encourage activity and social interaction.

The patient should sit in positions which will inhibit abnormal reflex development, prevent the formation of contractures, or joint stress, encourage awareness of body and the surrounding environment, and which will enable participation in activity.

It is a good rule never to pass a stroke patient who is sitting in an undesirable position, but rather to assist him immediately to improve it. Patients may not infrequently be seen, early post-stroke, slumped in a chair, with hemiplegic limbs dangling, head flexed to the affected side and rotated to the sound side. The therapist should rescue dangling limbs, assist head centring, position legs to take weight, and assist the patient to voluntarily push up and back in the chair (Fig. 5.28). Such assistance may be necessary many times each day.

2. Social stimulation

Patients should not be left in isolation in an unstimulating environment, nor should they be left in front of a turned on television, if they are not able to watch, make sense of what they see, turn it off, or ask for it to be turned off. It has already been initimated that gradual and specific use of television may be an excellent and appropriate treatment activity.

Patients should be seated near others who are able to initiate caring communication, and positioned so that they are able to use a table for looking at a magazine or newspaper, cope with a cup of tea or a meal, or be included in a simple activity such as a game of cards. If patients are responsive to such activities, aids to decrease frustrations due to dysfunction should be supplied, such as a book or newspaper rest, a marker system to cue visual scanning or a one-handed card holder.

Occupational therapists should stimulate inter-patient activity within the ward, enhance ongoing communication, so minimizing time available to the patient for unhealthy introspection, and maximizing feelings of belonging to a community. Structured group activities may be organised within small ward units, or include a wider group from other units. Activities may include exercise or relaxation groups, social or shared adult games such as bingo, board games, the viewing of a recorded film or sporting event shown too late to

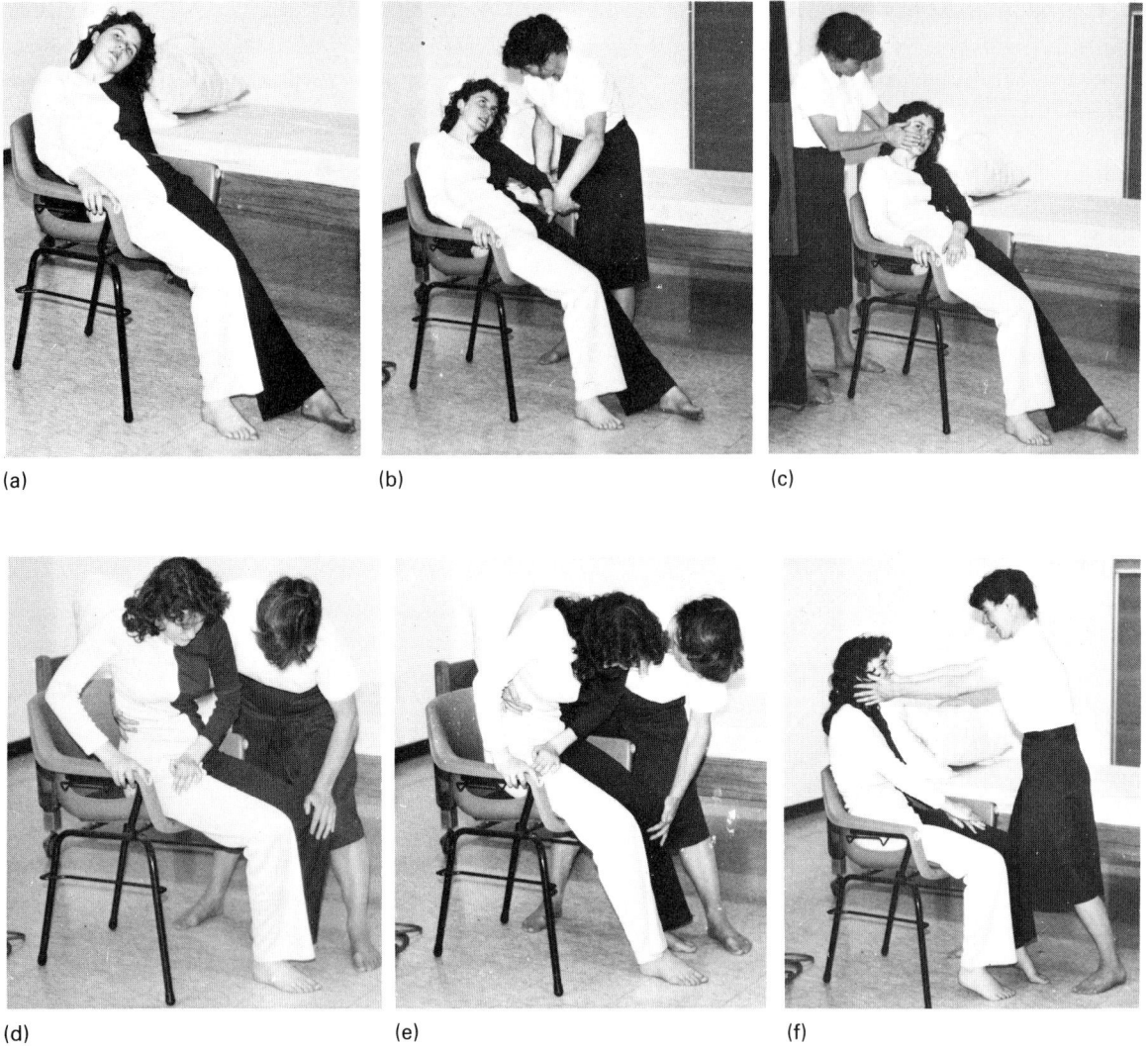

Fig. 5.28 Assisting the patient to sit up from a slumped position. (a) Typical position early post-stroke. (b) Dangling limbs are rescued. (c) Head centreing is assisted. (d) Legs are positioned close to chair. (e) Patient is assisted to lift up and back. (f) Patient is encouraged to look to hemiplegic side.

watch, or meal times which are pleasurable social occasions.

Activity is much more likely to be spread over the waking hours of the day if it includes inter-patient participation, rather than being dependent upon therapist/patient interaction. The promotion of an activity-oriented environment may be difficult and initially time demanding, but once facilitated may continue spontaneously and effectively, with only minimal time being needed to stimulate interaction and shared activity.

3. Dressing sitting in a chair

Techniques similar to those described for dressing in and on the side of the bed may be used, incorporating neurophysiological and neuropsychological aspects of specific treatment.

The amount of contact the patient needs will vary from support for the maintenance of balance and reflex-inhibiting patterns of movement, to verbal reminders of awareness of limbs and procedures.

Prior to dressing practice, facilitatory techniques may be used to maximize awareness, balance, movement and selective attention. These may include cutaneous stimulation of limbs about to be used, such as stroking or icing of the upper limb extensors, proprioceptive and kinesthetic stimulation through approximation and movement, visual and auditory stimulation by demanding visual attention to procedures used and by talking about them.

4. Eating

The cultural significance and implications of food and eating habits should be considered in treatment, for motivational reasons and to make use of previously learned skills, particularly when new learning is difficult.

Eating is best performed sitting in a chair, with food on a stable table directly in front. A symmetrical upright position facilitates swallow, and this position is easier for the patient to achieve and maintain out of bed. If, for medical reasons, patients are confined to bed they should be helped to sit up before mealtimes.

Several disorders following stroke may interfere with independent eating. These include lack of functional movement of one hand, poor balance, homonymous hemianopia, visual inattention, contralateral neglect, oro-facial weakness and loss of sensation and dysphagia.

Occupational therapists have been traditionally responsible for teaching one handed and adapted eating techniques, providing tools and equipment to facilitate the feeding process, re-educating visual awareness, and teaching methods to overcome perceptual deficits.

(a) One-handed tools and techniques of eating

- Graded selection of food so that initially it is easy to eat with one hand, establishing confidence before the patient needs to learn new techniques, such as those required for cutting meat.
- Extraneous objects moved away from the immediate site of operation so there is room for manipulation.

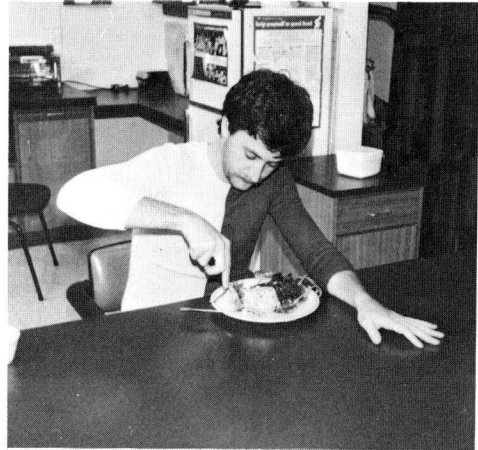

Fig. 5.29 One handed eating, using a non-slip mat, perspex plate guard and rocker knife. Hemiplegic upper limb is in a R.I.P.

- Non-slip place mats under plates, and between plate and 'hot compartment' if necessary.
- Hemiplegic arm, hand and fingers placed and maintained in a reflex-inhibiting position alongside the plate (Fig. 5.29).
- Food cut with a rocking rather than sawing action, using a special 'rocker' knife if needed (Fig. 5.29.)
- Provision of a perspex plate guard to assist with forking up the food, which is the least obtrusive and most 'adult' of aids available (Fig. 5.29).
- If any functional upper limb movement is possible it should be facilitated and utilized during eating procedures.
- Patients may prefer to eat food they can manage with one hand using 'normal' utensils.

(b) Techniques to overcome visual and perceptual disorders

Patients should be encouraged:
- To choose their own menu, ticking off selected items on provided lists.
- When the meal arrives, to name and visually locate food items chosen, to take items off the serving tray and set out on the dining table, to increase spatial awareness of position of food and items.

The therapist should:
- Supervise the meal, be aware if food is ignored on the side of the plate contralateral to the

lesion, and if this occurs either direct verbally visually or tactually scanning and head movement to locate the remaining food, or suggest the patient rotates the plate, and discovers the remaining food.

- Keep the immediate dining space uncluttered to lessen visual confusion.
- Give manual guidance, and step-by-step verbal input if apraxia prevents sequential, functional manipulation.
- Ensure regular, repetitive reinforcement to effectively increase awareness and skill, so if necessary relatives, friends and other staff may be taught the chosen procedure.
- Teach compensatory methods if patients are unable to understand remedial techniques, simplifying layout and placing items within intact visual and attention fields.

(c) Oro-facial weakness and dysphagia

In the early days following stroke, patients may experience difficulties in lip closure, voluntary tongue movement, swallowing, appreciating the presence of food in the mouth, normal chewing action, and in controlling saliva.

Social aspects of eating are of significance in most cultures, so unacceptable eating habits may cause embarrassment and acute distress to patients, relatives and friends. Help with difficulties should commence as soon as possible to alleviate psychological problems developing. Early intervention may also negate or reduce the need for nasal-gastric tube feeding in cases where drooling, aspiration and dysphagia result in a poor nutritional state (Carr & Shepherd, 1982).

The responsibility for re-education of oro-facial function tends to differ from hospital to hospital, being performed by either speech pathologists, physiotherapists or occupational therapists, according to treatment programs, schedules and individual expertise. It is immaterial who assists the patient with these problems as long as effective intervention takes place regularly, and expertise between therapists is shared for ultimate patient well-being.

Intervention techniques:
- Distraction-free environment.
- The patient should be seated in an upright symmetrical position with head slightly flexed so that the oesophagus is open, the airway is narrowed, and gravity assists peristalsis (Syms, 1982).
- The therapist's head should be, as far as possible, directly in front of the patient to prevent unwanted rotation, extension, or flexion of the head (Syms, 1982).
- Food choice graded from jelly, through thick vitaminized food, textured puréed food, fork mashed food, soft foods such as scrambled eggs and mornays, to a normal diet demanding chewing (Syms, 1982). Liquids are more difficult to swallow and easier to aspirate (Larsen, 1972; Carr & Shepherd, 1982).
- If the patient wears false teeth, the therapist should check they are in place correctly. If the patient has difficulty positioning false teeth, gum awareness can be increased by brisk rubbing (Carr & Shepherd, 1982).
- Ice, manual pressure and touch are suggested as pre-feeding facilitatory modalities, although Carr and Shepherd advise that icing may cause numbness leading to a decrease in awareness of tongue, lip position and mobility. If ice is used, fast icing may be applied to external lower cheeks and mouth area, and a flavoured ice-block on a stick may be sucked briefly to stimulate secretions.
- To facilitate swallow, the patient may need to be prompted, verbally and tactually, to close teeth and lips. This should be reinforced during treatment programs whenever the patient's mouth falls open. Closure may be facilitated by firm, but gentle, stroking around the lips, applying stretch or pressure above the lips, or sucking through a straw. When possible, patients should be taught to apply facilitatory techniques for themselves.
- When lip closure is achieved, the patient should be told to touch the roof of the mouth with the tongue, hold the food momentarily, think about swallowing and then swallow (Syms, 1982). The actual swallow may be facilitated by various interventions, including a slight pinch to the larynx (Gaffney & Campbell, 1974), upward or downward stroking of the digastric muscle, ice to the sternal notch, or turning the head sideways.

- Patients may practise dry swallow at other than mealtimes, by learning to briefly finger-press the anterior portion of the tongue downwards, or under the side of the tongue inwards and upwards before swallowing.
- After meals a check for any food residue should be made, and the patient should remain sitting up for 15 to 30 minutes, to assist digestion and prevent regurgitation.
- Individual treatment to encourage weak facial musculature is recommended, including self-care tasks of a facial/tactual nature, breathing exercises and awareness of facial expression in relaxation sessions, and short suck-puff games such as blow football. Overuse of intact musculature should be discouraged.

5. An example of an individual treatment activity

Individual treatment may be carried out within the ward, and in the early post-stroke period it is advisable to include activity which is pleasurable, promoting feelings of well-being and self-esteem, as well as facilitating body awareness and physical recovery. A self-care activity to meet these objectives, and suitable for women, is shown in Figure 5.30. Similar gains for male patients may be achieved by shaving.

Method

The patient is seated in front of a mirror, close to a table, with the hemiplegic upper limb positioned

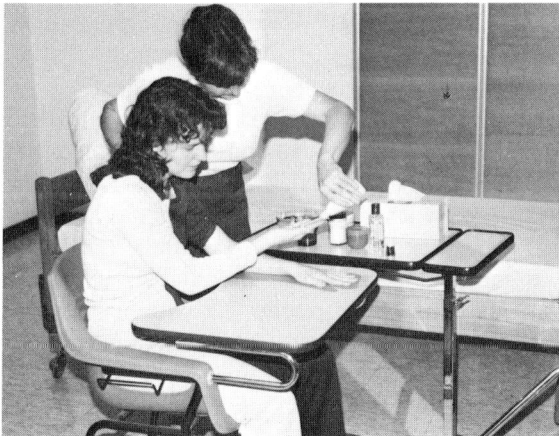
(a)

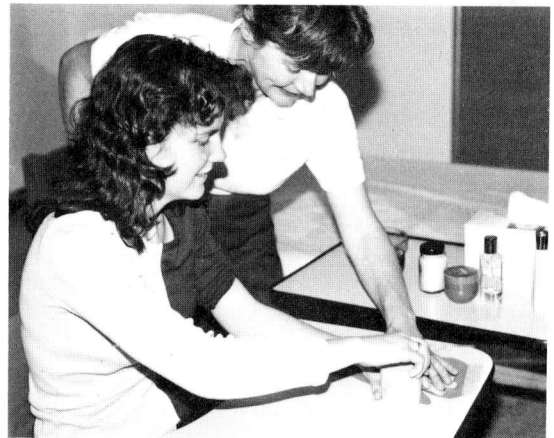
(b)

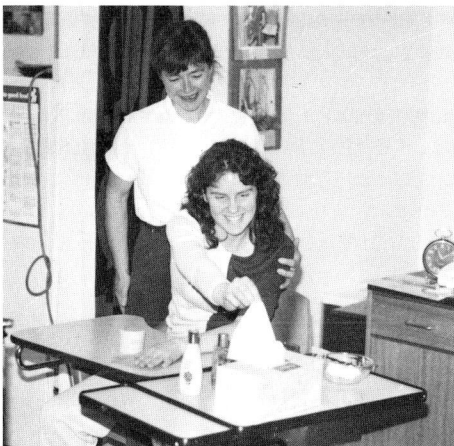
(c)

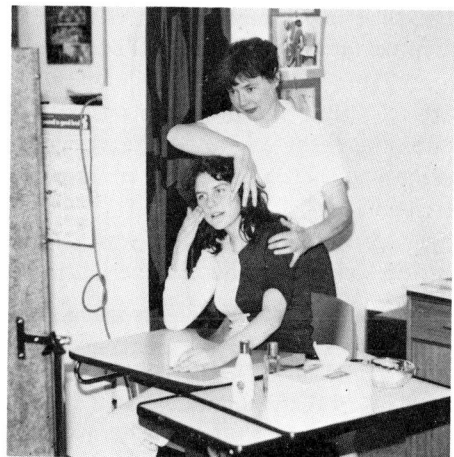
(d)

Fig. 5.30 An example of an individual treatment activity. (a) About to apply cream to extensors of hemiplegic arm and hand. (b) Using web space to stabilize jar to open the lid. (c) Crossing the midline to reach requirements. (d) Therapist makes sure cutaneous stimulation is applied to the hemiplegic side.

in a reflex-inhibiting pattern, shoulder protracted, and fingers extended. A coloured paper cut-out of a hand and arm taped to the table gives visual information to the patient of where and how to maintain the position of hand and arm. An array of creams and lotions are placed to the hemiplegic side. The patient is encouraged to select requirements from the table, reaching across the mid-line with sound hand, and rotating shoulder on pelvic girdle. The web space of the affected hand may be used to stabilize jars or bottles for opening. The patient may then rub a pleasant smelling cream over the extensor surface of the arm and hand and apply cream or make up to the face. The therapist may need to assist with balance, prompt procedures, or awareness of neglected body parts through tactile, verbal, or visual stimulation.

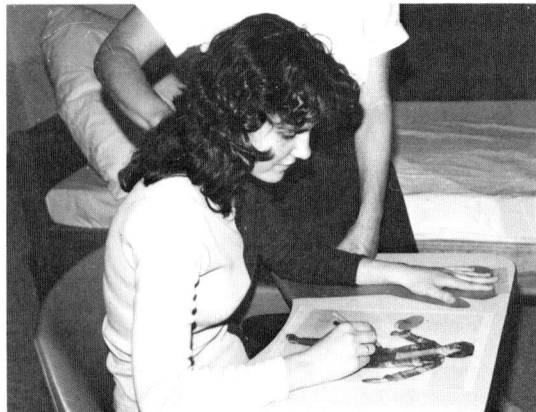

Fig. 5.31 Patient outlining a 'figure' design for a batik project.

Therapeutic rationale

• Tactual, visual and olfactory stimulation will increase awareness of the hemiplegic side. The patient is likely to feel more attractive, and as it is almost certain that other people will comment on her appearance, these feelings will be extended and enhanced, increased awareness of face and body parts continuing beyond the period of the actual activity.

• A pleasurable, relaxing activity incorporates movement and balance re-education, and purposeful self-applied tactile stimulation.

• Activity of this nature may be used as continuing evaluation of impairment, particularly of perceptual motor disorder. The procedures involve visuo-spatial understanding and recognition of objects and their position, spatial and tactile awareness of self, concept of body scheme, and sequential, familiar skilled movements.

Other tasks and activities which may be included in ward programs for specific individual treatment gains include table and wall games with specific visuo-spatial components, reading and discussion of newspaper articles, simple creative projects, and designing and drawing for future projects. Figure 5.31 shows a patient outlining a design for a proposed batik project. The design is a human figure, to reinforce body awareness concepts being practised in functional tasks.

AS MOBILITY IMPROVES

1. End of bed exercise

End of bed exercise, which uses the rail on the end of a bed as an aid to standing and balancing, was developed to utilize available equipment before the necessity for activity programs for geriatric hospitals was recognised. It is an extremely functional retraining exercise which is suitable for stroke patients and may be carried out within the ward. If the bed rails are unsuitable for this purpose, a strong rail fixed to a wall under a window is an excellent substitute. The activity may be used as an alternative transfer technique, and to aid standing when adjusting clothing.

Patients respond well to this activity, perhaps because it enables them to stand on their own feet with safety very soon after stroke. Despite widespread acceptance of the efficacy of an ontogenetic sequence of re-education following stroke, many therapists feel that there is strong clinical evidence to support the usefulness of 'standing' as a treatment modality as soon as the patient is allowed out of bed.

This particular technique to aid standing is in fact a method used by infants before they achieve independent balance, to stand in cots or play-pens by pulling themselves upright, and may therefore be regarded as part of the functional ontogenetic sequence.

Even if this were not so, as, in stroke one hemisphere usually remains intact, knowledge of how it feels to stand remains, which allows adaptibility of approach, and suggests a rigid ontogenetic approach may be inappropriate for adult treatment. Early standing does not preclude the use of the developmental sequence.

Method

The patient sits on a chair facing the end of bed rail. (Fig. 5.32).

A portable block positioned on the floor across

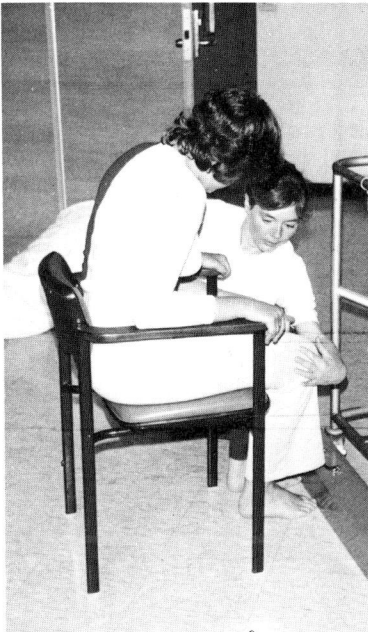

(a)

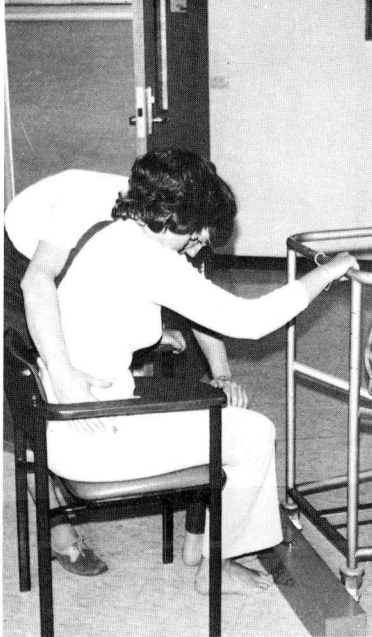

(b)

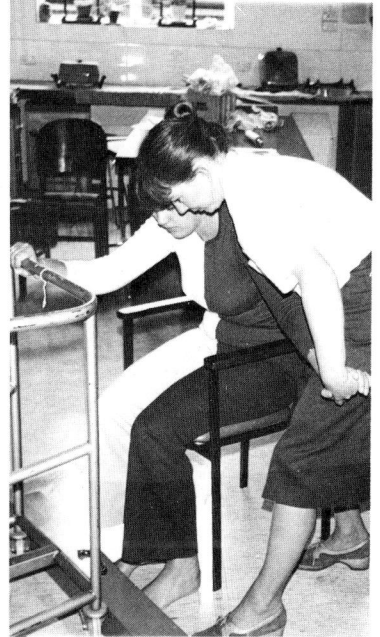

(c)

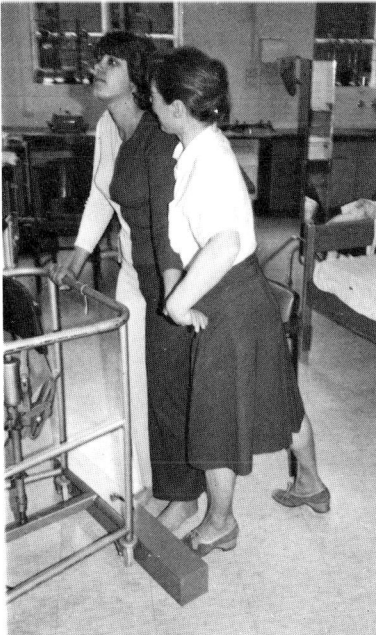

(d)

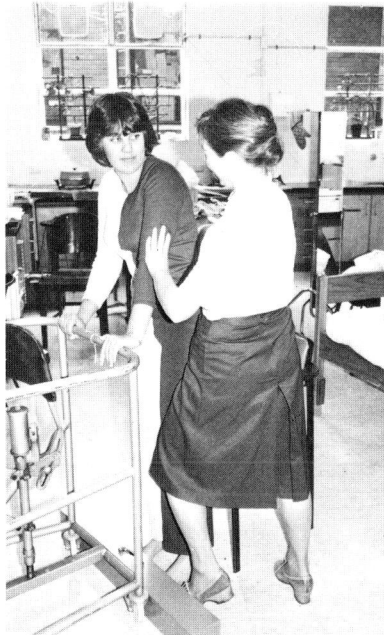

(e)

Fig. 5.32 End of bed exercise. (a) Feet are positioned. (b) Patient puts sound hand to rail, therapist applies approximation through hemiplegic leg. (c) Patient leans forward ready to stand. (d) Patient stands and is encouraged to look up, and put both hands on rail. (e) Therapist gives support to upper and lower limbs as patient is encouraged to look around.

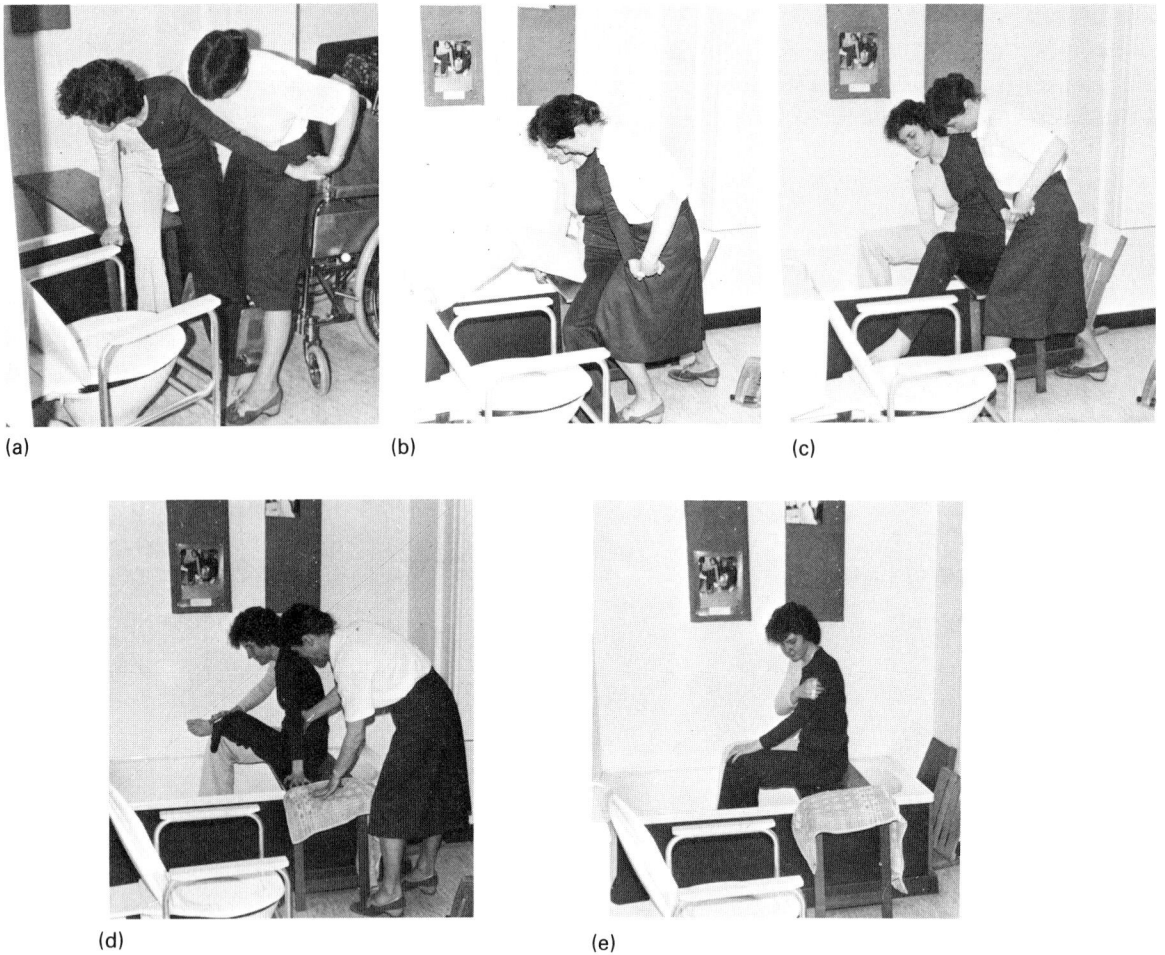

Fig. 5.33 Assisting transfer from a wheelchair to a bath, using a bathboard.

the foot of the bed, positions the feet away from the bed, allowing space for the body to assume upright standing. It also prevents feet from slipping fowards, and gives tactual and visual clues about appropriate foot placement. The patient sits symmetrically with feet apart.

With those who have gross dysfunction, are possibly overweight, old, confused, and likely to be discharged early to dependent care, it is suggested that foot, and sound hand placement, should encourage weight bearing on the sound side. The hemiplegic foot should touch the leg of the chair, the sound foot should be placed centrally, and the sound hand should hold the rail well to the sound side (McIntyre & Mort, 1973).

The patient holds the rail with the sound hand, the shoulder in slight abduction and elbow extended.

The therapist holds the hemiplegic hand and arm in a reflex inhibiting position and promotes forward shoulder movement by body/shoulder pressure. Forward leaning is encouraged verbally and by the therapist's other arm across the back with the hand on the patient's sound hip.

Instruction is given to lean forward and stand up, the therapist moving with the patient.

Once standing, the patient should be encouraged to take weight symmetrically, to sway, to rotate and to view the environment. Sitting slowly and standing is repeated several times.

Therapeutic rationale

- Clinical experience has found this to be a highly motivating activity for the patients.
- It assists the natural re-establishment of physiological and balance mechanisms.
- It is a safe and effective method of early balance re-education.
- It is an excellent technique for orderlies and aides, when transferring patients from chair to wheelchair or to toilet chair, if chairs are exchanged whilst the patient is standing. The risks of secondary dysfunction occurring as a result of faulty handling are largely negated and the patient feels much less dependent on others for mobility.
- Scanning and identification activities are incorporated in the standing exercise to retrain visual and attention deficits.
- Repetitive use of end of bed exercise for those being discharged to dependent care offers retraining in simple mobility, helps normalize

physiological processes such as circulation, bladder and bowel control, digestion, and prevents deterioration of joints and bones through lack of weight bearing.

2. Bathing and showering

It is becoming increasingly common for occupational therapists to assist patients with showering and bathing activities, as soon as the patient is medically able to undertake these tasks with assistance. In hospitals where more suitable facilities are available in the rehabilitation unit, patients may perform hygiene tasks away from the ward.

The highly cutaneous sensory nature of bathing and showering make these activities invaluable for sensory re-education. Techniques to enhance sensory motor performance should be used, during daily participation of these self-care tasks, which will also promote early independence in them.

Methods of transfer similar to those already

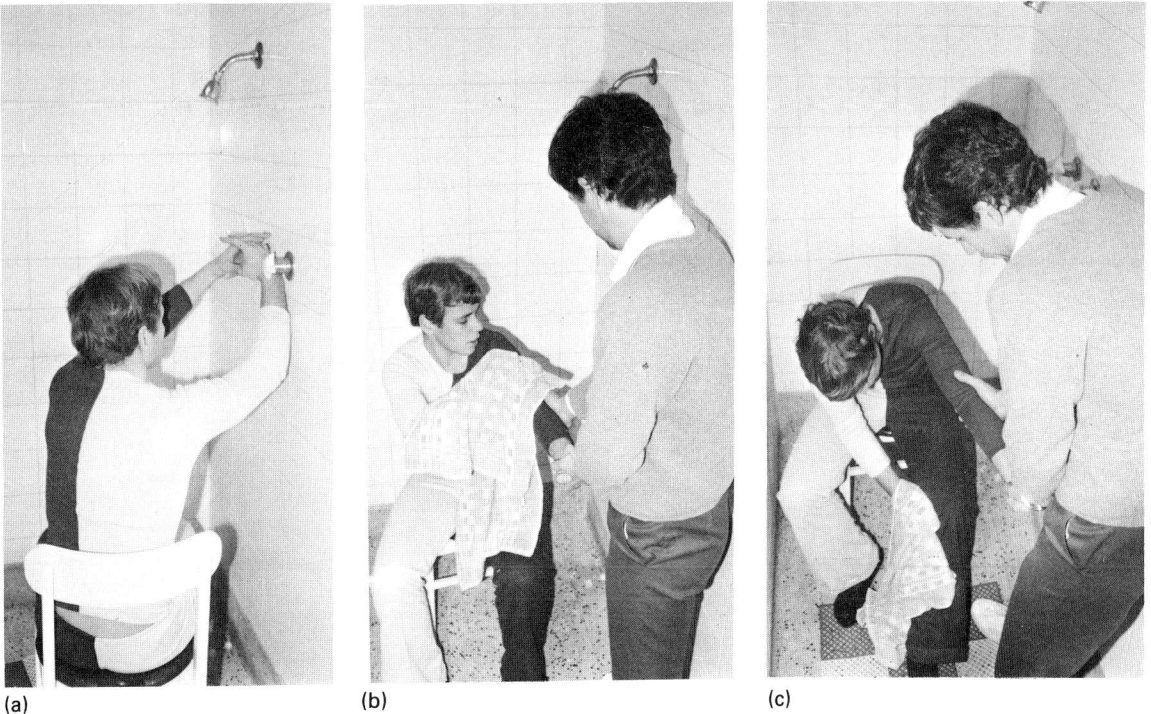

(a) (b) (c)

Fig. 5.34 In the shower: (a) Using bilateral grip to turn off shower water. (b) The patient is encouraged to watch and towel the hemiplegic upper limb. (c) The patient is supported in R.I.P. as he leans forward to towel the lower limb.

described may be used for transferring a patient to bath or shower, as demonstrated in Figure 5.33. Techniques to maintain balance and safety, promote normal tone by the use of reflex-inhibiting positions and rotation, increase visuo-spatial abilities and sensory awareness can be included as the patient handles a manual shower head, soaps, brushes, or towels body parts, or turns off the tap (Fig. 5.34). Unless there is a manual shower head which may be safely positioned, taps should be turned on prior to the patient getting into a shower so that water temperature can be regulated, to prevent burns.

Mobility and independence skills may also be taught when assisting the patient to use a lavatory. This will be discussed further in later Chapters.

SUMMARY

Intervention, early after onset of stroke, is important to facilitate recovery processes. Activities of a personal nature, directly relating to the body are suggested to promote awareness and enhance sensory motor re-education.

Neurophysiological and neuropsychological treatment should be included with activities of daily living and those of a social nature. These may take place in the ward to promote appropriate day-long programs, ensuring maintenance of patients' intact ability, as well as maximal utilization of treatment opportunity. Individual interests, cultural differences and discharge plans should be considered from the first treatment.

REFERENCES

Bobath B 1978 Adult hemiplegia evaluation and treatment, 2nd edn. Heinemann Medical Books Ltd, London
Cailliet R 1980 The shoulder in hemiplegia. F A Davis Co, Philadelphia
Carr J, Shepherd R 1982 A motor relearning programme for stroke. Heinemann Medical Books Ltd, London
Gaffney T W, Campbell R P 1974 Feeding techniques of dysphagic patients. American Journal of Nursing 74:12
Hebb D O 1961 Distinctive features of learning in the higher animal, In: Delafresnaye J F (ed) Brain mechanisms and learning. Oxford University Press, London
Held J P 1975 The natural history of stroke, In: Licht S (ed) Stroke and its rehabilitation. Waverly Press, Baltimore, ch 2
Hewson L 1982 When half is whole. Dove Communications, Blackburn, Victoria
Hurd M M, Farrell K H, Waylonis G W 1974 Shoulder sling for hemiplegia, friend or foe? Archives of Physical Medicine and Rehabilitation, Nov 55(11): 519–522

Johnstone M 1978 Restoration of motor function in the stroke patient, a physiotherapist's approach. Churchill Livingstone, Edinburgh
Knott M, Voss D E 1968 Proprioceptive neuromuscular facilitation, 2nd edn. Harper and Row, New York
Larsen G L 1972 Rehabilitation for dysphagia paralytica. Journal of Speech and Hearing Disorders 37:2: 187–194
McIntyre B, Mort M 1973 Geriatric retraining the Newcastle method as applied to hemiplegia. Rehabilitation in Australia, ACROD, Oct
Mossman P L 1976 A problem oriented approach to stroke rehabilitation. Charles Thomas, Springfield, Ill
Syms A 1982 Early feeding intervention with brain injured adults. Conference Proceedings 12th Federal Conference Australian Association of Occupational Therapists, 45–62
Tobis J S 1957 Post hemiplegic shoulder pain. New York State Journal of Medicine 57(8): 1377–1388
dysfunction, 2nd edn. Williams and Wilkins, Baltimore

RECOMMENDED READING

Cailliet R 1980 The shoulder in hemiplegia. F A Davis Co, Philadelphia
Dardier E 1980 The early stroke patient. Cassell Ltd, London
Hewson L 1982 When half is whole. Dove Communications, Blackburn, Victoria

McIntyre B, Mort M 1973 Geriatric Retraining the Newcastle method as applied to hemiplegia. Rehabilitation in Australia, ACROD, Oct
Syms A 1982 Early feeding intervention with brain injured adults. Conference Proceedings 12th Federal Conference Australian Association of Occupational Therapists, 45–62

6

When balance and gross mobility are priorities

Whichever treatment method is followed the re-education of balance and postural mechanisms is an important primary consideration. The amount of emphasis differs from technique to technique, as does the rationale and specific procedures used. Major differences are found between therapists using a developmental approach, those using a remedial functional approach, and those using a compensatory approach.

DEVELOPMENTAL APPROACHES

Not all therapists will feel comfortable about, or wish to use a developmental approach. When treating the elderly, who frequently have other disorders, such as those of a cardiovascular or muscular skeletal nature, some of the positions suggested as part of the treatment progression may be impossible, or inappropriate. Therapists who use activities in developmental positions suggest that the number of elderly people who respond favourably to this type of treatment, both physically and psychologically, is surprisingly high. However, all patients need to have individually tailored programs, and the therapist needs to feel confident in techniques chosen for use.

It may not be necessary to start a patient at the beginning of the sequence, this being dependent upon the extent of the dysfunction and abnormal responses. Nor is it necessary to stay rigidly within one stage; patients may progress through several stages rapidly in one session or extend gains made, by using them in different positions. This is called 'overlapping'. As seen in the previous Chapter, rolling and propping activities may be commenced early whilst the patient is in bed, and related to bed mobility. In the rehabilitation unit progressive postures may be practised dynamically on a mat or large plinth.

113

Methods

1. On a plinth

(a) Sitting to prone

It is easy to position a patient on a plinth, as he may simply be transferred from a wheelchair to the side of a plinth and, taking weight either through the hemiplegic or sound upper limb according to ability, or therapist choice, and with appropriate support, swing both legs onto the plinth. Patients are then assisted to roll into prone, away from the edge of the plinth and supported on a wedge or cushions (Fig. 6.1).

A brief, simple activity, or part of an ongoing project using the sound hand, ensures that body weight applies intermittent joint approximation to the hemiplegic limb, which is maintained in a reflex-inhibiting pattern.

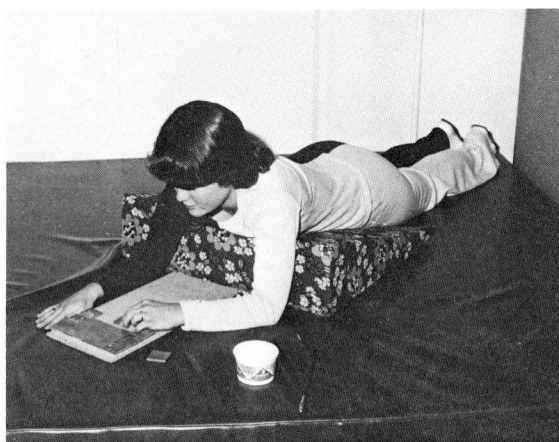

Fig. 6.1 Simple activity in a prone position, using a wedge to support the trunk.

(b) Bridging

Alternatively the patient may move to the middle of the plinth by using bridging (described in Ch. 5). When balanced in a bridged position the patient is asked or assisted to swing the pelvis away from the edge of the plinth before lowering, and then adjusts shoulders, head and both legs into a symmetrically aligned position ready to bridge once more until the desired location on the plinth is reached. This should be done slowly, step by step to prevent unwanted effort causing increased abnormal tone.

(c) Side sitting

To move from supine to side sitting the patient rolls onto the hemiplegic side (as described in Ch. 5) and is asked or assisted to take weight, and push up on the hemiplegic arm and hand, and then to bend both legs closer to the body.

To progress from prone to side sitting (Fig. 6.2), the therapist kneels facing the patient beside the hemiplegic side, supports the hemiplegic arm and assists either sound shoulder or pelvis as the patient rolls onto the hemiplegic side and back to the therapist. The legs are allowed to flex naturally as the roll occurs, and the patient is instructed to bend both legs closer in to the body. The therapist gives support to the hemiplegic arm as the patient presses up on the hemiplegic hand. Weight may be taken by the sound hand as the patient does this.

When in side sitting and weight bearing on the hemiplegic arm, the therapist may need to assist maintenance of the position by approximation through the correctly aligned upper limb by manual contact and cutaneous sensory stimulation of extensors of the upper limb (Fig. 6.3), or by use of an air pressure splint as the patient is involved in an activity which promotes rotatory movement of the trunk.

Examples of activity include reading the newspaper, table games, simple crafts and watching television.

(d) Four point kneeling

The patient may be progressed from either side sitting or prone lying to four point kneeling, i.e. a crawling position.

If the patient is in side sitting the therapist kneels close to the patient, maintaining support to the hemiplegic arm in extension throughout the exercise. Figure 6.4 illustrates the therapist using both legs to support the hemiplegic limbs. The patient is asked to place the sound hand parallel with the hemiplegic one, and the therapist assists the sound buttock upwards with the other hand, and moves with the patient so that the hemiplegic thigh is supported by that of the therapist. The patient is asked to move each leg to be in line with the upper limbs, whilst the pelvic girdle is controlled between the therapist's leg and

(a)

(b)

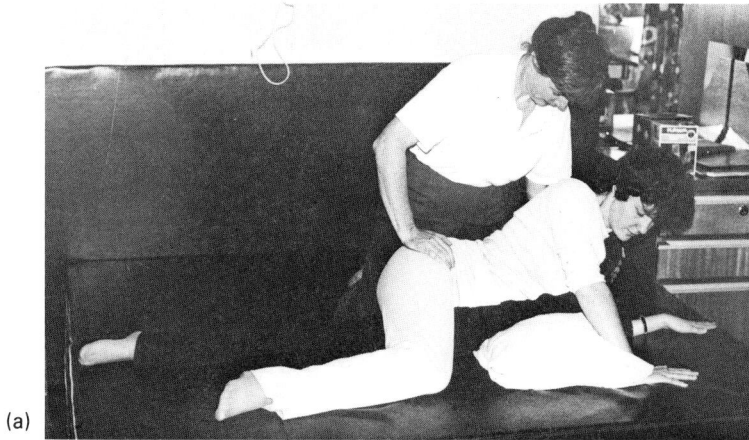

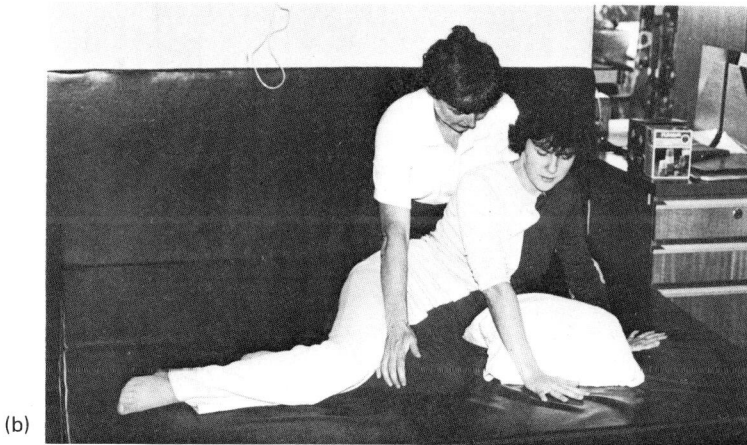

Fig. 6.2 Assisting a move from prone to side sitting.

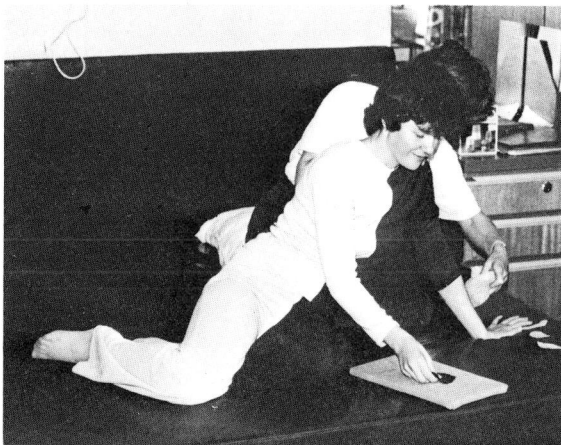

Fig. 6.3 Application of ice to the upper limb extensors whilst the patient is engaged in a simple activity involving trunk rotation.

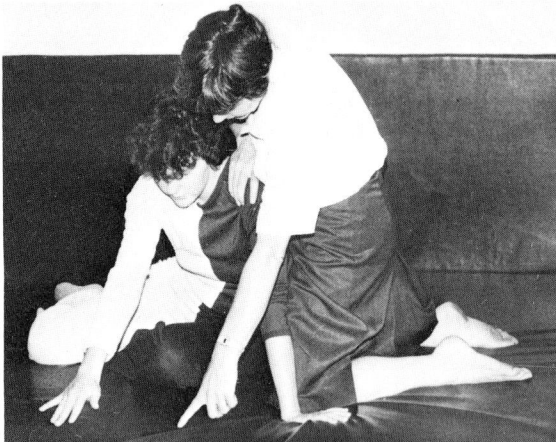

(a)

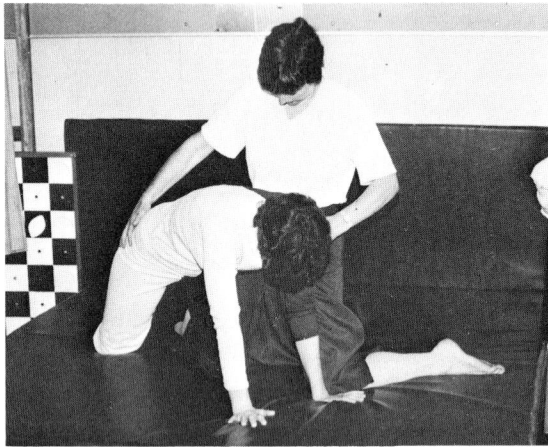

(b)

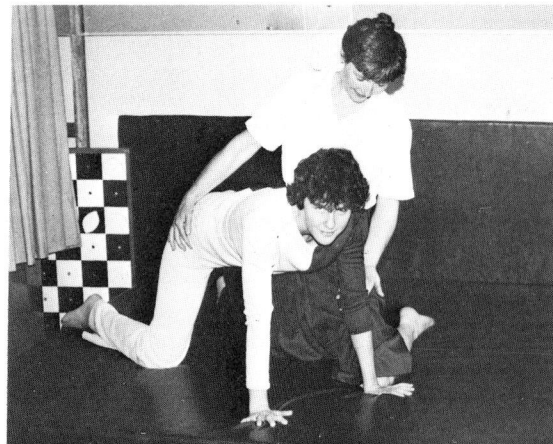

(c)

Fig. 6.4 Assisting a move from side sitting to four point kneeling.

body on the hemiplegic side, and the hand on the sound side.

To assist the patient from prone lying to four point kneeling (Fig. 6.5), the therapist kneels on the hemiplegic side, asks the patient to roll slightly towards the sound side and assists the hemiplegic knee forwards. The patient is then assisted to roll towards the hemiplegic side, the patient's thigh being supported by that of the therapist, and is asked to bring the sound knee forwards. Supporting the hemiplegic arm, the therapist asks the patient to move the sound hand parallel to the shoulder and push up, whilst the therapist assists the hemiplegic shoulder upwards, and the arm to extend.

This position promotes proximal stability at hip and shoulders. Before asking the patient to use the sound arm in simple activity, the patient should experience rocking and swaying, side to side, backwards and forwards, and diagonally, to experience weight bearing and facilitate stability, with manual contact, approximation and assistance being given as required. This position is usually only naturally assumed briefly in transition from one position to another, as in getting up from the floor, or in making a move in a game when played by a group around a board on the floor, or in such daily activities as scrubbing the floor, looking under items of furniture for something lost, working in the garden or playing with an infant or pet. However, therapists may use simple activity of the sound hand, providing it is fairly brief (Fig. 6.6), or incorporate four point kneeling into activity which demands changes of position. This will provide the patient with practice in moving into and out of the position, which may be helpful in developing eventual normal, rather than limited, patterns of mobility.

(e) Kneeling

Patients may be assisted to move backwards from four point to two point kneeling (Fig. 6.7). The therapist kneels on the hemiplegic side, holds the hemiplegic hand in handshake hold, maintaining the arm in extension, and asks the patient to lift head and shoulders backwards into an upright position.

Kneeling may also be assumed easily from side

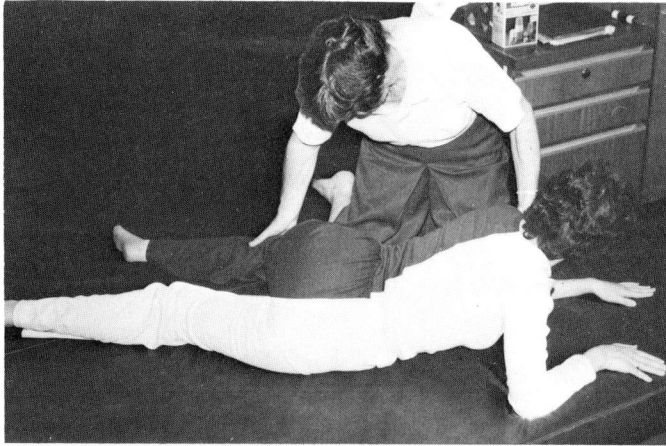
(a)

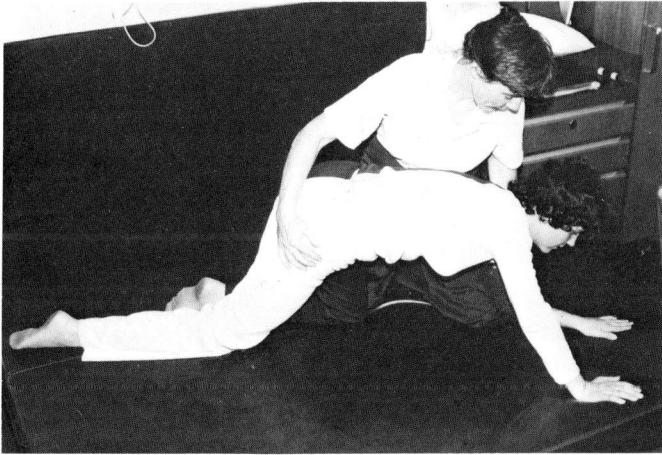
(b)

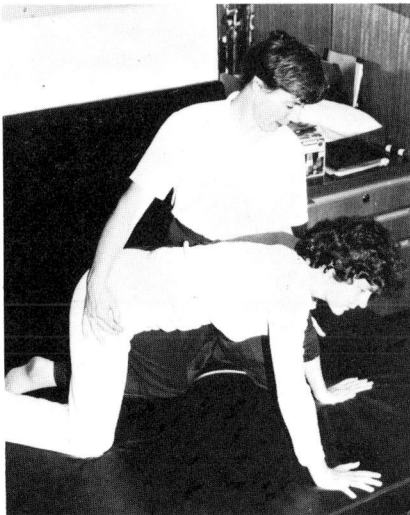
(c)

Fig. 6.5 Assisting a move from prone lying to four point kneeling.

sitting in a similar way, the therapist asking for sideways rather than backwards movement. When kneeling, simple activity incorporating rotation may be used, balance demands being graded by the position of materials, as illustrated in Figure 6.8. With support on the hemiplegic side patients may progress to half kneeling.

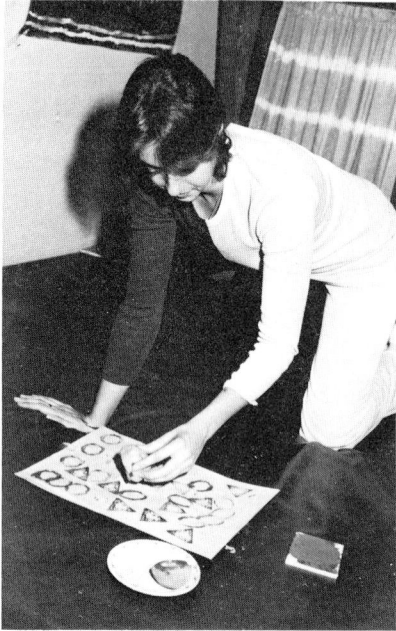

Fig. 6.6 Simple activity in four point kneeling.

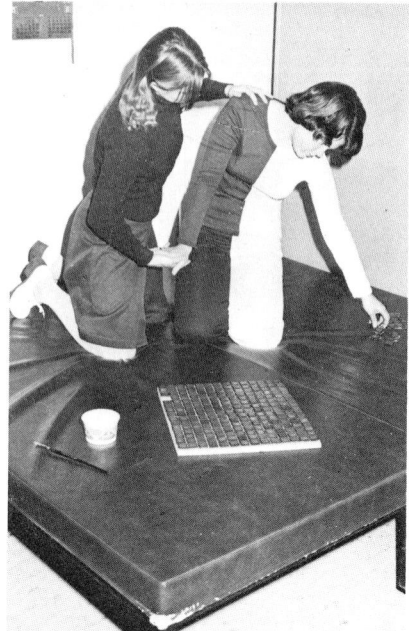

Fig. 6.8 Activity in kneeling.

(f) Sitting

Other positions which may be used on a plinth are those of long and short sitting, during which the patient may alternate between weight bearing through both upper limbs, leaning slightly back-

wards, and leaning forwards to participate in unilateral or bilateral activities.

Patients may sit on the side of the plinth instead of a chair, to practise balance without back support, whilst engaged in activity demanding rotation or leaning, as illustrated in Figure 6.9.

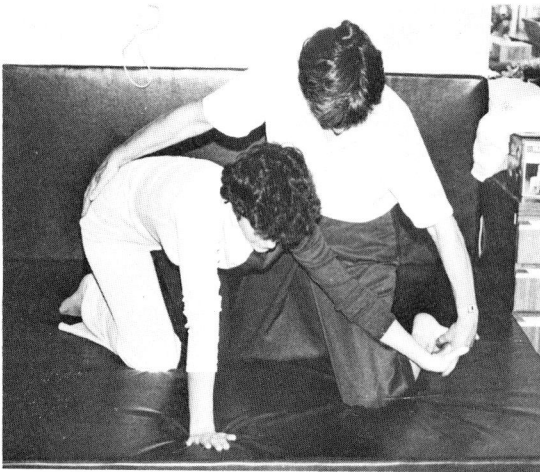

(a)

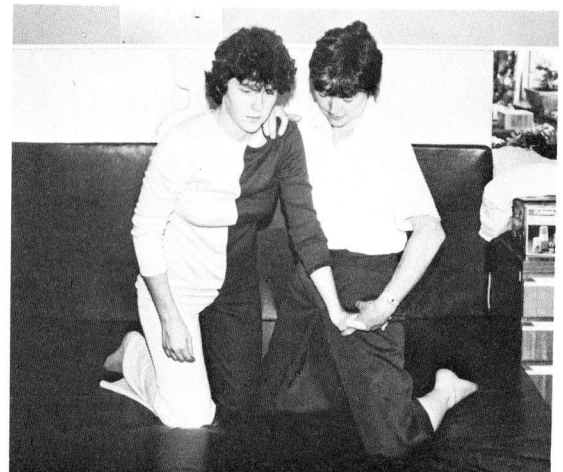

(b)

Fig. 6.7 Assisting a move from four point kneeling to two point kneeling.

(a)   (b)

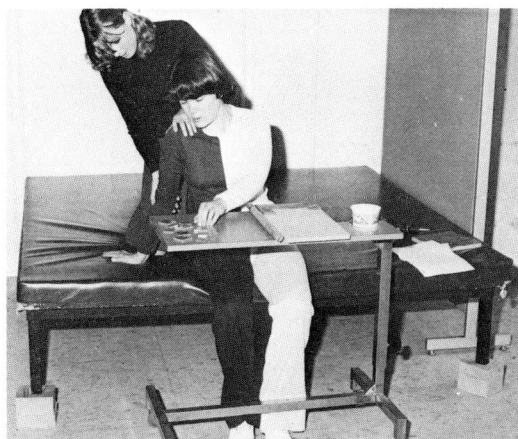

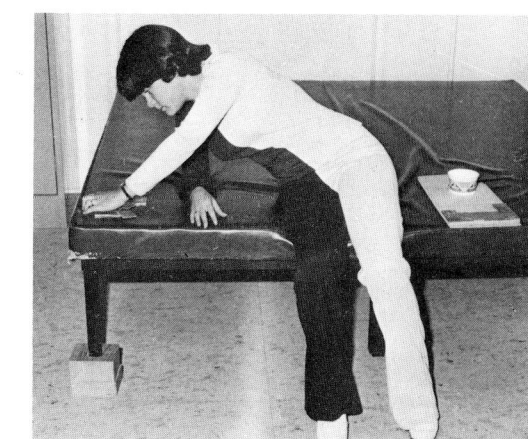

Fig. 6.9 Activity sitting on the side of the plinth to encourage propping on the hemiplegic side, or rotation.

2. On a floor mat

(a) Getting down

Regular training which demands getting down to and up from the floor is useful to provide experience and familiarity with such movements, for daily activities such as getting in and out of a bath normally, and for getting up off the floor should a fall occur. Getting down calls for more control than getting up, and until patients feel comfortable about getting down, they may need help and encouragement to tackle the movement.

A technique which may be used early in treatment is for the therapist to lower the patient to the floor from behind. This is a surprisingly easy procedure as long as the patient is able to relax and has confidence in the therapist.

The patient stands back to the mat, hands clasped in midline. The therapist stands behind the patient supporting the trunk and both arms and hands, as in Figure 6.10. The therapist asks the patient to relax, moves slowly backwards, bending at the knees, until the patient is sitting on the mat. Arms are then positioned so the patient is sitting safely in long sitting.

When patients feel confident, they may be helped to get down to the floor in reverse developmental sequence, from standing to half kneeling, sound leg kneeling, two point kneeling to side sitting, as in Figure 6.11.

(b) Activities

When on the mat, patients may participate in activities demanding gross reaching and rotation, with the therapist providing stability through approximation as necessary. This is illustrated in Figure 6.12, in which the patient is working on a batik project. The subject of the batik is the figure of a boy, which the therapist may discuss to increase input pertaining to body parts. Safe handling of the heat source may be preparatory to, or compatible with, retraining in household tasks.

Therapists may also use games which are played at floor level, such as skittles, floor draughts or bowls, assisting patients to assume different developmental positions as they participate. Figure 6.13 shows bowling being used in this fashion. These games are also useful in retraining visuo-spatial, motor planning and attention skills whilst providing an enjoyable social situation.

As balance improves patients may be encouraged to try out the redeveloped skills in unassisted activity (Fig. 6.14).

In order to feel confident in the use of developmental positions during activity, students and therapists should practise on each other to gain confidence, and experience, in how to use body and hands to control patient mobility, so that patients may feel secure. This will enhance patient participation, and reduce risks of abnormal reflex

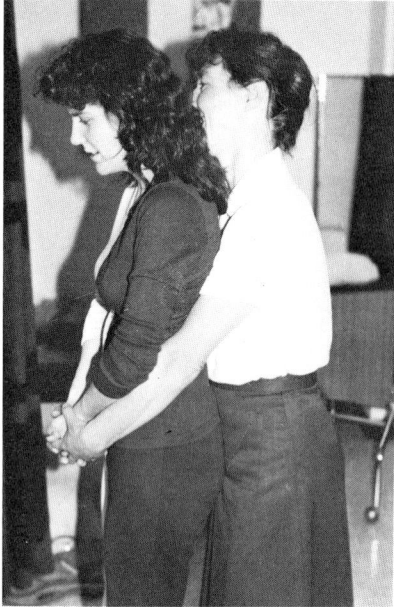

(a)

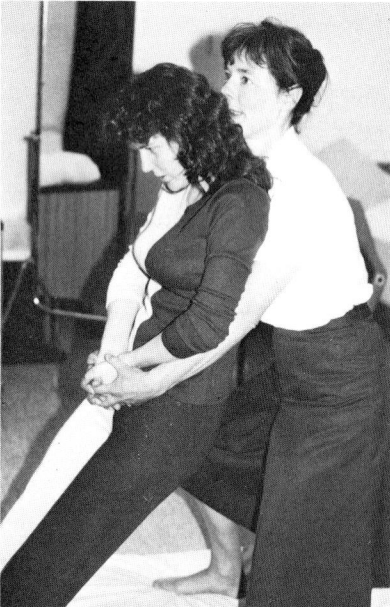

(b)

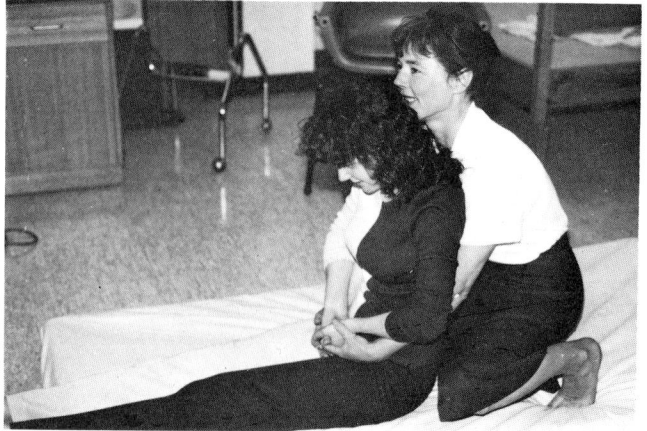

(c)

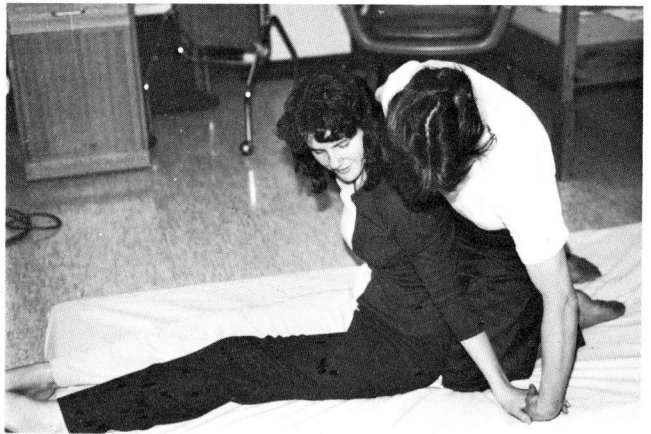

(d)

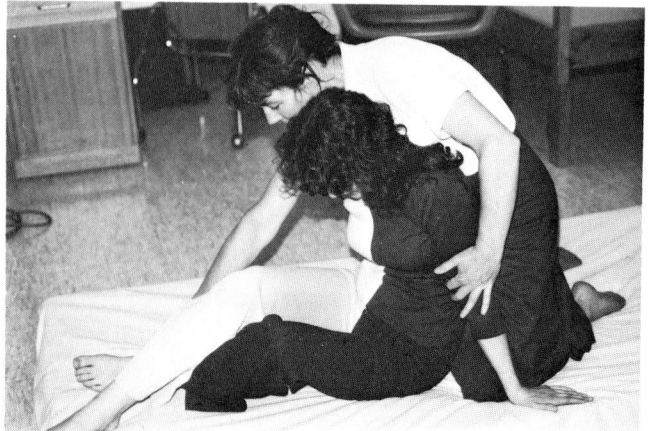

(e)

Fig. 6.10 Lowering a patient backwards on to a floor mat.

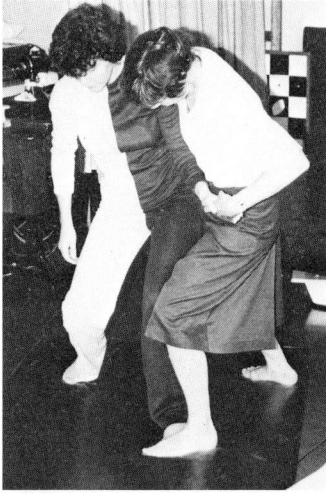
(a)

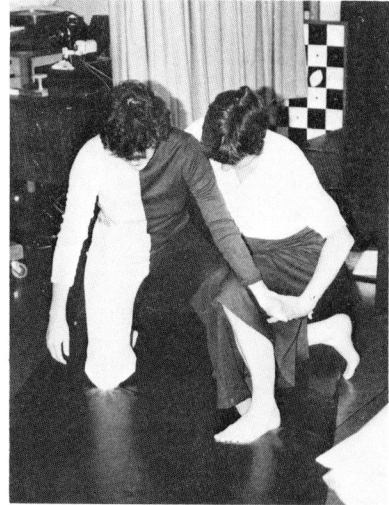
(b)

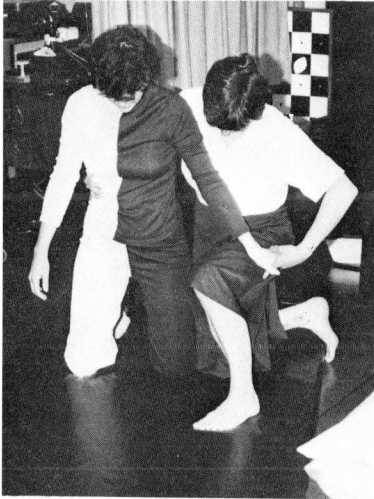
(c)

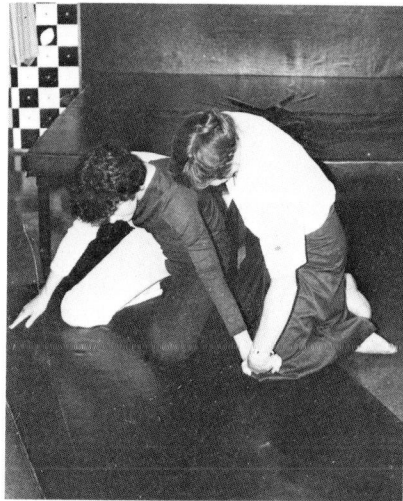
(d)

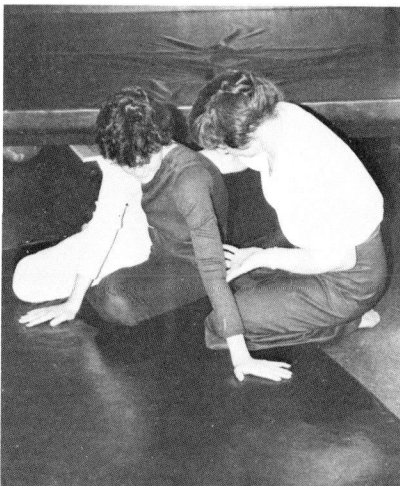
(e)

Fig. 6.11 Assisting the patient to get down to the floor from standing using a normal sequence of movement.

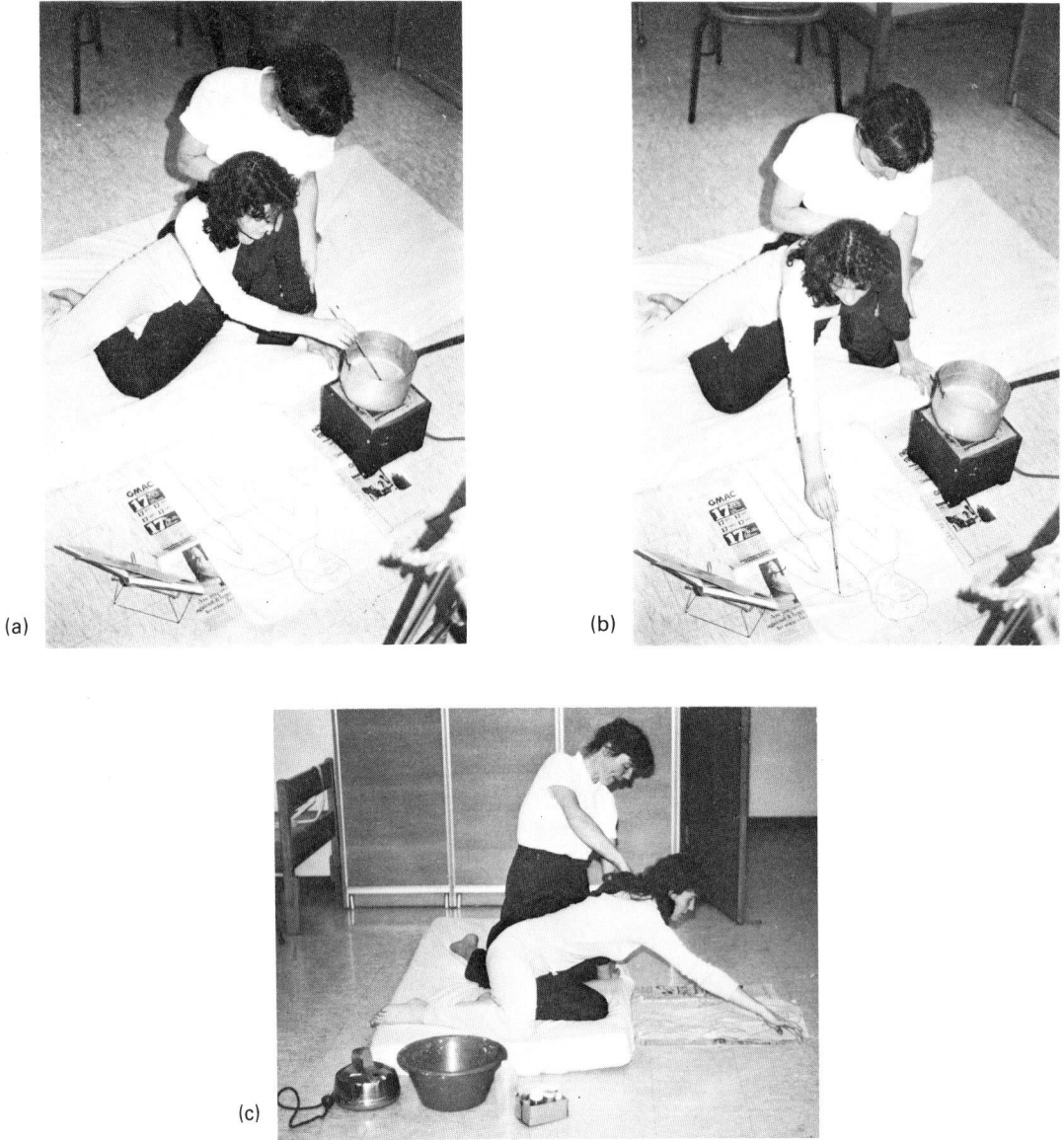

Fig. 6.12 An activity on the floor mat demanding gross reaching and rotation. The design was enlarged by projecting the transparency outlined in Fig. 5.31 and drawing around it, providing continued opportunity to introduce body awareness training.

behaviour occurring because of stress and unnecessary effort.

Choice of activities used during developmental sequencing should, as far as possible, reflect patient interests. In some cases 'pretend' activities in appropriate positions may be used if the activity itself is not viable. For example, planting vegetable seedlings in the garden, bathing a dog or playing with a child may be activities in which the patient naturally assumes 'developmental' positions, but which may not be possible in the occupational therapy department. 'Pretend' activities may be contraindicated for apraxic patients. Therapists may find it helpful to discover if the patient uses

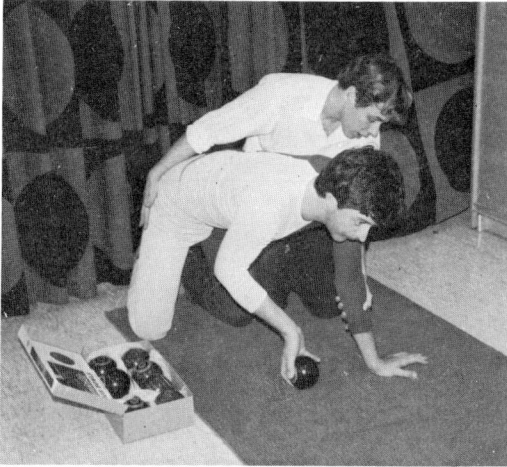

(a)

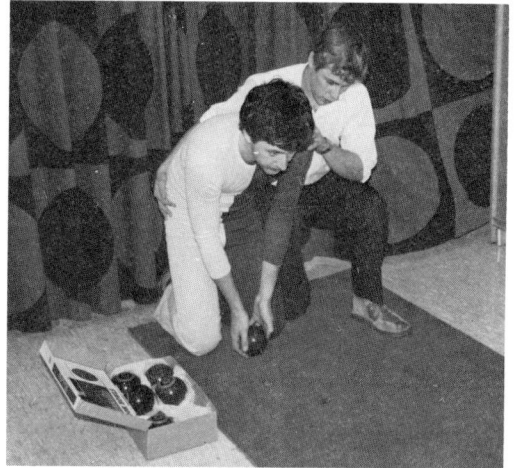

(b)

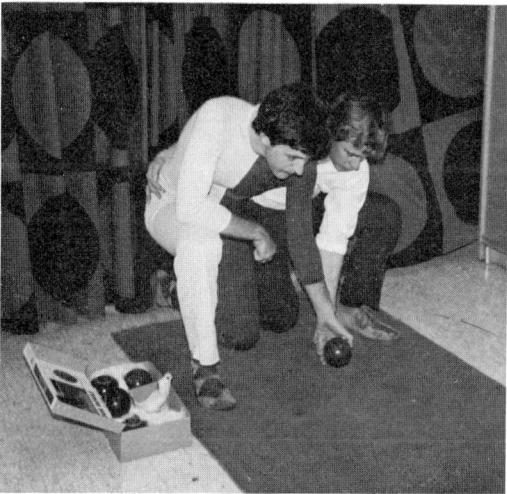

(c)

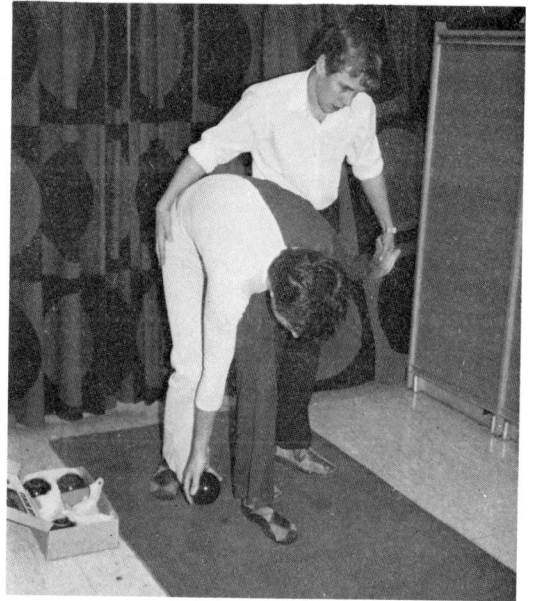

(d)

Fig. 6.13 Indoor bowls being used as an assisted activity during retraining using developmental positions.

any developmental positions habitually, and relate retraining to such activities.

Activities used should also be applicable to other impairment such as higher cortical dysfunction. For example, menu planning for a proposed cooking session may be carried out when the patient is side sitting; short writing practice or word games may be used when a patient is supported by a wedge in prone; or facial, hair care sessions or dressing practice, to increase sensory and body awareness, may be used during long sitting.

Patients may also be included in group activity or discussions whilst experiencing developmental positions.

It is important for patients' attention to be

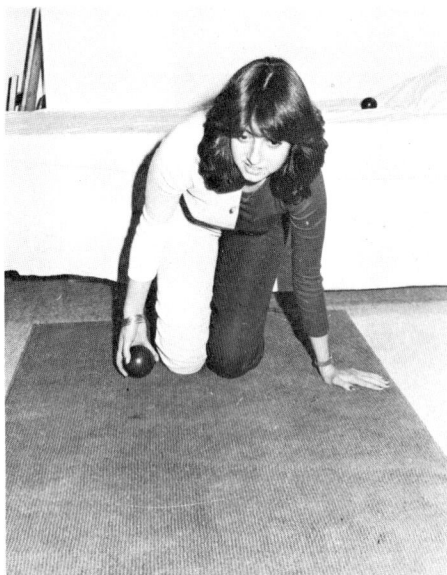

(a)

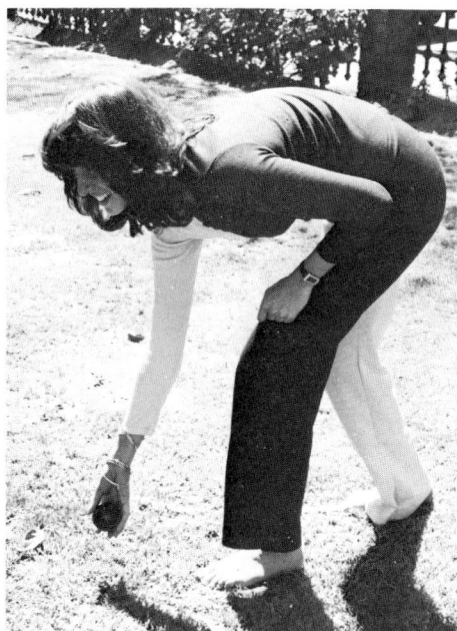

(b)

Fig. 6.14 Patients using relearned balance skills in unassisted activity.

diverted from conscious consideration of movement patterns and positions, in order for these to become part of the patient's automatic repertoire.

Therapeutic rationale for activity in developmental sequence:

- Provides a theoretical framework for treatment progression.
- Provides inhibitory patterns of movement for upper limb, lower limb and trunk.
- Provides early weight-bearing activity to develop proximal stability.
- Provides trunk rotation and facilitation of equilibrium reactions.
- Provides a wide, stable base and low centre of gravity for early balance and equilibrium reactions, and simple upper limb activity.
- Provides proprioceptive input to hemiplegic upper and lower limbs, helping with body awareness and tactile sensory loss.
- Prepares for lower limb weight bearing without total extension synergy.
- Prepares for the upper limb to respond in protective extension when necessary.
- Encourages visual scanning and attention skills, depending on choice and position of activity.
- Provides a logical sequence for the treatment of higher cortical skills (see Ch. 8).

'UNSTABLE BASE' APPROACH

Once stability in sitting balance has been reached, demands on balance and equilibrium may be increased by the provision of an unstable base on which to perform activities of a reaching and rotatory nature.

This aims at promoting normal equilibrium responses in unexpected and demanding situations.

Methods

(a) Sitting on an unstable base

Patients are engaged in activity whilst sitting on an unstable base. They may sit astride or on the side of an abductor roller (Fig. 6.15), whilst participating in any activity demanding trunk and upper limb movement. The roller will move with the patient, causing the need for constant postural adjustment. Therapists sitting next to or behind the patient may control the movement of the roller whilst assisting patient movement and control. Examples of how it may be used are shown in Figure 6.15, and include the therapist supporting

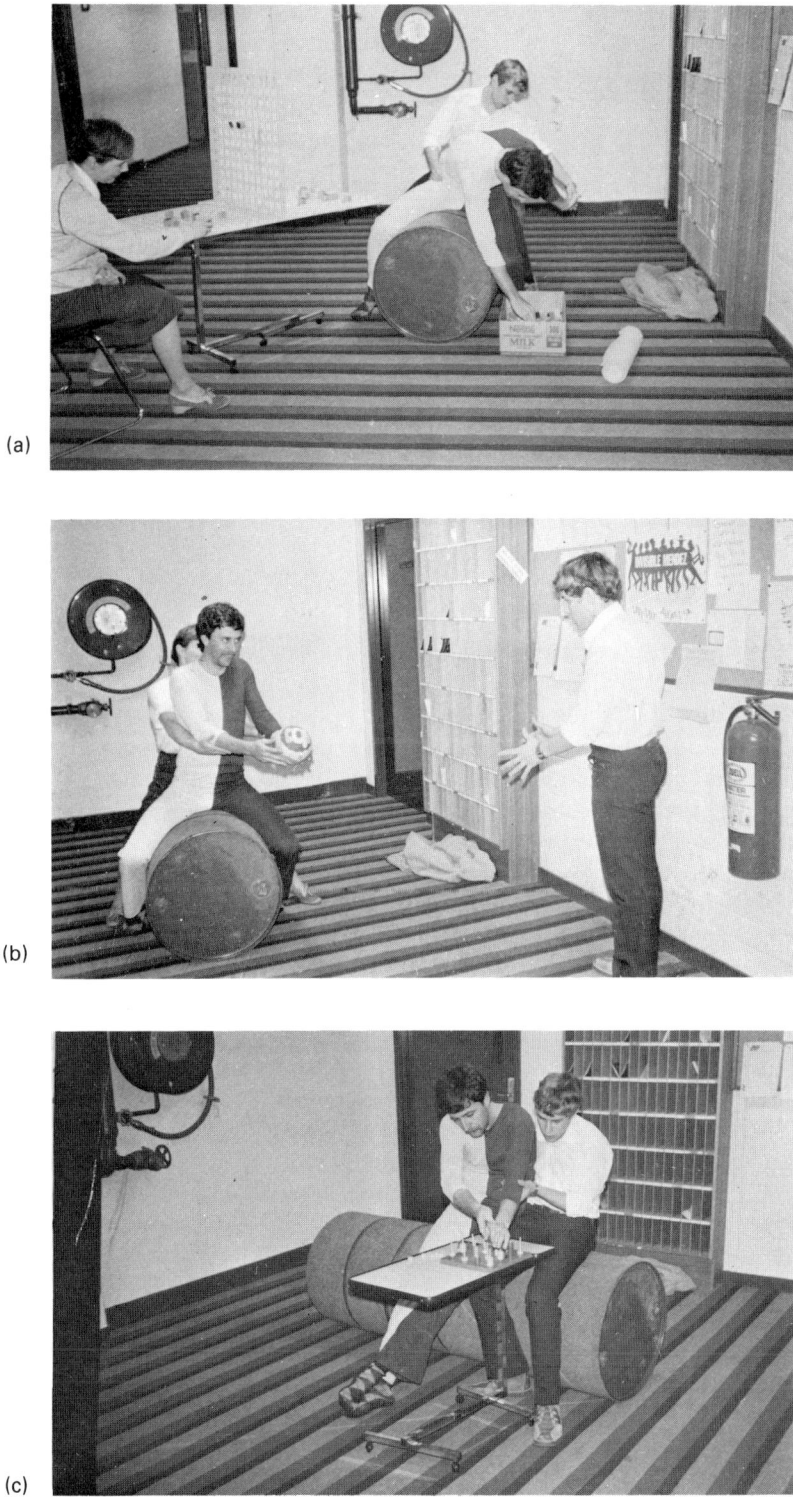

(a)

(b)

(c)

Fig. 6.15 Use of an abductor roller to promote normal balance reactions.

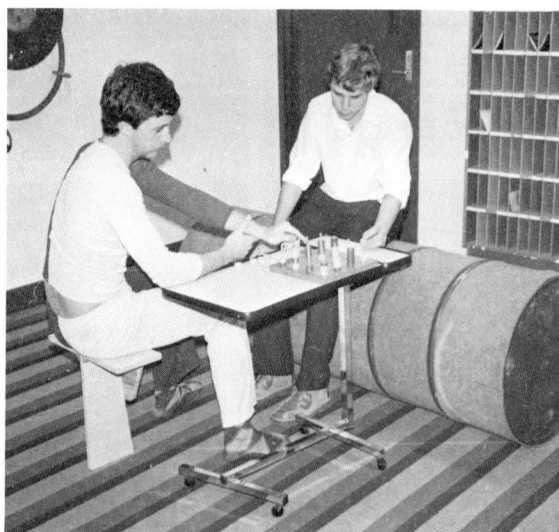

Fig. 6.16 A one-legged stool used in the final stages of balance retraining.

the patient's trunk bilaterally, from behind, as the patient uses the sound or impaired upper limb; promoting trunk rotation and leaning towards the hemiplegic side using an upper limb reflex-inhibiting pattern and trunk support; and providing unilateral or bilateral upper limb support to reduce patient effort so that functional hand movement is possible. The therapist's feet on the floor control the amount of sideways movement of the roller.

A small roller of chair height may replace a seat for many tasks such as weaving, printing, painting etc. A one-legged stool (Fig. 6.16) may also be used in the final stages of balance retraining when the patient has control over trunk and lower limb movement, to facilitate normal equilibrium and righting reactions. Maintaining a safe position whilst involved in an activity demanding concentration, such as 'Four in a Row' illustrated in Figure 6.16, progresses the act of balancing from conscious to an automatic level. Patients are likely to need practice in using the one-legged stool, with the therapist available to support the patient on the hemiplegic side if necessary. Use of a mirror to give the patient visual feedback may be useful.

(b) Standing and walking on an unstable base

Patients are engaged in activity whilst standing or walking on an unstable base.

They may stand or move on a floor mattress or rocker board whilst engaged in activities requiring throwing or rotation. The therapist should stand behind, supporting the trunk and upper limb when required, to ensure safety. The unstable base should be by a wall so that patients may use upper limb protective extension to steady themselves.

When possible, appropriate unstable base training should extend into the community, with the patient gaining practice in activities and environments they are likely to encounter after discharge, such as gravel paths, uneven cambers on roads, the golf course and the beach.

Therapeutic rationale for advanced balance retraining:

- Provides reflex inhibitory patterns of movement for lower limb, trunk and upper limb.
- Provides vestibular stimulation.
- Facilitates more normal equilibrium reactions and protective extension of upper limb.
- Provides experience in reacting to unexpected changes in position.
- Provides bilateral tactile and proprioceptive lower limb input to increase body awareness and cutaneous sensation.
- Encourages visual scanning and attention skills, depending upon choice and position of activity.

FUNCTIONAL BALANCE RETRAINING APPROACH

This approach seeks to encourage improvement in balance during the performance of functional activity. Tasks used are those seen as necessary for daily living, or for treatment for other aspects. of dysfunction. Balance retraining of a functional nature is inherent in the bed mobility and self-care activities described in the last chapter, and this may be extended to sitting, standing and walking activities accomplished in the rehabilitation unit.

Carr and Shepherd (1980), who follow a re-medial functional approach, indicate that the rationale for using a developmental progression to treat impairment which occurs after central nervous system maturation, has not been substantiated, and that damage to the adult central nervous system should be considered differently to impairment of an immature central nervous system.

It is reasoned that use of functional activity motivates patients because they understand, and want to do what is required of them, and no transfer of learning is necessary from a specific exercise to necessary task. Positions that are difficult and undignified for many elderly persons are unnecessary.

The importance of head control, trunkal stability and rotation, the ability to move against gravity and develop normal equilibrium reactions is appreciated, early sitting, standing and walking being stressed as important in the development of these mechanisms. Carr and Shepherd (1982) believe that patients should take a very active role in rehabilitation, and be made aware of specific deficits interfering with normal balance and movement, so that they may work to correct them, in co-operation with the therapist.

One of the common manifestations of balance and stability impairment seen during acute care is leaning to the hemiplegic side (see Fig. 5.28), particularly left hemiplegics who have impairment of spatial perception. This causes the patient to perceive they are vertical when, in fact, they are deviating to the left. Brunstrom (1970) suggests the complication of a spatial perceptual disorder may account for the fact that the trunk muscles of the sound side fail to counter the deviation away from upright, as would normally be expected.

She also describes investigations by Beevor (1903) which suggest that patients with left hemiplegia who lean to the left and have no control of movement to that side, have control of movement to the right of midline and bilateral simultaneous trunk movement, such as flexion and extension.

If disorders of balance and posture are caused by impairment of spatial perception, with patients having difficulty in appreciating verticality, attention should be focussed on improving spatial judgment as part of balance retraining, initially providing verbal reinforcement and visual clues. Brunnstrom (1970) suggests that kinesthesis, light touch, pressure and rhythmic rotary movements of the trunk and head, may be useful techniques to employ in such cases.

Carr and Shepherd (1982) suggest that a patient who has impaired sitting balance early post-stroke may actually be having difficulty with visual control, and that the relationship between head and eye movement and postural control should be considered, the patient being given tasks which involve locating and fixating on specific objects.

During all functional activity, normal sequence, timing, and movement, and correct joint alignment should be aimed at. Patients should be encouraged to practise moving from asymmetrical to symmetrical positions, and symmetrical to asymmetrical positions on both sides, reaching sideways, downwards, and up, rotating, and reaching to the extent of each patient's ability, but not beyond their point of balance and control. Activities which may be useful for repetitive reaching and rotating, include those of daily living such as dressing and showering, and creative tasks such as weaving or woodwork.

Methods

1. Activities in sitting

(a) Symmetrical sitting

Patients should be encouraged to sit symmetrically and take care of hemiplegic limbs, particularly if they are flaccid, and impaired cutaneous sensation and contralateral neglect are complications.

Peripheral stimulation and cortical input should be applied, and the therapist should encourage normal sequence and timing of movement during activities. If therapists are unsure of the sequence and timing of a particular activity chosen for its lifestyle relevance, they should try out the activity for themselves, analysing which part of the body leads the movement, and the sequence of movement components.

Each time patients begin to lean to the hemiplegic side they should be reminded to sit upright by the use of tactile and verbal cues. The symmetrical position should be verbally and visually reinforced by use of a mirror, and by cueing the patients to help them recognise the relationship of environmental objects to themselves. Patients should be told when they are straight and asked to maintain the position using the visual cues, and then to think about the feel of the position.

Once sitting symmetrically, patients may be

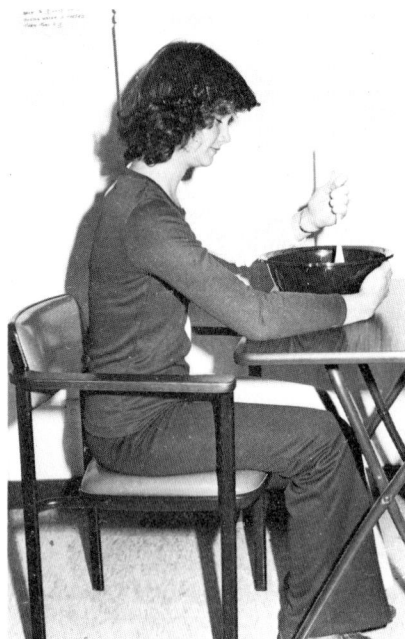

Fig. 6.17 Maintenance of symmetrical sitting in simple cooking activity.

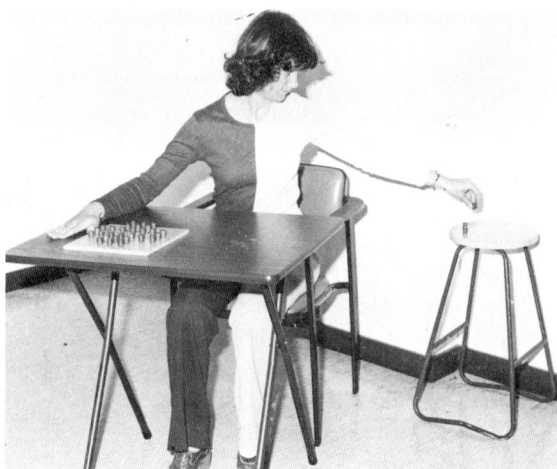

Fig. 6.18 Simple activity with components positioned so that trunk rotation is demanded.

given tasks which involve visual exploration and fixation, and are of interest to them. Activities relating to the human form, such as people jigsaws, games, drawings, and discussion of current affairs 'people' pictures, or personal 'people' photographs, may be useful. Maintenance of symmetrical sitting may also be a major aim during early group activities of a social nature, such as simple cooking or creative activity which may be performed in the midline of the body (Fig. 6.17).

(b) Trunk and upper limb movement

Activity may be graded to include first flexion and extension of the trunk and, as a cognitive awareness of upright is developed, activity which calls for trunk rotation and lateral flexion may be introduced. This may be achieved simply by the placement of objects. Figure 6.18 shows solitaire being used for this purpose, whilst obviously also demanding cognitive and perceptual skills.

Trunk movement including rotation and controlled asymmetry to the hemiplegic side, may be included in dressing practice, as illustrated in

Figure 6.19. The therapist standing behind the patient's chair, assists propping with hand or leg, cues rotation, and encourages reflex inhibiting patterns throughout the procedure.

Sitting balance retraining should also include particularly difficult activities, such as maintaining balance when using toilet paper whilst sitting on a lavatory. Patients are usually forced to lean to the hemiplegic side as, in many cases, the sound hand has to be used to hold and manipulate the paper, because of motor and/or sensory loss of the hemiplegic hand. This activity may be graded. Initially the patient should sit well on to the toilet so that the seat gives some support around the buttocks, with feet firmly on the ground and apart. The legs may, for patients with gross balance problems, be positioned so that the sound leg is to the midline (Fig. 6.20(a)). When it is safe, legs are positioned to either side of midline, and the patient should be instructed to lean forward to use the paper, rather than take weight on the hemiplegic leg (Fig. 6.20(b)).

As balance improves, normal positioning and transfer of weight on the lavatory is encouraged.

Other difficult balance activities in sitting may include self-care tasks which cause temporary occlusion of vision, such as putting on overhead garments, or showering when water spraying the face results in automatic eye closure. Verbal or tactual cueing to maintain or retain balance may

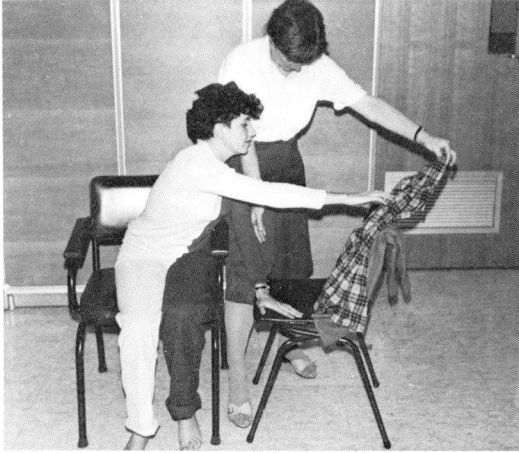

(a)

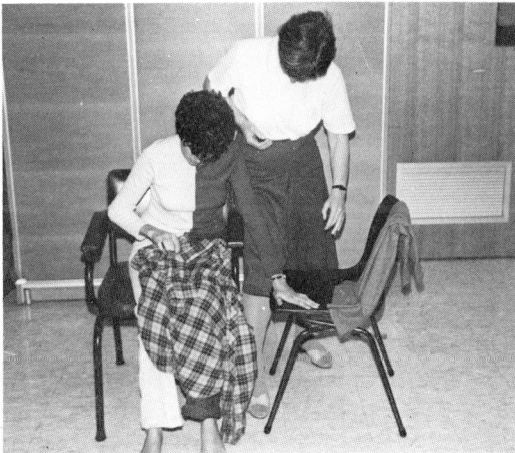

(b)

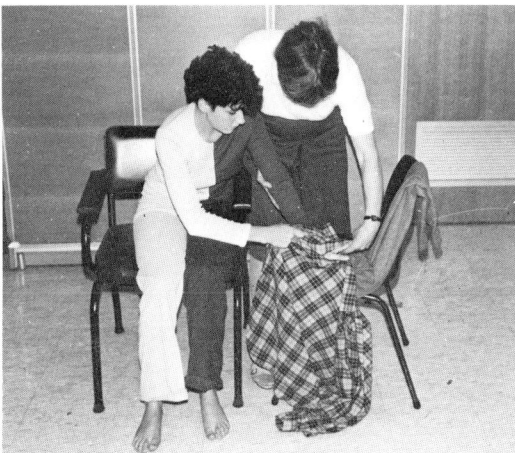

(c)

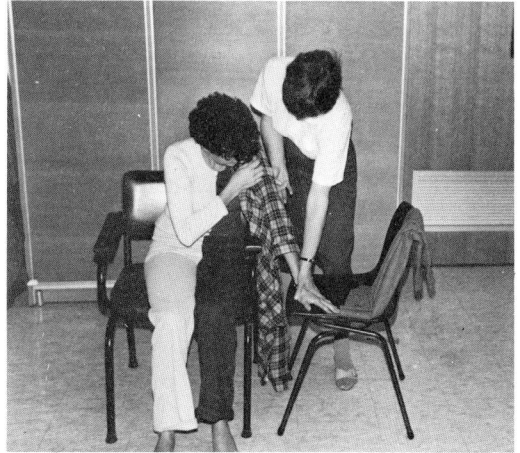

(d)

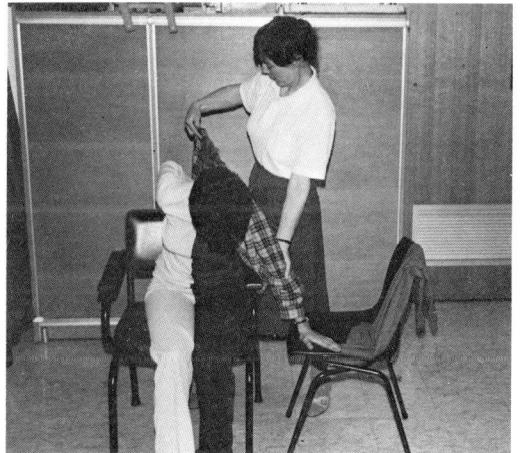

(e)

Fig. 6.19 Demonstrating dressing as an activity to promote automatic sitting balance and equilibrium reactions. Weight is taken through the hemiplegic side in R.I.P. Rotational movements are increased by the placement of the clothes, and visual attention and peripheral stimulation are maximized on the hemiplegic side.

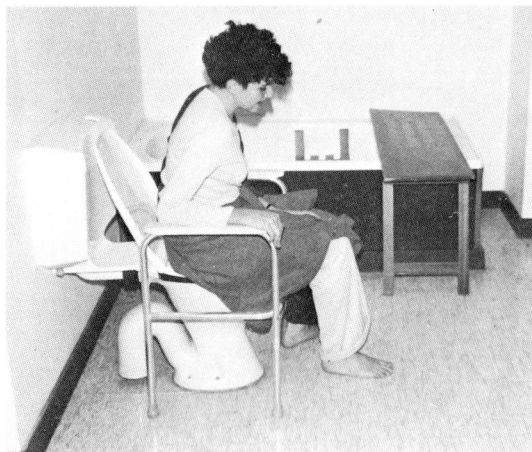

(a)

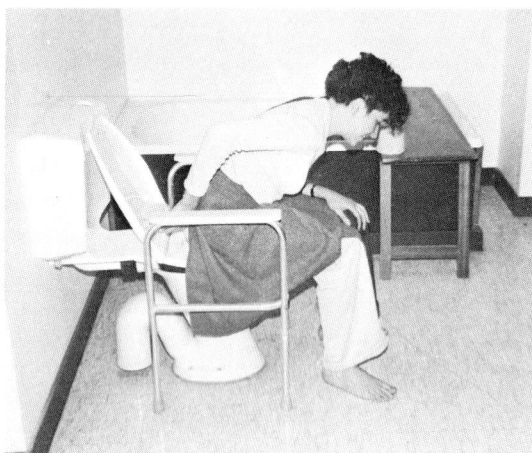

(b)

Fig. 6.20 (a) When balance is grossly impaired, initial use of a lavatory may encourage weight over sound limbs by asymmetrical foot position, graded to (b) Feet symmetrically placed, forward rather than lateral flexion being suggested when the patient uses toilet paper.

be necessary. If patients continue to have balance problems when unable to use vision, alternative methods may have to be recommended, such as repositioning a shower head or making sure a light is available and usable by the patient for night care activities.

2. Activities in standing

(a) Symmetrical standing

Balance in standing activities may also start early

in treatment. Unless the patient is to be manually transferred from bed to chair to wheelchair, standing will be a necessary part of the patient's functional mobility. Nor is sitting balance a necessary prerequisite for standing, practice in both being needed for the patient to redevelop good control over either position.

To stand up at a table, patients may support their forearms on the table with both hands in the midline, and lean forward over the table, supporting weight on the forearms. When the buttocks are off the seat, the patient pushes up on the arms and hands (Fig. 6.21). To sit down the procedure is reversed.

Patients may stand at a window, with a suitable rail for them to hold, whilst being encouraged to orient themselves and to visually scan the environment, locating and naming objects, buildings etc. that they see. The therapist stands either behind or on the hemiplegic side, so that the patient's vision is unobscured, supporting as necessary for safety. The patient is assisted with gentle swaying, bilateral weightbearing and correct joint alignment at hip, knee and ankle.

(b) Trunk and upper limb movement

The patient may stand to perform an activity. Work tables should be high enough for a comfortable working position. Therapists may use manual contact to emphasize symmetrical posture, as in Figure 6.22(a); applying approximation through the hips with the heel of the hand as weight is taken through the hemiplegic lower limb, all joints correctly aligned, as in Figure 6.22(b), and controlling unstable joints by positioning of body, legs and hands as the patient moves during activity, as in Figure 6.22(c).

Standing activity with application to home requirements should be used in treatment, including those which may be safety hazards, such as ironing (Fig. 6.23), making a cup of tea, cooking a meal, showering, or mopping a wet floor (Fig. 6.24). Support, peripheral and cortical input should be graded from virtually moving with the patient to facilitate smooth normal action, stimulating, cueing, and prompting to promote success, to simply observation of independent balanced activity.

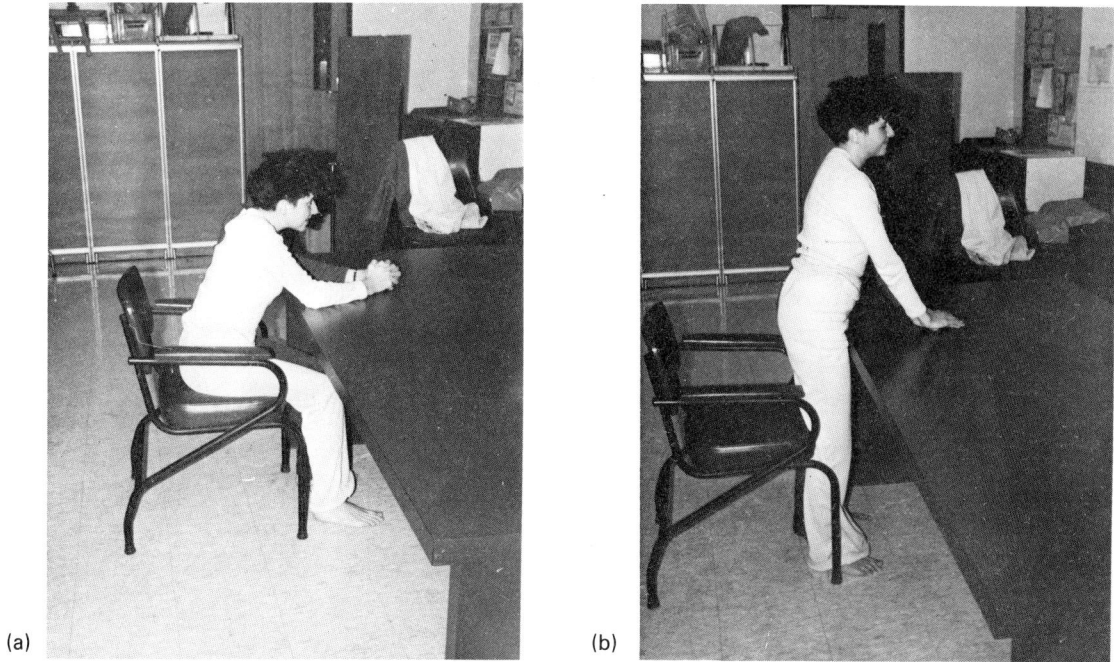

(a) (b)

Fig. 6.21 Symmetrical standing using a table for support and to promote forward leaning as a necessary step to standing.

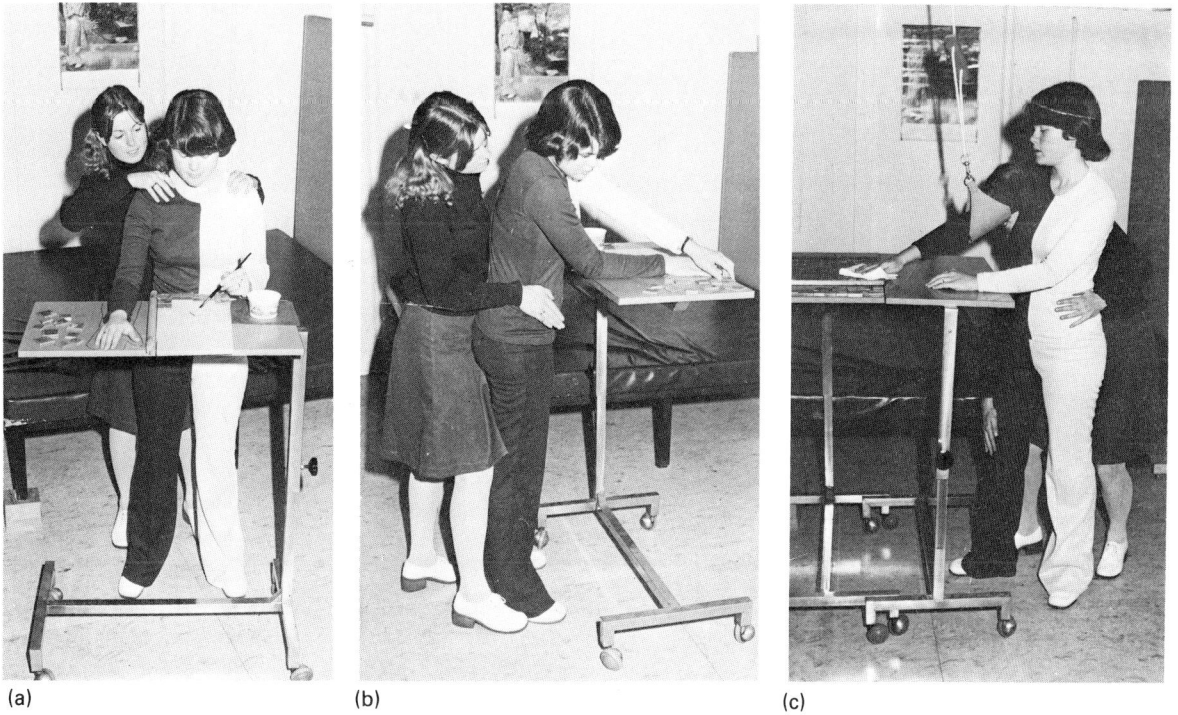

(a) (b) (c)

Fig. 6.22 (a) Manual contact to encourage symmetrical standing. (b) Providing proprioceptive input through lower limb approximation, as weight is transferred in the normal course of activity. (c) Control of unstable joints as the patient transfers weight during activity.

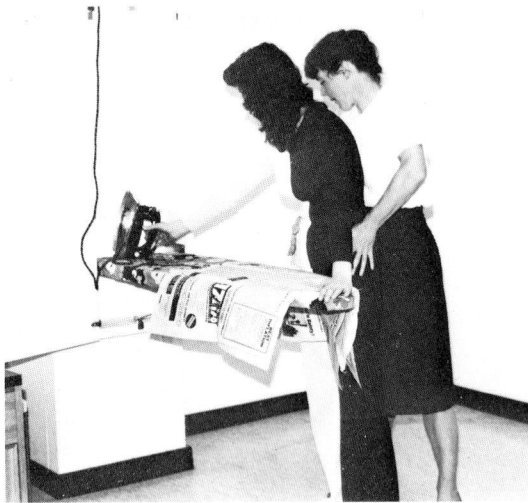

(a)

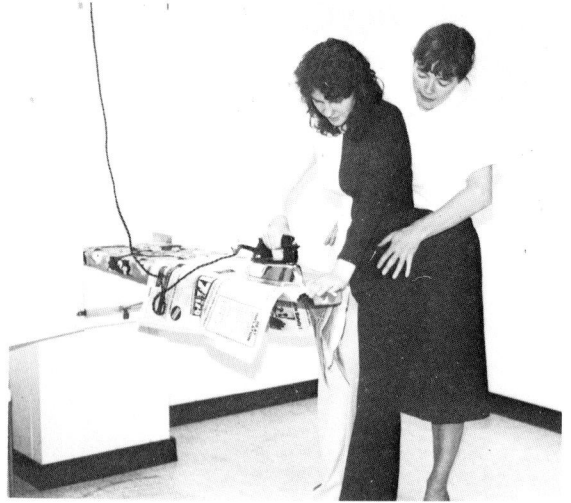

(b)

Fig. 6.23 Standing activities required in the home, such as ironing, need assistance and practice. The newspaper on the ironing board covers a wax batik, an alternative when domestic duties do not appeal to the patient.

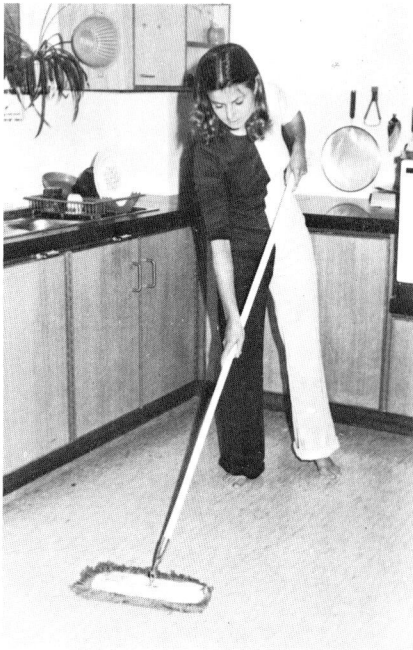

Fig. 6.24 Practice of potentially dangerous standing activities, such as mopping a wet floor, should be supervised.

3. Functional activity incorporating position changes

Carr and Shepherd (1982) suggest that 'balance training should not be considered as separate from training in everyday activities' and that it should 'enable the learner to regain the dynamic components necessary for each individual function'.

(a) Dressing and personal care

It is suggested that instead of trying to decrease balance requirements, in this approach it is useful to look for activities which require position changes, and postural adjustments, and use them in treatment. Dressing and personal care tasks are obvious choices, if components to increase balance requirements are utilized, rather than finding ways to compensate for impairment.

Putting on 'over feet' garments may be particularly demanding even if some of the task is performed sitting down, as bending, rotation, alternate weight bearing, sitting and standing, are all required. The amount of assistance given by the therapist will be dependent on patient ability. In Figure 6.25 the patient's balance and movement patterns are controlled and assisted by the therapist, whilst in Figure 6.26 the patient puts on socks and trousers with mainly verbal cueing from

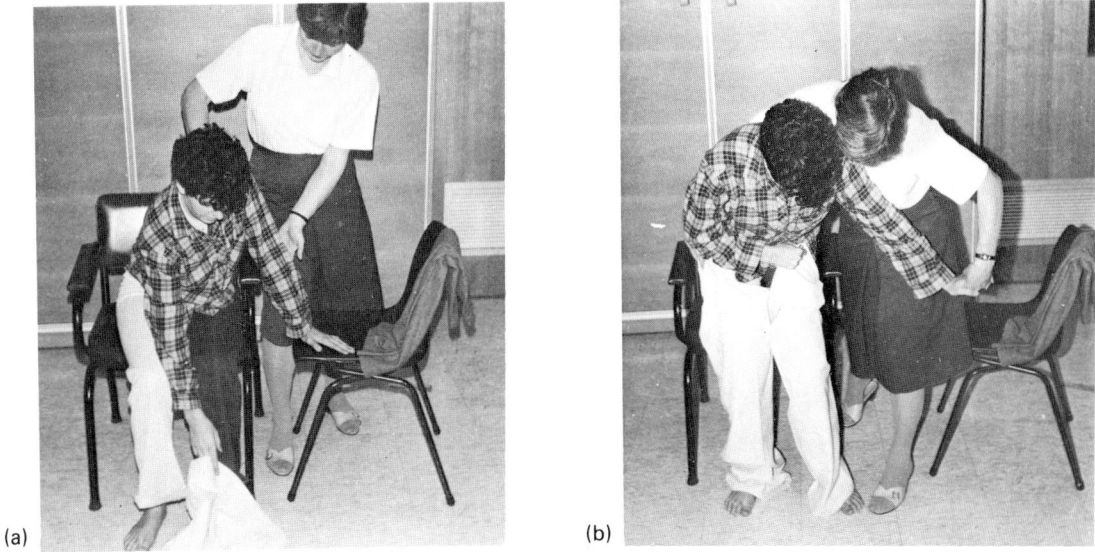

(a)   (b)

Fig. 6.25 Early balance in forward leaning and standing are controlled by the therapist.

the therapist, who stands to the hemiplegic side to ensure patient safety.

If patients are unable to bend far enough, to reach their feet without overbalancing, the therapist may downgrade the demands by using a footstool to raise the foot level as in Figure 6.27, or have the patient cross legs to raise the foot level, as in Figure 6.28. A hemiplegic leg may slip off the sound knee unless it is higher than the pelvis.

Therapists may also promote forward balance prior to the activity, by encouraging the patient to lean forward to the point of 'loss of balance' with one or two hands (upper limb in extension) being supported and/or resisted by the therapist, as in Figure 6.29.

Adjusting clothing when using the lavatory is another demanding balance activity.

Jay (1979) suggests for women, that legs should be apart, that panties should be pulled down, not too far, and that the back and sides of the skirts should be tucked into the waistband or belt. Panties should be readjusted before the skirt.

For men, braces kept hooked over the arm are recommended.

Elastic waisted slacks such as those of track or leisure suits may be suitable garments to recommend for early retraining purposes, both for men and women. They have several advantages: the elastic waistband clings to parted legs during getting on and up from the lavatory, and may be pulled up quite easily with one hand, without too much effort, so that stress and subsequent loss of balance, or detrimental changes in tone, are minimized.

Getting in and out of a bath in a normal manner is one of the most difficult personal care, balance tasks. Progressing through several position changes, in a limited amount of space, and on a slippery surface, is an impossible task for many stroke patients. However, for some who experience good progressive recovery of sensory motor function, this activity may be appropriate for balance retraining, initially using a bathboard, and aiming towards using a bath normally. Repetitive practice in a bath, with a non-slip mat, and without water is recommended.

(b) Getting into a car

Getting into and out of a car also makes high demands on postural adjustment and balance, and is a desirable activity for many patients, whether they will drive again or be passengers only. For those who reach a high level of postural stability and adjustment, helping the patient to motor memorize the usual timing and sequence of getting

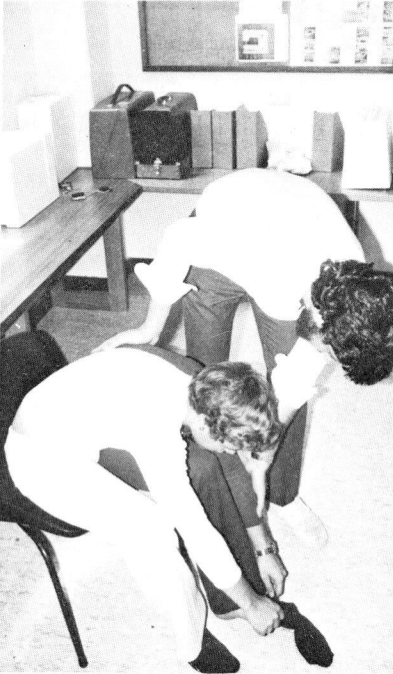

(a)

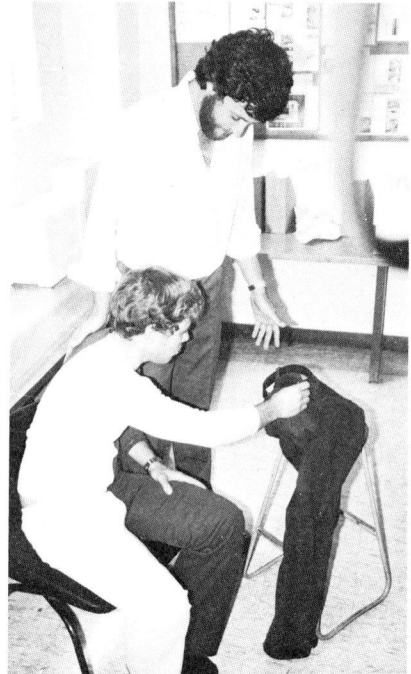

(b)

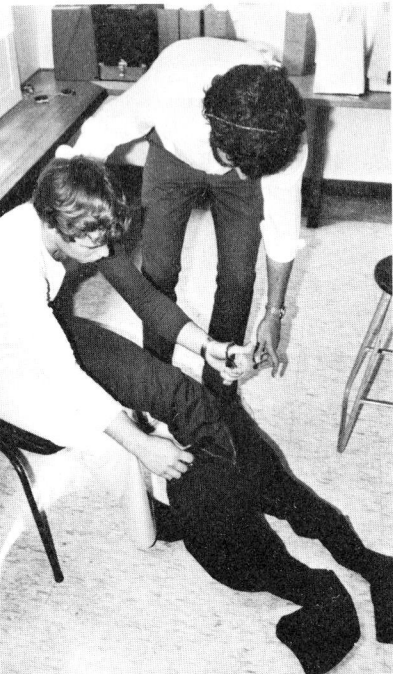

(c)

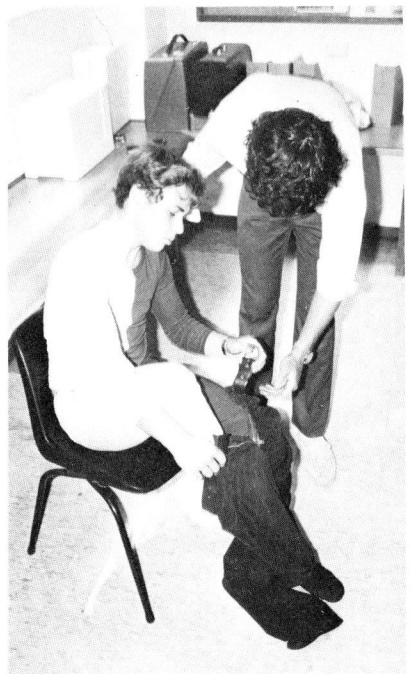

(d)

Fig. 6.26 Putting on socks and trousers in a normal sequence of movement supervised by the therapist. The patient will need to stand to complete the task.

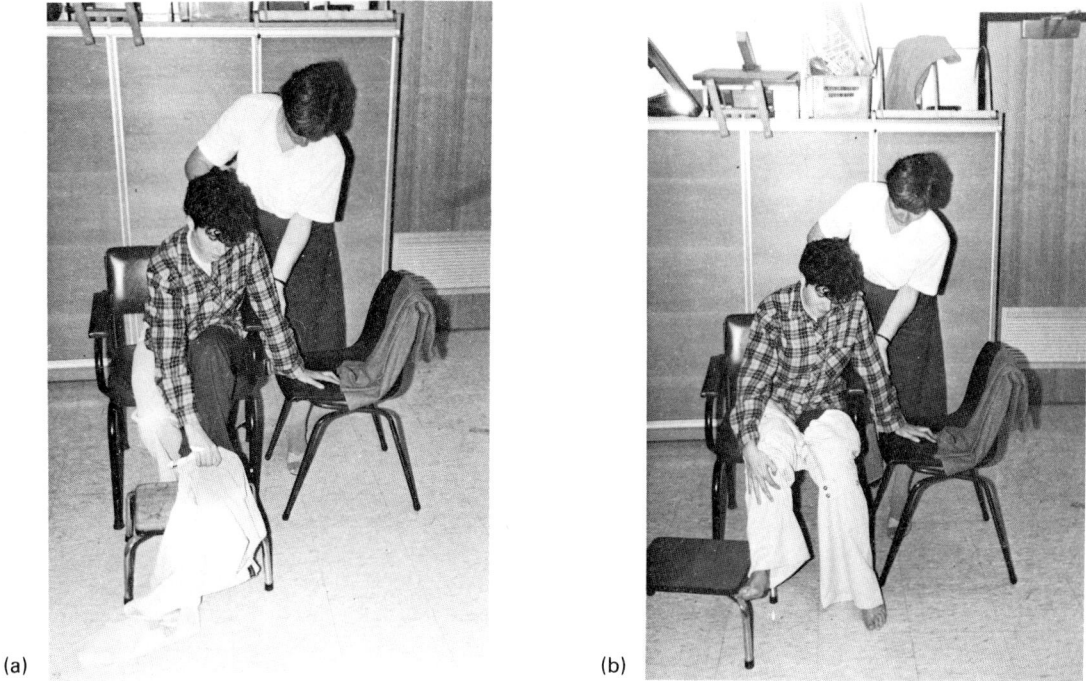

(a)

(b)

Fig. 6.27 Balance demands of forward flexion reduced by using a footstool.

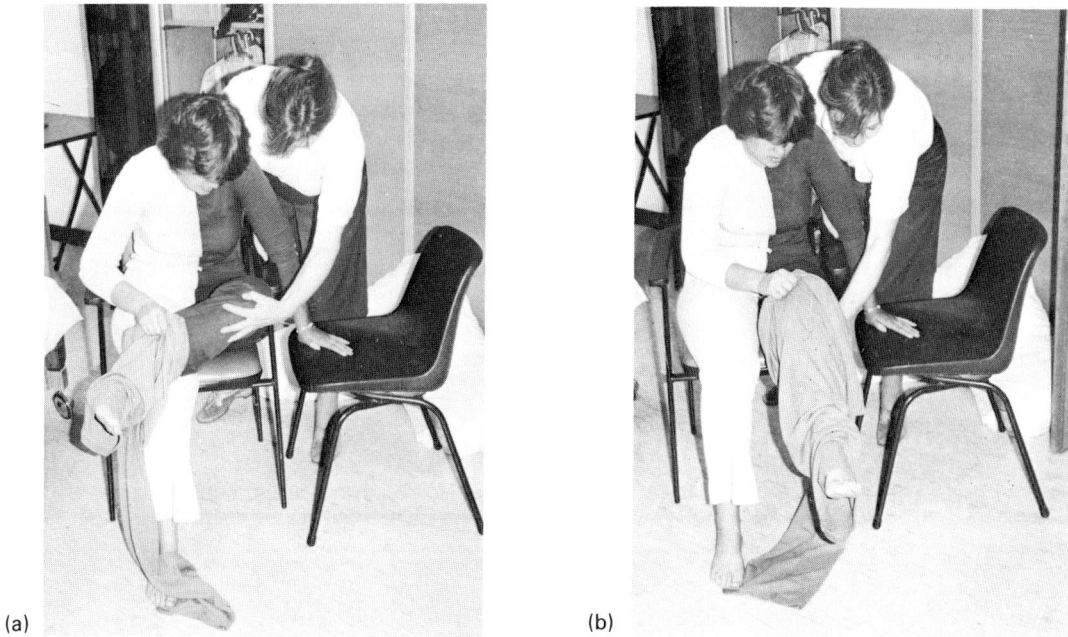

(a)

(b)

Fig. 6.28 Balance demands of forward flexion reduced by the patient crossing the hemiplegic leg. Help may be needed initially, as the leg may slip off unless higher than the pelvis.

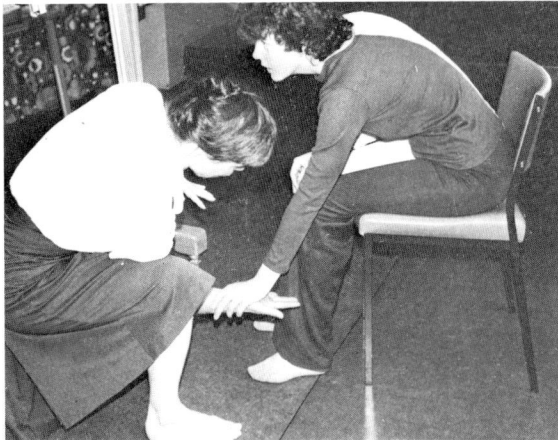

(a)

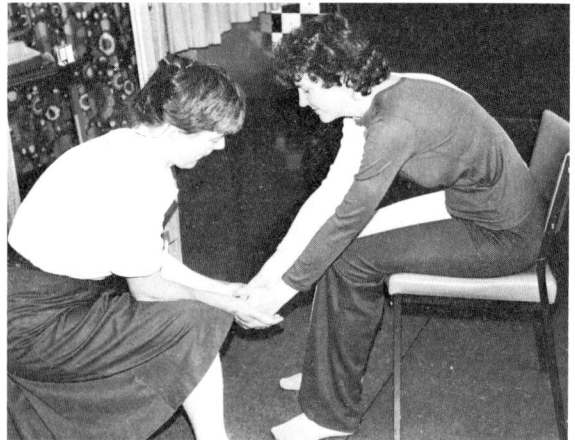

(b)

Fig. 6.29 Promotion of forward balance, prior to overleg dressing activity, by support or resistance to the point of balance (a) unilaterally and, (b) bilaterally.

into a car will be helpful (Fig. 6.30). Demonstration and verbal cueing may be helpful.

(c) Workshop and recreational activities

Workshop and recreational activities may also be used as retraining modalities for balance, particularly when aiming at automatic adjustments, necessary for successful and 'normal' task completion. Suitable treatment activities require repetitive and rhythmical weight transference such as planing (Fig. 6.31), leaning over and weight bearing through the hemiplegic limbs, as when using a jigsaw (Fig. 6.32), and tasks which alternate bilateral and unilateral lower limb weight bearing, such as using a printing press (Fig. 6.33), or the one handed vice (Fig 6.34). Activities of significance to the patient which demand good control of balance should be introduced, whenever possible, into the program, such as in Figure 6.35, where sideways transfer of weight is assisted during 'putting' practice.

In later stages, use of community resources, such as the Horse Riding for the Disabled organisation, recreational club facilities or commercial enterprises, such as ten pin bowling alleys, may be appropriate.

For patients with a background of different cultural practice, care should be taken to try to meet daily living balance needs. An example that springs readily to mind is of people who have meals sitting on, or low to, the ground.

(d) Walking

Techniques taught by the physiotherapist should be reinforced and practised during functional activity.

Therapeutic rationale for functional balance retraining:

- It is motivating and understandable to patients because it is related to real problems.
- It is gradeable by patient ability, rather than predetermined progression.
- It can include rotation and reflex-inhibiting patterns according to choice of activity.
- It is individually tailored, and only limited by the level of recovery reached.
- Functional skills increase as balance improves, without transfer of training.
- It can incorporate functional perceptual and cognitive retraining.
- Early lower limb weight bearing is thought helpful to bladder and bowel continence.

PROPRIOCEPTIVE AND TACTILE SENSORY LOSS

Motor problems will be compounded by proprio-

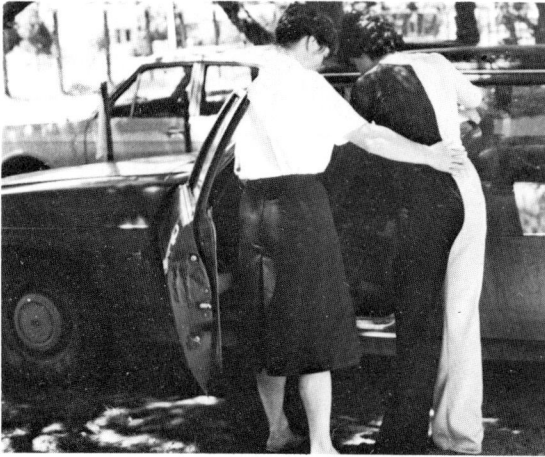

(a)

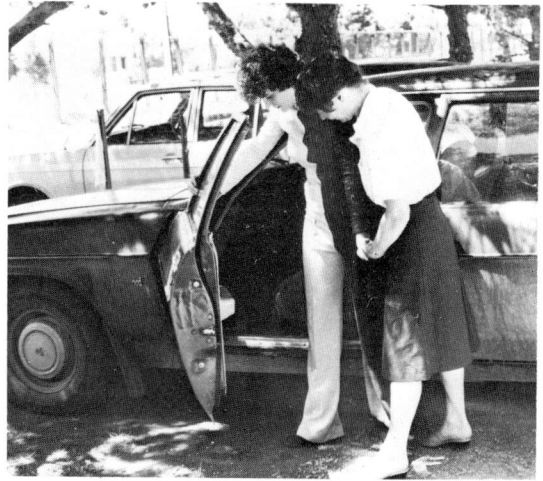

(b)

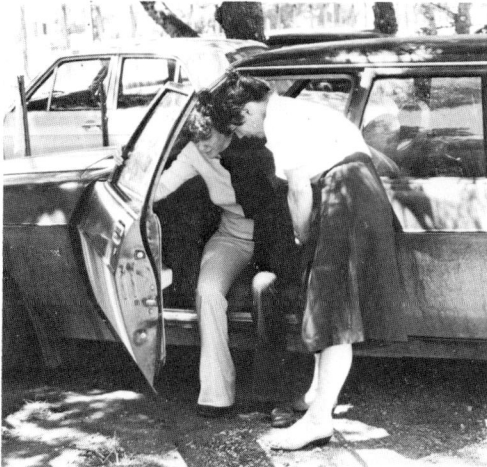

(c)

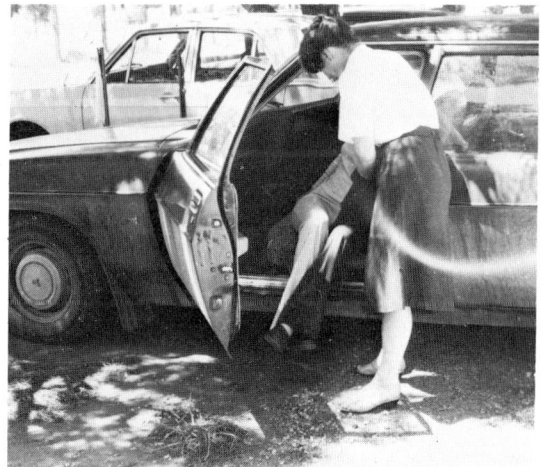

(d)

Fig. 6.30 Getting into a car — helping the patient to motor memory the normal sequence of managing door, turning, and sitting.

ceptive and tactile sensory loss, and a poorer prognosis is likely. The approaches described earlier may be used with increased but controlled sensory input. Therapists should be prepared to try different sensory modalities, vestibular, tactile, proprioceptive, kinesthetic, visual, and auditory, in a systematic way, observing patient responses, asking for patient awareness and concentration on inputs, and consulting them about what they feel is most effective. Observations should be for immediate or delayed responses.

Direct peripheral stimulation may be used, or activities may be chosen or adapted, so that tactual input is increased and demanding, for example, different fibres may be combined in a weaving project, or interchangeable covers of different textures may be used on tool handles or table surfaces.

The position in which the patient works is also important, as proprioceptive input, using weight bearing or manual approximation should be encouraged, which should be dynamic, changing as the patient rotates or moves.

Patient awareness of position, and self-initiated

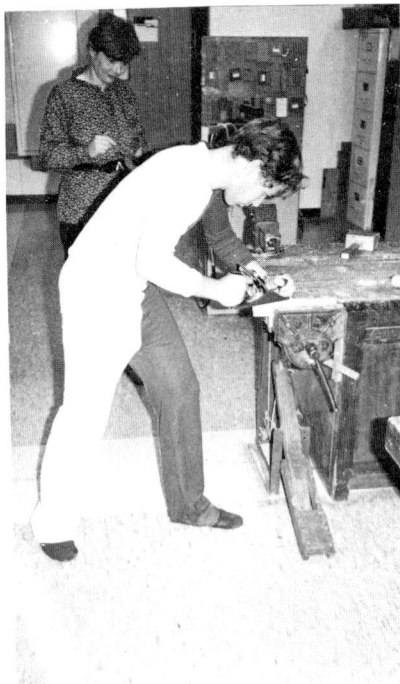

Fig. 6.31 Planing timber for repetitive, rhythmical weight transference.

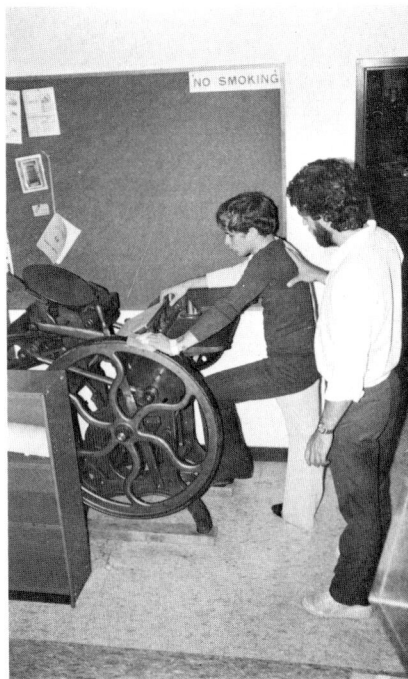

Fig. 6.33 Bilateral, alternating weight bearing or controlled movement of lower limbs.

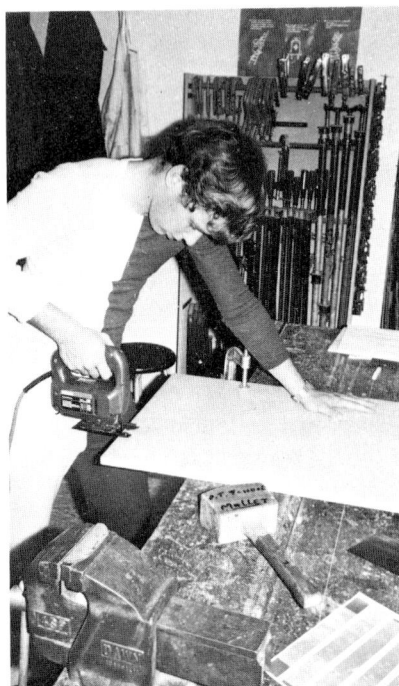

Fig. 6.32 Leaning and weight bearing through hemiplegic limbs using workshop tools.

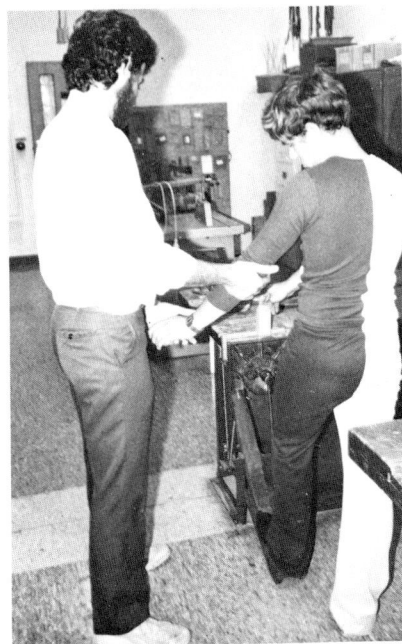

Fig. 6.34 Using an adapted vice in which leg movement is used instead of hand movement to close the jaws on the work (adapted from a vice designed at Queen Elizabeth Hospital, Adelaide).

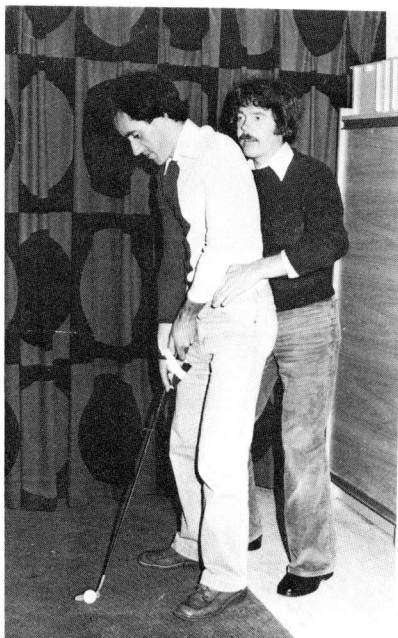

Fig. 6.35 'Putting' practice to encourage weight transference and relevant balance retraining.

position changes, should be promoted, plus encouragement to look at and touch the hemiplegic side. Activities such as skin care may be useful for this purpose.

INCONTINENCE

Incontinence of bladder and bowel may cause psycho-social problems for patients, resulting in shame, anxiety, and depression. It may disrupt rehabilitation programs but should not be the cause of withholding treatment, or only commencing retraining when control is regained. Facilities in case of emergency should be available (even the smallest departments can have a commode and curtain) and if accidents occur they should be dealt with quickly and quietly by the treating therapist.

Carr and Shepherd (1982) suggest that early standing and mobility assists patients to regain control over these functions.

If the patient is catheterised, and confusion is a complication, it is wise to make sure that the patient does not interfere with, or pull at, the catheter. It is also important to make sure that equip-

ment is safe when transferring or moving the patient during treatment procedures.

COMPENSATORY APPROACHES

Complete recovery of balance and pre-stroke mobility is not achieved by all patients. This is particularly true for patients with gross dysfunction, who are discharged early to dependent care (see Ch. 10), but is also true of many patients who return home.

For these latter it is necessary to look at safe, effective methods of compensation and adaptation for tasks they need or want to do. Occupational therapists should help to devise methods to suit individual requirements, and, most importantly, help patients practise these regularly in the treatment setting, and at home. It is not enough to advise on alternative methods, for the habits of years are hard to replace. Motor memory patterns need to be built for new ways of doing things, particularly when the patient is faced with a home environment set up to facilitate the old methods, and to jog older motor memory traces.

Generally an adaptive approach to poor balance and gross mobility will mean, in many cases, mobility support such as a four point stick, and adequate training in how to use such support; sitting instead of standing to tasks of daily living, such as those of personal care and food preparation; practice in pre-planning and simplification of tasks; emphasis on safety considerations and careful alteration of the environment to satisfy both patient needs, and those of others living with them.

If sensory impairment does not improve, it may be necessary to teach compensation for cutaneous sensory loss. Patients are taught routinely and repetitively to visually locate, and if necessary adjust the position of extremities. This may be an extremely important procedure, particularly if neglect, visual inattention, or memory impairment complicate the problem of sensory loss. Even when tackled with the utmost diligence, including involving the patient cognitively in the visual compensation, success may be limited, particularly at times when the patient's attention is attracted to another focus. This implies that compensatory training should commence during simple activity, in a distraction free environment, and progress to include those situations a patient may have to cope with in the home or future environments.

Methods

1. Mobility

The occupational therapist needs to reinforce, during retraining in compensatory daily living skills, the method of walking taught by the physiotherapist. As the patient moves about, thinking and concentrating on the task in hand, safety rules and walking techniques may be forgotten unless prompted and corrected whenever necessary. Eventually this may lead to automatic safe mobility. The occupational therapist should consider and make patients aware of where the walking aid should be positioned during tasks, and methods of transferring objects from place to place should be devised.

A sling to support the hemiplegic arm will assist balance and safety, particularly when the arm remains flaccid, (see Fig. 5.5 & 5.6). Standing and sitting with weight over the sound side may be the technique of choice, to prevent falls during position changes. Walking with a slight lean to the sound side may also be advisable. This does not mean the hemiplegic side should be neglected. Attention should still be given to increasing patient awareness of the position of hemiplegic limbs, at all times.

Ongoing education about hazards such as floor surfaces, rugs, loose obtruding objects, and unstable furniture within different environments, should be an integral part of the program. Regular group discussion time may provide a suitable setting for shared ideas and experience to reinforce individual learning.

Despite the most careful safety program, some patients will fall, and training in getting up from the floor should always be included prior to discharge home. A technique which utilizes furniture to compensate for lack of balance and mobility is usually suitable. Patients are taught to roll into side sitting, weight on the sound arm, and to move to a solid piece of furniture such as a bed or sofa; to push down on the furniture with the sound arm until up on both knees; to bend the sound knee forwards and upwards, to a kneel stand position; and push down on the hand whilst straightening the sound knee, gradually coming to a flexed standing position as the hemiplegic leg straightens. The patient should turn and sit on the bed or sofa gently, whilst breath and composure are regained

Some patients, or their relatives, may ask advice about wheelchairs for use around the home and community. A visit to an Aids Centre to try out various types is recommended, as wheelchairs are expensive, and often found to be less useful than expected.

2. Sitting, rather than standing to tasks

Using a bathboard over a bath may continue to be necessary. Patients may use a hand held shower attached to bath taps, or sponge themselves, if there is no shower over the bath. A non-slip bathmat must be used and 'soap on a rope', or soap in a pocketed mitten (or similar device) are suggested, to save the necessity of bending to find lost soap, as it escapes from grasp into the bath. Judiciously placed rails, soundly plugged to the walls, are likely to be useful.

If a separate shower is available, a permanent plastic chair, stool, or commode type seat may be used, or a let down seat may be fixed to a wall. Rails correctly positioned may assist getting in and out of the shower seat. Adjustment of water heat is important and should be done prior to getting into the shower, if thermostatic control is not available, or if the shower head is not easily adjusted. A hand held shower nozzle may replace a fixed head; water heat is adjusted before being aimed at the body. Non-slip mats in and out of the shower are necessary, and 'soap handling devices' are recommended.

Some patients may feel safer sitting at the wash basin (Jay, 1979), sponging rather than using bath or shower. A large, absorbent bath mat should be placed under the chair to prevent a wet, slippery floor, and patients should be taught not to use the basin to take body weight. Everything necessary should be within reach. To prevent unnecessary dressing and undressing, this may be carried out in the bathroom before going to bed, or after early morning personal care. Provision for collecting dirty clothing for laundry, and for hanging clothes to be worn, should be considered if there is sufficient space.

One sided dressing may be performed when sitting, using either hip hitching or occasional standing for clothing adjustment. In exteme cases dressing may be safer in bed. If temporary occlusion of vision causes problems, clothes which are put on over the head may be contra-indicated.

To use the lavatory, rails will be needed. A raised platform toilet seat with arms may be a useful alternative, if it is difficult to fix rails, and if the extra height helps the patient to get up or down, or if extra width helps with sideways safety. Position of toilet paper may need consideration, and adapted clothing may be advisable.

Meal preparation may be done sitting in a chair, or on a stool, and activities which may be safety hazards should be practised frequently, for example, taking dishes from the oven. Alternative table top cooking appliances may be recommended, such as an electric frypan, or small table oven, so that stooping is avoided and hot dishes may be placed easily on the table.

Depending on the home-maker status of the patient, that is whether living alone, likely to be a major worker in the kitchen, or simply a helper, rearrangement of equipment to eliminate unnecessary movement may be considered.

3. Lifestyle modification

House cleaning and maintenance is likely to pose extreme difficulties for those with poor mobility and balance, and should be considered specifically for each individual. Safe positioning, choice of equipment, elimination of unnecessary tasks, pre-planning and help in making use of local agencies who may assist with household tasks, are all aspects the occupational therapist should talk over with the patient and/or family. Opportunity for repetitive practice of those tasks considered by the patient to be necessary priorities should be offered.

Structured discussion groups to share problem-solving ideas, with participation of involved relatives, is recommended, followed by practical 'try outs' of ideas generated.

All aspects of the patient's proposed lifestyle may need consideration and modification, should balance and mobility remain a problem.

Therapeutic rationale for an adaptive approach:
- Is required by many patients prior to discharge from rehabilitation.
- Promotes maintenance of self-esteem and morale, by providing a means for patients to continue doing necessary tasks independently.
- Allows the patient to be relatively safe in mobility from an early date.
- Is time efficient.
- May include cortical and peripheral stimulation, such as positioning an arm in a reflex-inhibiting pattern to stabilise objects, and cognitive awareness of safe positions and care for the hemiplegic side.
- Other techniques have not been proven more effective in the long term.

REFERENCES

Carr J, Shepherd R 1980 Physiotherapy in disorders of the Brain. Heinemann Medical Books Ltd, London
Carr J, Shepherd R 1982 A motor relearning programme for stroke. Heinemann Medical Books Ltd, London
Beevor C 1951 Croonian lectures in muscular movement delivered in 1903, In: Brain. McMillan Co, New York
Brunnstrom S 1970 Movement therapy in hemiplegia, a neurophysiological approach. Harper and Row, New York
Jay P 1979 Help yourselves, a handbook for hemiplegics and their families, 3rd edn. Ian Henry Publications, Essex

RECOMMENDED READING

Carr J, Shepherd R 1982 A motor relearning programme for stroke. Heinemann Medical Books Ltd, London
Jay P 1979 Help yourselves, a handbook for hemiplegics and their families, 3rd edn. Ian Henry Publications, Essex
Johnstone M 1978 Restoration of motor function in the stroke patient, a physiotherapist's approach. Churchill Livingstone, Edinburgh

7

When upper limb retraining is a priority

INTRODUCTION

Unless the stroke is caused by an infarct of the anterior cerebral artery, the upper limb is usually affected more severely than the lower limb.

The manipulative role of the upper limb, in contrast to the supporting, weight-bearing and transferring role of the lower limb, requires much greater recovery to achieve close to normal ability. The close association between hand skills and praxic, perceptual and cognitive abilities affects the extent to which the hand may be used during and after retraining, and the importance of finely discriminative sensory ability for useful hand function complicates rehabilitation.

Sensory re-education is a prime consideration during all aspects of upper limb retraining, and the tactual sensory characteristics of activities must be considered at all times, and increased if necessary.

Upper limb retraining should not be isolated from redeveloping total person abilities and skills. Presentation is separate for the purpose of clarity.

A patient who requires either hand for support will be unable to make use of them in skilled movement. In order to develop dexterity and manipulative skills, the patient needs to be balanced, to control head movement, to have proximal stability, to be able to move from one position to another, and be aware of bilaterality. If any of these are impaired, patients will be inhibited in the use of free movement, excess strain may result, effort may be increased, and patients will be unable to respond naturally to activity and environmental input.

Balance, proximal stability, movement, and position changes are important aspects of treatment in preparation for upper limb skill development.

Control of the trunk in balanced sitting or standing, achieved through either developmental or functional retraining procedures, will leave the arms and hands free to move. Without stability at the shoulder, controlled, safe movement of the arm, to position the hand for tasks will be impossible.

Impairment of cutaneous and proprioceptive sensation, limits both input and feedback for selection, regulation and control of movement. Compensation by vision is necessary, an inadequate substitute, which causes objects to be gripped too hard, or not enough, and multifocus activity to be nearly impossible. Proprioceptive and tactile sensory loss need early treatment. Weight bearing, deep pressure and resistance to movement, plus cutaneous sensory input should be used appropriately. The personal care activities suggested whilst the patient is still bed or ward bound, are very appropriate for this purpose, and these should be continued, upgraded, and refined with skill development throughout treatment.

Visuo-spatial sensation and perception need to be intact in order for the patient to fully redevelop upper limb, goal-directed activity, and retraining may very well incorporate aspects of sensory motor retraining with perceptual motor retraining.

FLACCIDITY

Research indicates that patients demonstrating prolonged hypotonus have a poor prognosis for motor recovery (Gersten, 1975). When flaccid hemiplegia persists, authorities agree that a major aim of treatment is to increase (normalize) tone.

Flaccid limbs are prone to damage, so safety is the other prime treatment consideration. Joints are unstable and unprotected by surrounding musculature, and subluxation of the shoulder is not uncommon (refer to Ch. 5). Another complication may be shoulder-hand syndrome, also called causalgia, or reflex dystrophy, when the patients experience pain in the shoulder, and oedema, pain and vasomotor changes in the hand (Cailliet, 1981). Treatment of this includes encouragement of movement at the shoulder and hand despite pain, and reduction of oedema through elevation,

manipulative activity, and pressure distal to proximal. Relaxation may be useful, especially if the patient is experiencing pain which inhibits participation in treatment.

Methods to increase tone

1. Sensory stimulation

Trombly (1983) reports that therapists use various sensory stimulation techniques to facilitate motor neuron response, and refers to studies by Matyas and Spicer (1980) who elicited immediate response in muscles stimulated by 15 seconds of fast brushing; and by Sahrmann and Norton (1977) who demonstrated that a combination of stretch and voluntary effort enhanced motor response. Bobath (1978) recommends that stimulation, facilitation and voluntary activity be given to increase tone, plus demanding patient awareness of sensory motor experiences.

Johnstone (1978), who advocates following developmental progression, uses controlled, supervised weight bearing throughout flaccid and spastic stages of hemiplegia. She uses an air pressure splint for proprioceptive input, and to assist joint position and stability.

Before and during activity proprioceptive stimulation by positioning to promote weight bearing and approximation and use of air pressure splints, may be used with cutaneous stimulation such as fast icing, tapping or vibration.

2. Irradiation

Brunnstrom (1970) recommends facilitation of associated reactions in the hemiplegic limb to stimulate movement. A resisted movement of the sound upper limb has been found to evoke the same movement in the hemiplegic limb by a process of irradiation.

For example, therapists may involve patients in activity which resists upper limb movement of the sound side, such as pushing an object away from the body, in order to facilitate synergic extensor movement in the hemiplegic arm. As movement in all the muscles linked in the extensor synergy may be elicited, therapists will need to modify or control unwanted parts of the movement by manual contact and peripheral stimulation. The effects may be influenced by tonic neck reflexes.

Johnstone (1982) suggests that irradiation is assistive to postural reflexes, and supplies sensory stimulation, when using the hemiplegic arm as a prop, during a reaching activity, in which the sound hand and arm cross the midline of the body diagonally. She emphasizes that use of irradiation should be controlled by limbs being positioned in anti-spasm patterns, and that the effects of either upper or lower limb movement be monitored, and considered for effects of irradiation to the hemiplegic side.

Harris (1980) suggests that despite controversy about the use of irradiation, when there is diffuse weakness, it may, by producing an overt response, motivate patients because they observe that movement of hemiplegic limbs is still possible. He advises that local stimulation be selectively superimposed on the synergic movement patterns to facilitate contraction of specific muscles.

3. Self-ranging

Some therapists recommend self-applied range of movement (Pedretti, 1981; Trombly, 1983), but caution against overenthusiasm on the part of the patient which may cause pulling to occur at lax and unsupported joints, such as the shoulder, which may result in rotator cuff injury, subluxation of the shoulder, frozen shoulder, or shoulder-hand syndrome. Because of this, exercise using overhead pulleys is contraindicated.

It is recognised that patients need to be involved in the treatment process, and activity which will not result in damage should be emphasized, plus adequate and appropriate education about why the activities are recommended. Contraindicated activity should also be fully discussed.

Support

Slings (refer to Ch. 5) may be necessary at times when the arm is not being treated, or supported in other ways, to prevent the weighty, floppy arm from causing shoulder damage, particularly when standing or walking.

Arm supports which attach to chair arms (Fig. 5.2c) are suggested as an alternative to slings,

when the patient is sitting (Trombly, 1983). Arm supports are usually gutter shaped for the forearm, with the hand section flat, inclined, shaped as a functional resting splint, or incorporating a cone shape, the widest part to the ulnar side of the hand (Pedretti, 1981).

ACTIVITY TO ENCOURAGE UPPER LIMB EXTENSION

Duing retraining procedures used in the ward, the hemiplegic upper limb is shown being maintained in total or partial extension, to inhibit reflex flexor tone from dominating movement patterns. Peripheral stimulation applied by the therapist or patient is used in conjunction with reflex-inhibiting patterns, to encourage weak extensor muscles, so that more normal balance between flexors and extensors is promoted. This approach may be continued in the rehabilitation unit, in sitting or standing activities which emphasize extension of the upper limb.

Methods

1. Passive positioning

The hand and arm should be positioned in total or partial extension at all times, when not involved in activity processes. Visual cueing, such as an outline hand and arm on the table top (Fig. 7.1), may help patients to maintain upper limb extension (Bobath, 1978) when working in activity with the sound hand. Peripheral and cortical input may be used to facilitate relaxation of the flexors and/or activity of the extensors, should increased tone be evident.

2. Weight bearing

Johnstone (1978) considers upper limb weight bearing as a prerequisite for voluntary controlled finger extension. Extension of wrist and arm is encouraged whether the limb is hypertonic or hypotonic. Using the hand and arm to prop is inherent in the developmental positions, but it may also be used as a stabilizer or prop during activities in sitting or standing (Fig. 7.2).

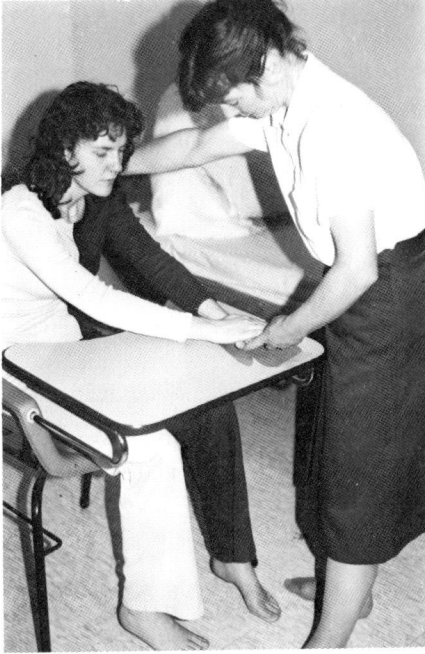

Fig. 7.1 An outlined hand and arm on the table top to cue patients about upper limb position.

3. Effects of gravity

Activity in standing may make use of gravity to assist extension of the arm, provided weak shoulder musculature is given appropriate support. When voluntary, but limited shoulder movement is possible, this may be used by the patient in activity which calls for extension of the upper limb assisted by gravity: for example, positioning paper for a screen printing project as shown in Figure 7.3.

4. Activity

Activities may be chosen because of inherent demands for extension of arm and hand, or different techniques may be utilized in selected activity to promote upper limb extension, as shown in Figure 7.4 demonstrating the use of a rolling pin. The finger extension mit (Jones, 1964) used with the rolling pin (Fig. 7.4c), was designed as a file holder, and is a useful aid for extension and abduction of the fingers. It also promotes wrist extension and rhythmical movement of the hemi-

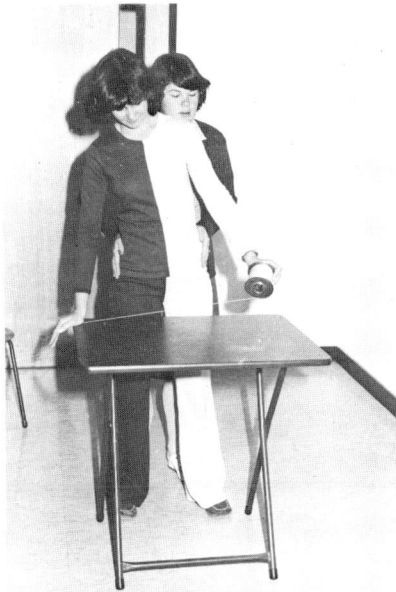

Fig. 7.2 Hand arm being used to prop and stabilize materials whilst standing to an activity.

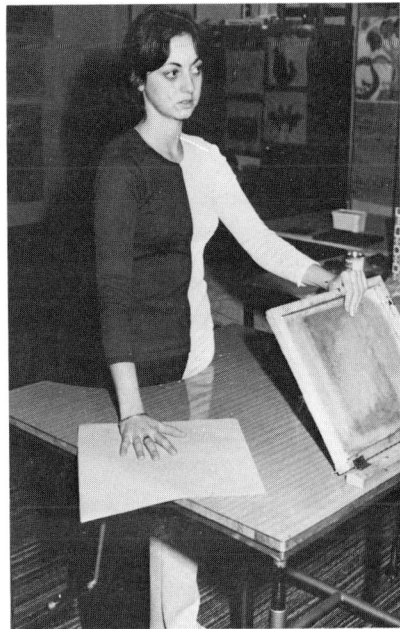

Fig. 7.3 Correct table height provides support to upper limb joints, as gravity assists the patient to maintain extension whilst positioning paper for screen printing.

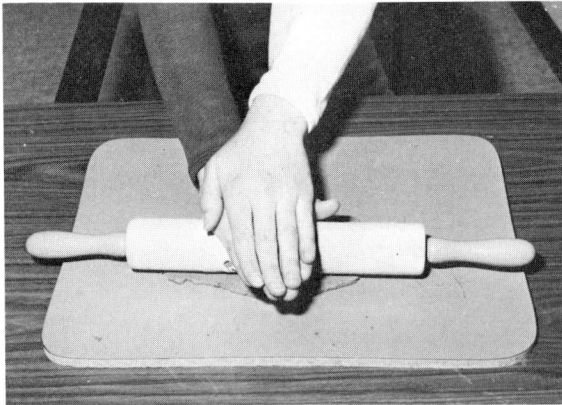

(a)

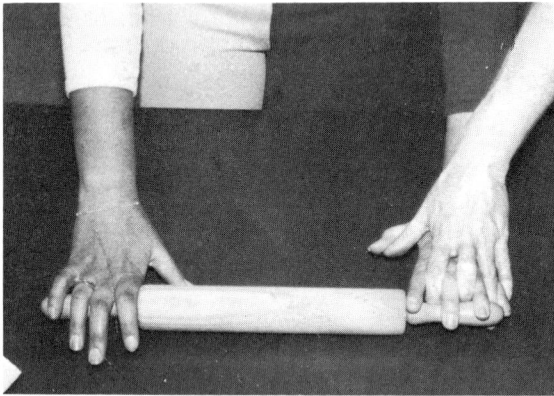

(b)

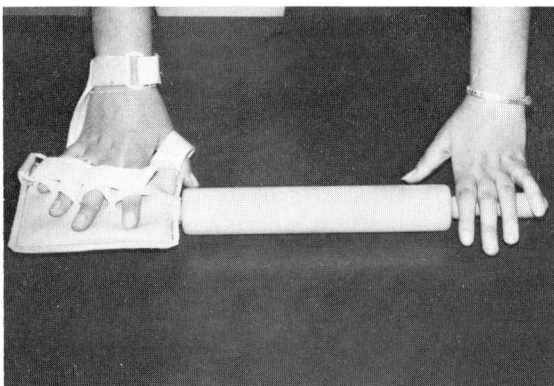

(c)

Fig. 7.4 Use of a rolling pin to encourage movement in upper limb extension. (a) Using the sound hand to help move the rolling pin mainly under the fingers, and avoiding the palmar surface. (b) Using a finger abductor grip the therapist assists movement of the hemiplegic arm. (c) Using a finger extensor mit (Jones, 1964).

plegic arm, as it moves in unison with the sound hand guiding the file.

Movement in extension enables patients to experience cortically the feeling of 'semivoluntary' movement rather than reflex movement, and may give patients a boost because they feel in control of the movement. As noted in the previous section, activity which demands active-resisted extension of the sound side is likely to be facilitatory to extensors of the hemiplegic side (Brunnstrom 1970).

Figure 7.5 illustrates two examples of activity utilizing and assisting extensor movement. In one an adapted squeegee enhances bilateral symmetrical movement, and in the other a flexion mit maintains a patient's continuous grasp of an iron, allowing proximal musculature to guide side-to-side movement. The handle may need building up to provide pressure on muscle insertions to inhibit flexor spasticity in the hand. The material used for building up should be hard, not soft (Dayhoff, 1975; Farber, 1982).

Patients should, when possible, be shown how to apply peripheral stimulation to themselves, in order to facilitate upper limb extension for independent activity, apart from treatment. Tapping is the easiest form of cutaneous input for patients to self-apply, and pictures showing where to tap, plus drawing on the patient's arm may be useful. These will not only supply information about where to apply stimulation, but will also act as a tactual, visual and cognitive reminder of the hemiplegic arm. Washing off the drawing at night, and reapplying in the morning, will be an excellent reinforcer. Non-toxic body paint may be used for this purpose. Tapping in time to a known piece of music may be successful in promoting patient understanding of the need to vary the tapping pace and to only use it for a few moments before a pause.

A.D.L. and activities of significance to the patient's lifestyle may be adapted to decrease demands for upper limb flexion and increase upper limb extension, before being included in retraining.

As voluntary movement increases, activity may be used which gradually introduces flexion of the upper limb; however, occupational therapists should constantly monitor whether the patient can voluntarily relax flexors to achieve extension. If

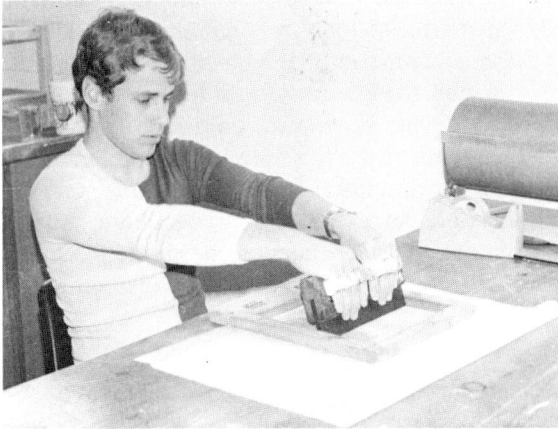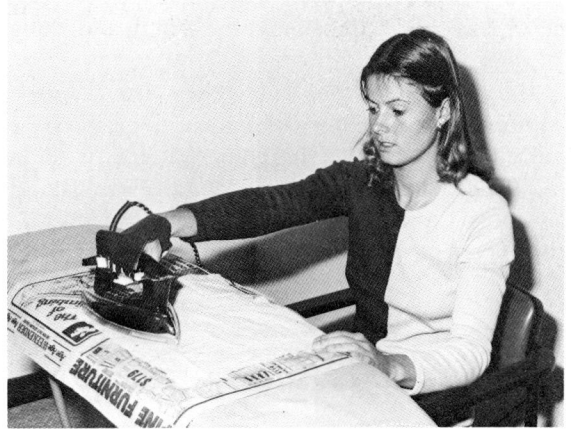

(a)   (b)

Fig. 7.5 (a) Bilateral symmetrical movement utilizing an adapted squeegee. The fingers are separated and held by velcro loops. (b) A flexion mit enables the patient to use proximal musculature to guide side-to-side movement of the extended upper limb. Shoulder elevation should be inhibited.

they are not able to do this, flexion components of the activity should be reduced, or peripherally inhibited, during the task. Alternatively, extensors may be stimulated cutaneously.

Therapeutic rationale for activity in extension:
- Helps to control and modify dominant and restrictive upper limb reflex activity.
- Assists in strengthening weak upper limb extensors.
- Encourages the patient to make functional use of limited movement in a manner thought by many as essential to recovery.
- Promotes awareness of hemiplegic side.
- Provides a basis for further recovery.

USE OF UPPER LIMB SUPPORT MECHANISMS

To promote purposeful use of limited upper limb movement, slings or support mechanisms may be used to maximise movement. Weak contraction of individual muscles may be insufficient to maintain the arm against gravity and move it directionally. As the patient makes more effort, muscles may begin to contract in synergic patterns, which may prevent the achievement of the desired activity, at least in normal sequence and timing. Weak contraction needs assistance, and synergic activity needs control. Suitable support may provide such assistance, minimising the need for patients to put effort into the control of unwanted abnormal movement. Weak isolated muscle contraction about the hand may be used in activity, if the effort of maintaining and moving the whole arm against gravity is reduced.

In many cases recovery of involuntary and voluntary movement returns in a cephalo-caudal direction, that is proximal before distal: however, this is not always the case, some patients experiencing recovery of distal before proximal musculature (Gersten, 1975); for example, involuntary thumb movements may occur before anything else. Patients become very excited over evidence that an apparently paralysed limb is still capable of movement, and it is psychologically important for the therapist to respond positively to the movement experience. Reducing the effort of other parts of the limb by eliminating gravity, cutaneously stimulating the muscle involved in the movement, and restricting possible increased tone which may prevent weak movement, are realistic interventions which should be continued to promote more movement.

The use of overhead slings to eliminate gravity and yet allow the patient's arm and hand to move freely, has decreased in recent years. Slings or other support mechanisms may be of considerable value in allowing patients to make functional use of specific hand movements, which they are unable to do otherwise, because additional control and effort is required to maintain the arm in a working position.

Slings, skateboards, and other arm support equipment may allow the patient to experience movement in a reflex-inhibiting pattern, without dependence upon another person, give mechanical advantage to weak muscle contraction and provide the opportunity to be involved in bilateral activity.

(c) Maintain the shoulder forward and the hand up, so that it may be used as an assistant to the sound hand. Function of the hand is assisted by a dynamic splint (Fig. 7.6c).

Sprung slings, suspended from overhead mesh, may be used to provide forward movement at the hemiplegic shoulder, and the maintenance of upper limb extension against gravity, so that movement of the hand may be used in activity such as the weaving project shown in Figure 7.7.

Methods

1. The 'O.B. Help Arm' may be used to:

(a) Support the hemiplegic arm and wrist, maintaining upper limb extension as the extended hand is used in activity such as rolling clay (Fig. 7.6(a)). Movement is assisted by the sound hand which helps provide rhythmic and relaxing impetus.

(b) Support the forearm and hand, maintaining wrist extension and thumb abduction in gentle trunk rotational activity (Fig. 7.6b), and,

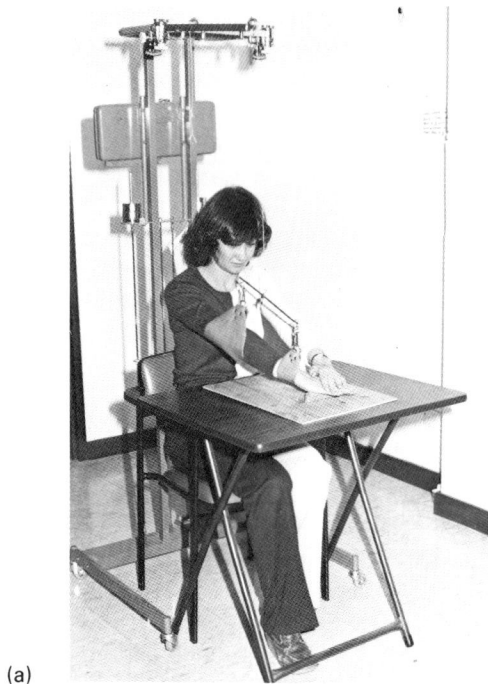

(b)

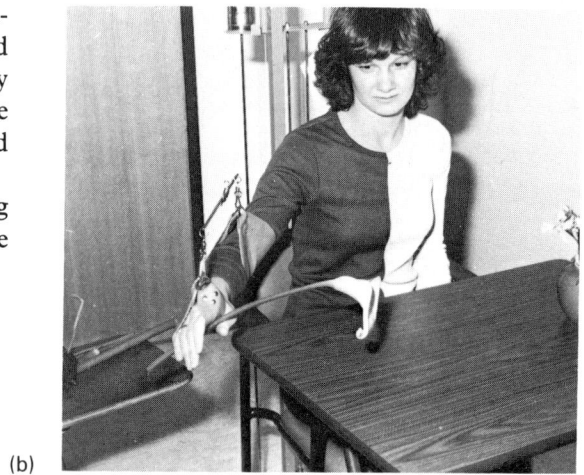

(a)

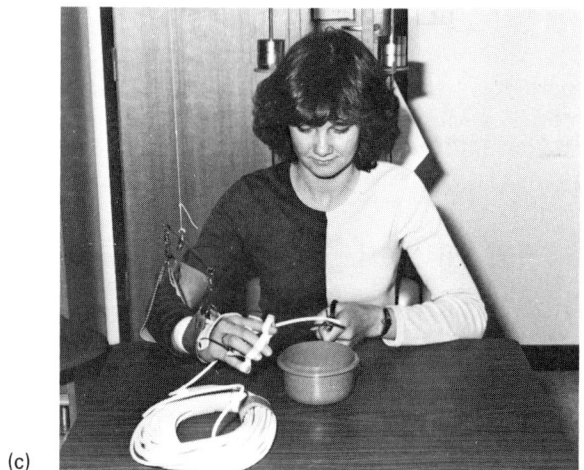

(c)

Fig. 7.6 Use of the O.B. help arm; (a) To support and maintain the upper limb in extension during activity. (b) To support forearm and hand maintaining extension of the wrist and thumb abduction. (c) To maintain hemiplegic limb position as an assistant to the sound hand during activity.

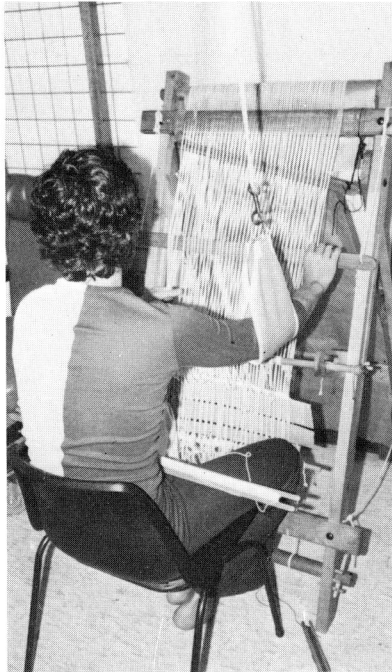

Fig. 7.7 Overhead sling promoting forward movement at the hemiplegic shoulder and support of limb against gravity.

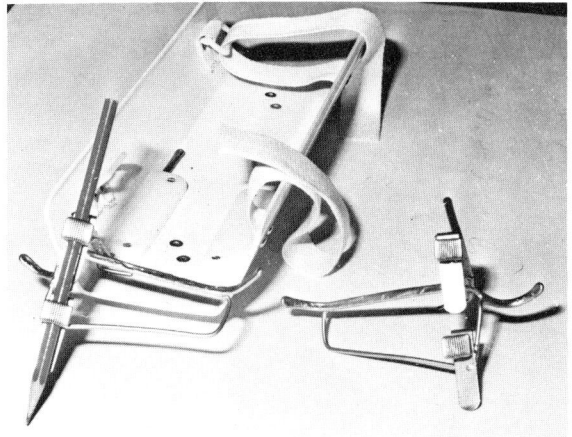

(a)

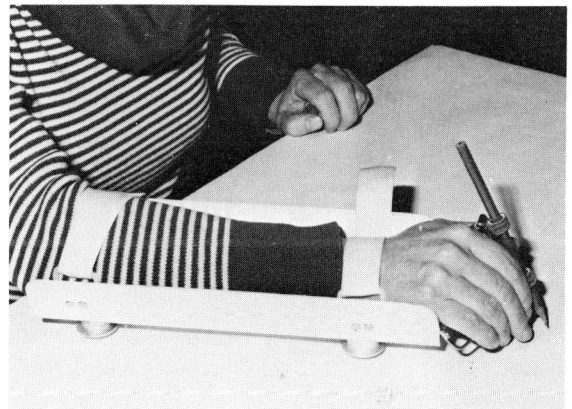

(b)

Fig. 7.8 Table top mobile gutter support designed for writing and art work whilst maintaining the forearm, wrist and phalanges in a functional R.I.P.

2. Gutter supports

(a) Gutter supports may be an alternative to overhead slings. They are less obtrusive, and not dependent on a fixed structure such as overhead mesh. They may be of several types, such as a table top support, mobile, or static floor types. The table top mobile gutter shown in Figure 7.8 was developed for writing and art work. It is made from a length of plastic guttering with four small, ball-bearing feet fixed. to the base. The gutter is low to the table to provide a more normal relationship between arm, tools and task. A removable hand and pencil support fits into acrylic sockets for either left or right hand use. 'D' ring and Velcro fastenings are used to maintain the forearm in the correct position. The hand piece was designed to position the wrist in extension and slight supination, and the hand in a 'functional' position in relationship to the working tool. The gutter is simple to make, and effective in moving with proximal control. Patients remain in a useful reflex-inhibiting position and appear to experience much satisfaction out of 'voluntary writing'.

(b) An extendable mobile gutter to support the upper arm when the patient is involved in a standing activity is illustrated in Figure 7.9.
(c) The horizontal, static floor support (Fig. 7.10) has a long horizontal track which is height adjustable. It supports a gutter which traverses the track as the patient moves in activity. This support was designed specifically for use with a piano (see Fig. 7.29) but has application for many other table top or bench activities.
(d) A ball-bearing wrist support (Fig. 7.11) has application for patients who have reasonable return of upper limb function but are unable to move the arm smoothly across a table top when involved in fine, complex activity such as writing.

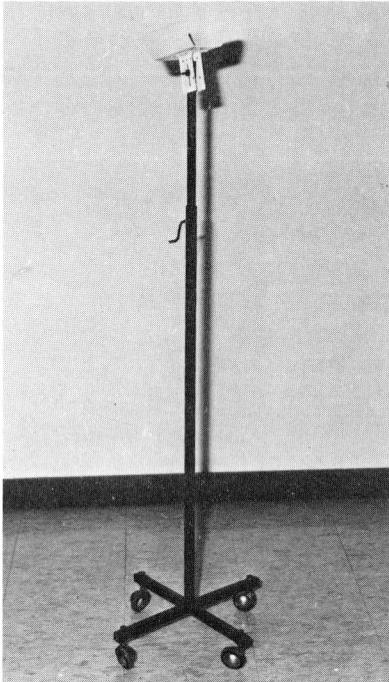

Fig. 7.9 Extendable mobile gutter support for work in standing.

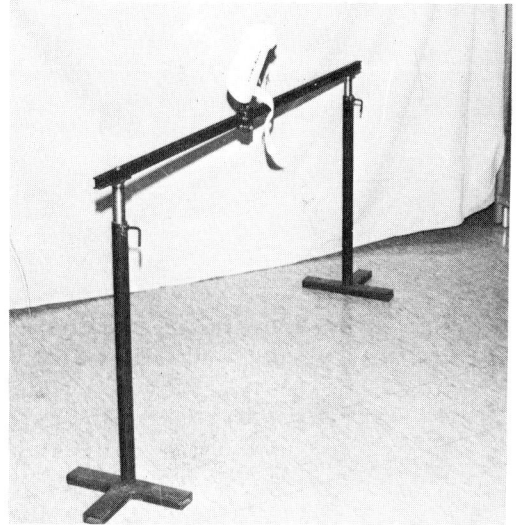

Fig. 7.10 A static floor support with gutter which traverses a horizontal track as the patient moves in activity.

The model shown was made from two of the three sections of a 'thrust race', held together with a thin slice (approximately 1 cm) of acrylic tubing and adhered to a small piece of acrylic formed to support a wrist. The weight of an arm maintains it in contact with the table.

Therapeutic rationale for support mechanisms:
- Promotes purposeful use of limited upper limb movement and weak muscle contraction.
- Supports upper limb against gravity, reducing effort and stress, and unwanted reflex activity.
- Allows proximal movement to direct distal movement.
- Provides assistance for control and modification of upper limb synergies.
- Promotes activity in upper limb reflex-inhibiting patterns.
- Is highly motivating and stimulating to the patient.

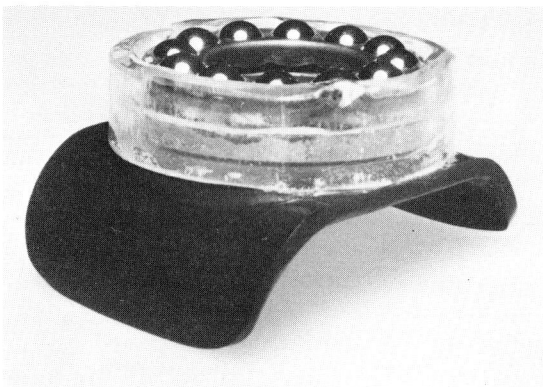

(a)

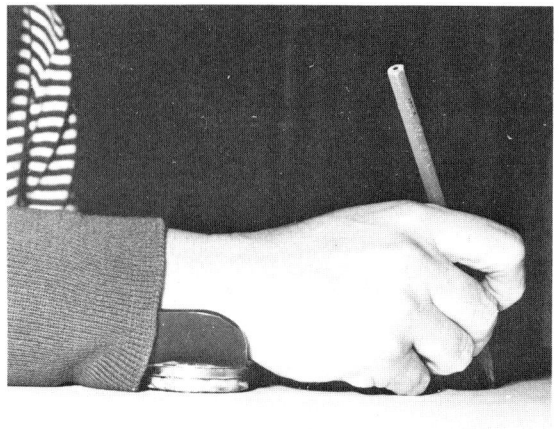

(b)

Fig. 7.11 A ball-bearing wrist support designed to assist smooth movement across a table for activity such as writing.

MODIFICATION OF SYNERGIES

The typical hemiplegic posture of the upper limb, when there is increased tone, is a combination of the strongest components of flexor and extensor

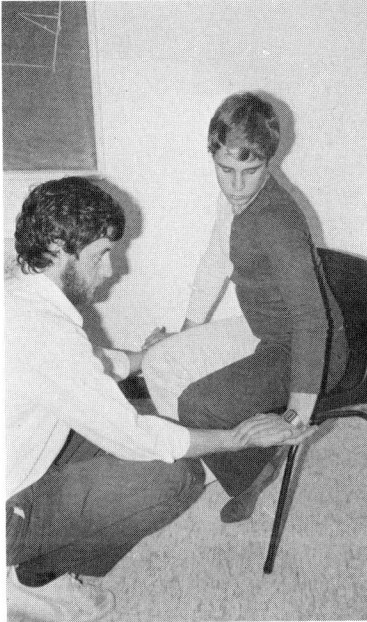

(a)

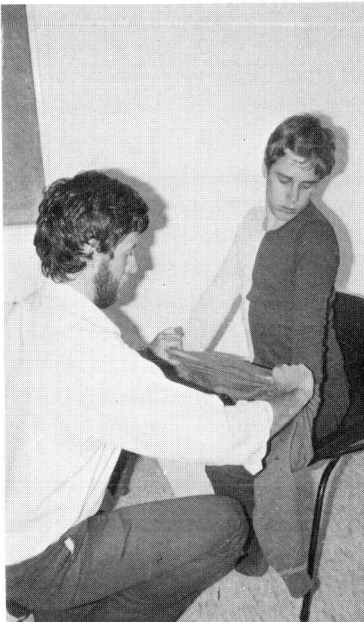

(b)

Fig. 7.12 Using the extensor synergy to assist with putting on a garment (Brunnstrom, 1970).

synergies, particularly elbow flexion, the strongest component of the flexor synergy, and adduction of the shoulder by pectoralis major, and pronation of the forearm, the strongest components of the extensor synergy.

Modification of synergies involves making use of flexor or extensor patterns, and assisting them to combine in functional movement, different to the typical hemiplegic posture.

Methods

1. Extension

Therapists usually seek to elicit upper limb extension before flexion. Because the strongest component of the extensor synergy is pectoralis major, in which tone usually develops early, Brunnstrom (1970) suggests that when synergies are dominant, triceps may only be contracted with pectoralis major, and that when elbow extension is first elicited it is seen in conjunction with shoulder adduction and forearm pronation, indicating that

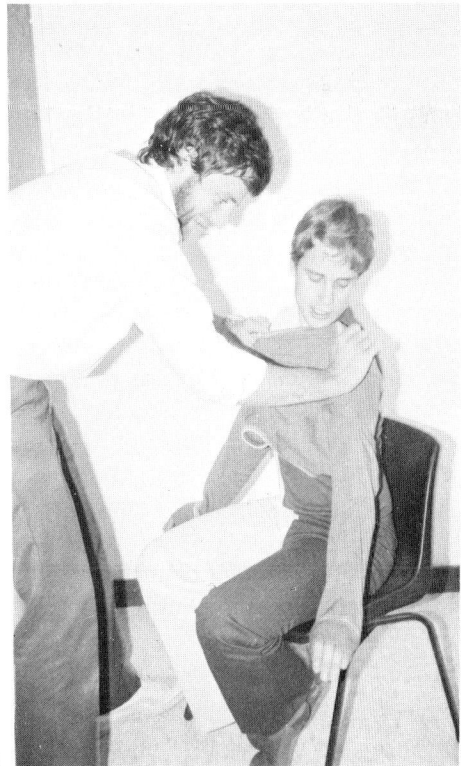

(c)

extension of the upper limb may initially be facilitated downwards and inwards. This movement may be used in activities such as putting on a sweater, as in Figure 7.12. Upper limb extension is reinforced by head rotation to the hemiplegic side, forearm pronation, trunk rotation to the sound side, cutaneous stimulation of the triceps, and, prior to putting on the sleeve, having the patient push into extension against the therapist's hand. To modify the early combination of pectoralis major and triceps, the extensor movement must be gradually guided laterally, and used functionally in bilateral or unilateral activity (Brunnstrom, 1970).

2. Flexion

Elbow flexion is usually one of the first components over which the patient gains voluntary control, and Brunnstrom (1970) suggests it may be incorporated into procedures to encourage shoulder movement. For example, if the patient's affected arm is supported in elbow flexion, whilst firstly bilateral, then unilateral shoulder elevation and lowering is assisted, gradual forward shoulder abduction may be facilitated. The therapist passively alternates supination and pronation of the forearm, as elevation and lowering occur, so introducing external rotation of the shoulder, which is required for abduction of the shoulder beyond the horizontal. Head rotation towards the sound side may assist relaxation of the pectoralis major. The patient is requested to reach up and straighten the elbow, after turning the head towards the hemiplegic side, to facilitate elbow extension, and awareness. The patient may use the extended elevated arm position to prop against a wall whilst engaged in activity positioned vertically (Fig. 7.13). This type of movement is encouraged to organise and develop the flexor synergy and increase the range of movement at the shoulder. It includes some aspects of the extensor synergy which are then emphasized in other activities. Movement and integration of both flexor and extensor synergies are thus encouraged.

3. Combining flexor and extensor synergies

As the synergies modify, flexion and extension

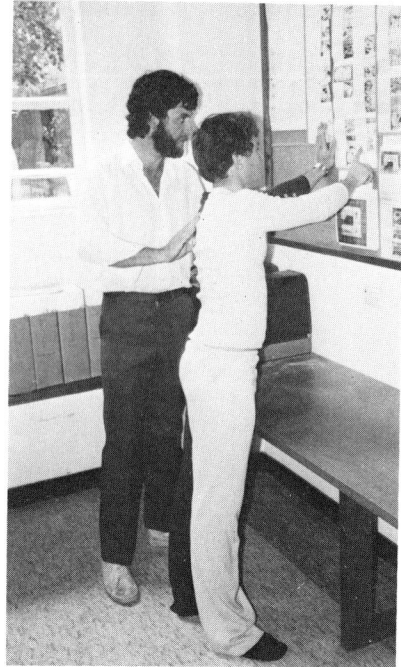

Fig. 7.13 Use of extended elevated arm position to prop against a wall.

may be combined in activities such as polishing, dusting, sanding, sweeping, printing or weaving.

Brunnstrom describes two methods of combining the flexor and extensor synergies, so the hemiplegic hand and arm may reach to the back for tasks such as washing or tucking in clothing.

Either the patient elevates the shoulder girdle, abducts the arm and flexes the elbow, so that the back of the hemiplegic hand touches the hip, then pushes downwards across the back (Fig. 7.14), when the therapist may resist the downward push: or, the patient may be encouraged to extend the upper limb, pushing forward, then obliquely sideways, downwards and backwards, whilst the therapist facilitates with repetitive, rhythmical, and verbal encouragement. The movement may be practised immediately before being used in an activity such as towelling the back (Fig. 7.15), and should be incorporated into daily hygiene and dressing tasks.

As the patient becomes able to learn easy variations from the basic synergies, but control of individual joint movement is difficult, activity may be used which has flexor and extensor character-

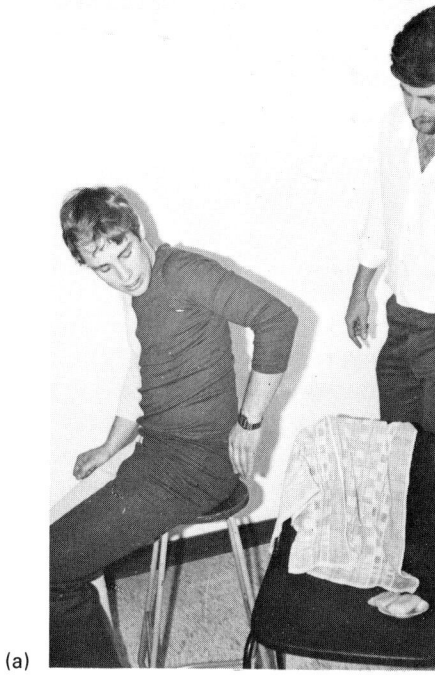

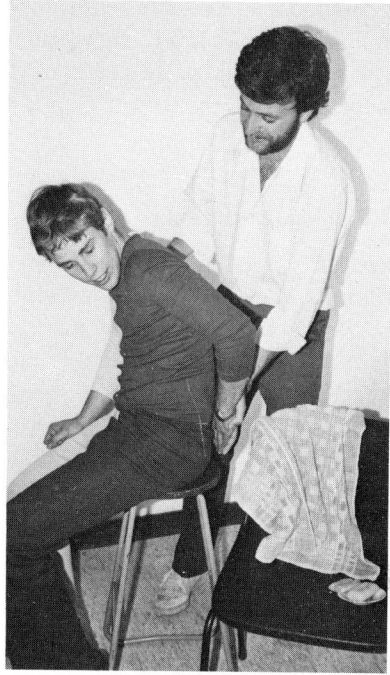

Fig. 7.14 Utilizing the flexor synergy to assist the patient reach to the back.

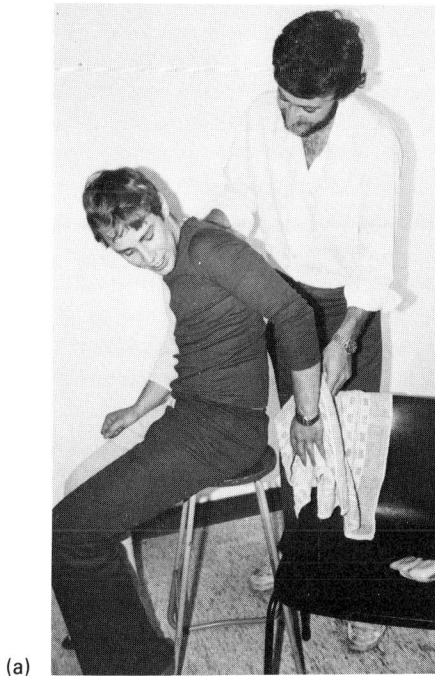

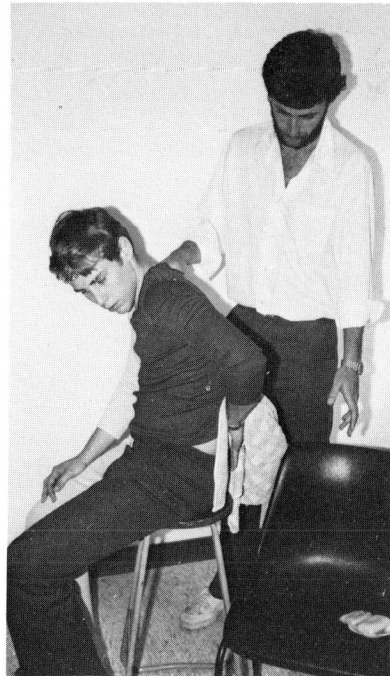

Fig. 7.15 Utilizing the patient's ability to reach to the back in personal care activity.

istics, such as those of self-care requiring hand to mouth, to shoulder, or to head, movement. Repetitive guided movement may be necessary prior to the functional activity.

4. Spiral diagonal patterning

Spiral, diagonal, upper limb patterns of movement combine flexor and extensor synergies, and may be used in activity such as the dressing method, using 'diagonal 2' patterns, illustrated in Figures 5.23 and 5.24.

Activities utilizing the 'diagonal 1' pattern may be introduced in such activity as combing hair, initially using the sound hand, then using the hemiplegic hand.

Therapeutic rationale of synergy modification:

- May be considered an essential part of the recovery process.
- Maximizes patient participation in use of hemiplegic limb, and is therefore motivating and encouraging.
- Movement is functional if or when recovery plateaus.
- Enables patients to experience the feel of movement, other than reflex patterned.
- Stimulates kinesthetic and tactile sensation.
- Increases awareness of bilaterality.

GRASP-RELEASE ACTIVITIES (COMBINED WITH FOREARM AND WRIST MOVEMENT)

When gross movement of the upper limb is possible, but it is difficult for the hand to voluntarily relax, functional use of the arm movement is limited. Functional use of the upper limb is also limited if arm movements are not sufficiently refined to facilitate movement of the hand.

Bobath (1978) points out that wrist extension, finger and thumb extension and abduction, are difficult when the arm is pronated and flexed, because grasp-release activities utilize normal forearm and wrist movement.

Methods

1. Pronation and supination

Bobath suggests that patients may be able to grasp objects when the forearm is pronated, and release objects when the arm is supinated; may find grasp is easier with wrist extended, and release easier with wrist flexed; and that return of digit movement usually begins on the ulnar side, patients being able to extend the little, ring, and middle fingers, but not the thumb or index finger.

When patients are seated, the arm supported in front of them, they should be encouraged to pronate and supinate the forearm. If the patient is unable to achieve this voluntarily, they should be shown how to assist the hemiplegic arm and hand with the sound one.

In such activities as hand and arm washing, during daily hygiene tasks, after meals, workshop activities, or to 'warm up' the limb to assist relaxation prior to treatment, patients should be taught to include pronation and supination of the hemiplegic upper limb by position and movement of the sound hand (Fig. 7.16).

If some grasp release is possible, activity which involves selecting and turning over objects may be used, for example 'pairing' or 'concentration', where the cards are replaced by masonite or wooden plaques which do not bend. Therapists should inhibit shoulder elevation should it occur, and try out different combinations of forearm movement with grasp-release activity.

Use may be made of activities such as macrame (Fig. 7.17), or weaving, because the gentle, repetitive movement of picking up, pushing through, retrieving and putting down the shuttle includes wrist and forearm movement with grasp release.

A 'FEPS' attachment to raise or lower the weaving shed may be useful, especially if a handle is made to include a cone shape, at right angles to the body (Fig. 7.18), so that pronation and supination is required repetitively.

2. Cone shapes

The use of cones, and cone-shaped handles to facilitate grasp-release movements, has become common in the last few years, because it is thought

(a)

(b)

(c)

Fig. 7.17 Macrame used for pronation, supination, grasp and release activity.

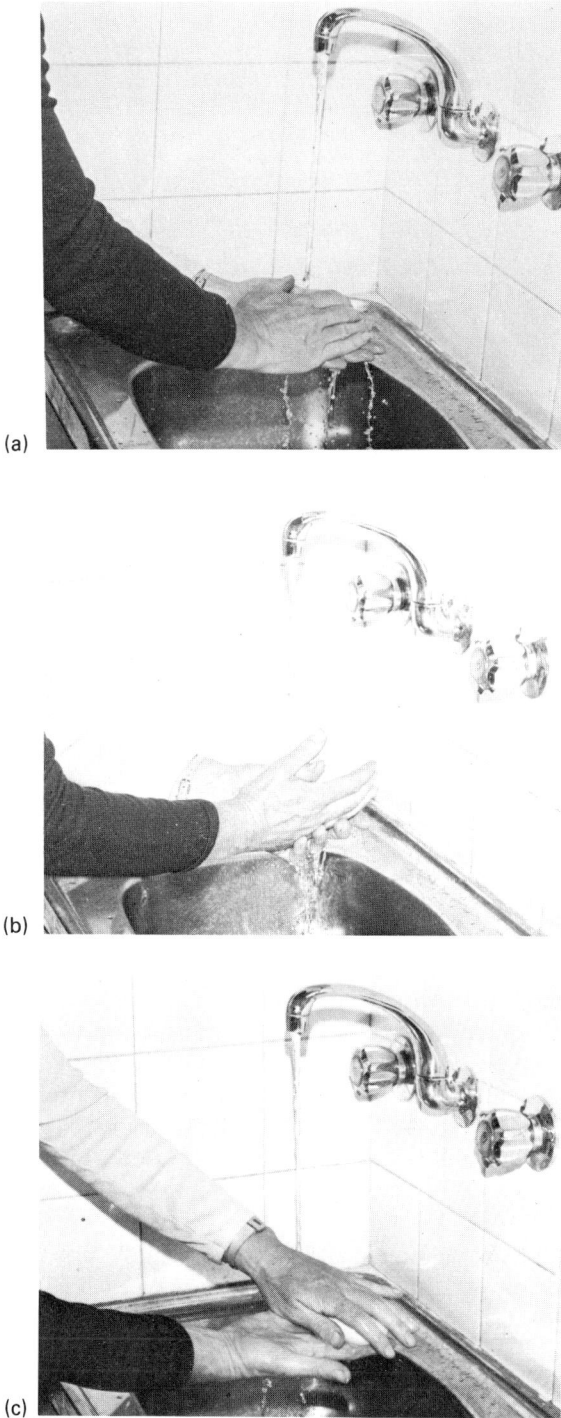

Fig. 7.16 The sound hand used to promote forearm pronation and supination whilst washing hands. The hemiplegic arm may need to be supported if unable to maintain a position briefly against gravity.

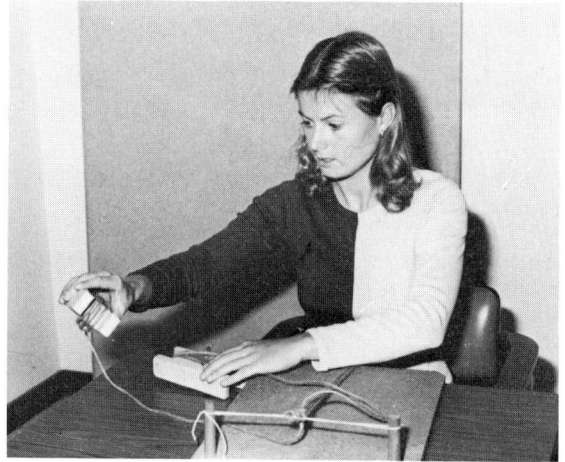

that firm pressure over muscle insertions produces an inhibitory effect, in this case of the finger flexors (Pedretti, 1981; Farber, 1982), to prevent grasp reaction dominating hand movement. Padded or soft handles are thought to increase flexor activity, and are therefore contraindicated (Dayhoff, 1975; Pedretti, 1981). The shape of the cone, with the greatest diameter to the ulnar side, allows most pressure to occur on the outer fingers where grasp-release movements begin, and encourages wrist extension and radial deviation. Johnstone (1978) notes that the shape encourages good opposition of thumb and index finger. Cones of yarn may be used for weaving projects (Fig. 7.19), and as draught or chess pieces on a large table board (Fig. 7.20). They may be attached to a polishing, sanding or printing block which is moved during activity with clasped hands, abducting fingers, as illustrated in Figure 7.20,(a). Cones may also be attached to a heavy base, and used for the patient to hold, maintaining a reflex-inhibiting position, during other activity. Tools may be fitted with cone-shaped handles (Fig. 7.20(c)) which will allow the patient to re-lease the handle with greater ease when the task is completed.

3. Manipulation

When release is difficult, or a hand is tightly flexed, manipulation prior to, and perhaps during

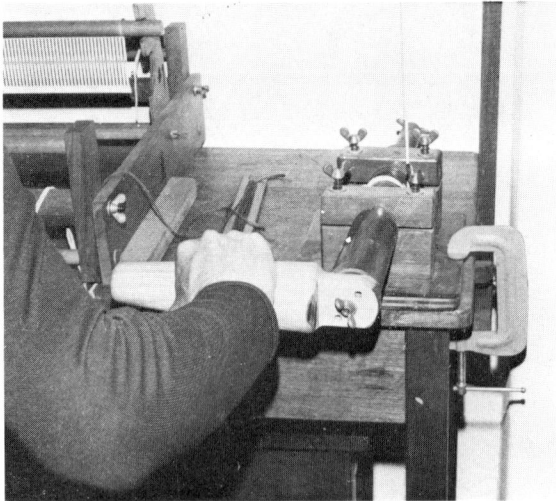

(a)

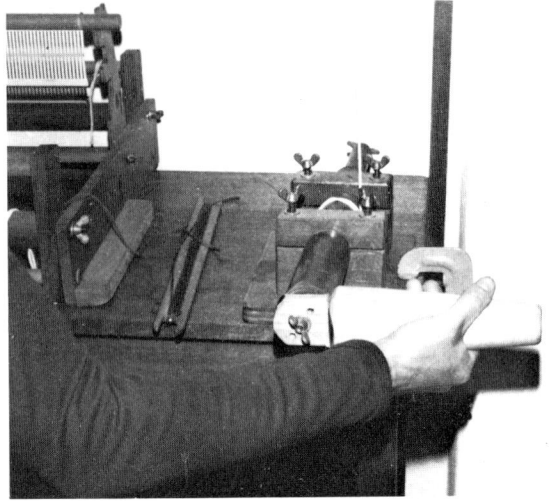

(b)

Fig. 7.18 A cone-shaped handled fitted to FEPS to raise or lower a weaving shed.

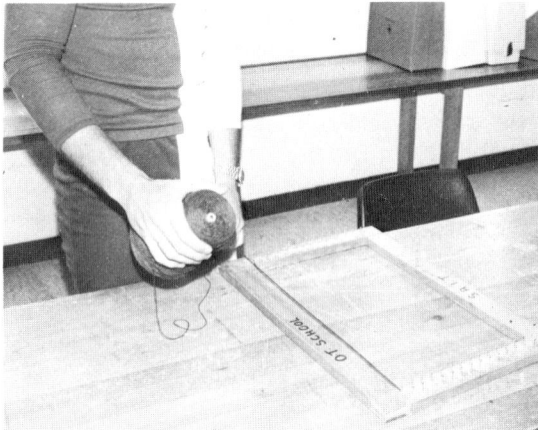

Fig. 7.19 'Cones' of yarn used for weaving projects.

activity, may be useful, so that passive-assisted extension of the fingers alternates with active grasp (Brunnstrom, 1970). This is illustrated in Figure 7.21 with the therapist manipulating the patient's hand prior to drinking from a cup. The therapist strokes or taps the thumb extensors before pulling the thumb proximally outwards, and supinating the forearm. Passive alternate forearm pronation and supination may be useful. Rapid proximal to distal stroking over finger extensors is performed until flexor tone is relaxed. The hand is assisted to grasp a large cup and the patient encouraged to lift it to the mouth to drink. The patient should be told,

or assisted, to keep the upper arm in contact with the trunk to avoid elevation of the shoulder with abduction of the arm.

4. Functional activity

Carr and Shepherd (1982) suggest patients practise, with assistance if necessary, holding a cylindrical object such as a jar, forearm in mid-position, wrist radially deviated and extended, lifting, pronating and supinating the jar. These movements may be used in activities such as cooking, where measured amounts are tipped into a mixing bowl. The sound hand may be needed to assist control of the tipping movement, and for safety. Ingredients can be measured and put into a suitable jar or, when appropriate, tipped straight from a container. Containers which are slightly larger in diameter at the base may enable utilization of the 'cone shape effect' (Fig. 7.22).

Taking the lid off a jar uses the hand in bilateral asymmetrical activity to stimulate voluntary wrist movement. As shown in Figure 7.23, the patient's extended hand is assisted to lightly grasp the lid, the hemiplegic wrist extended, without ulnar deviation (Carr & Shepherd, 1982), as the sound hand turns the jar in the opposite direction.

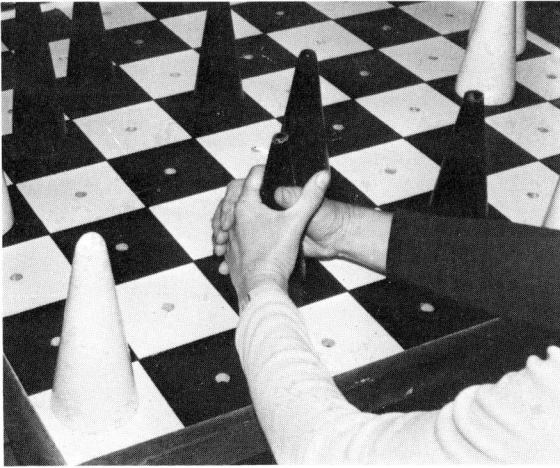

(a)

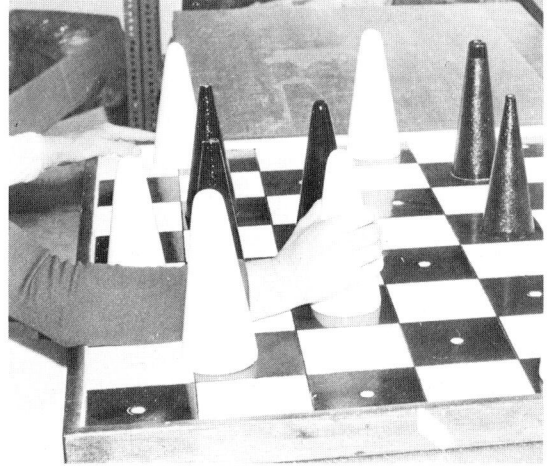

(b)

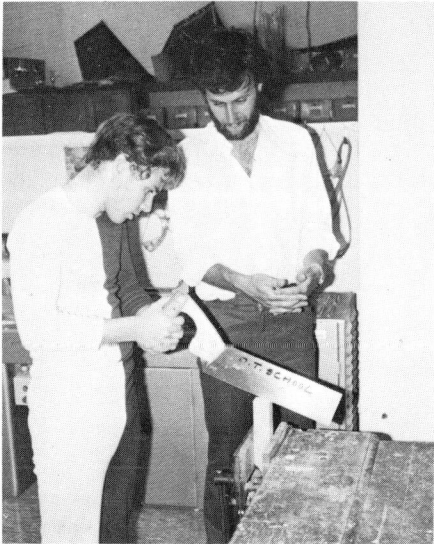

(c)

Fig. 7.20 Yarn cones used as draught pieces with (a) a bilateral abductor grasp, or (b) hemiplegic hand alone and, (c) another use of cone shapes — a saw fitted with a cone-shaped handle.

5. Elevation of the arm

Use of movement reactions, such as Souques' phenomenon, (Marie & Foix, 1916) in which involuntary extension and separation of the fingers occurs, when the arm is elevated more than 90°, will encourage release following grasp. Supination after elevation assists extension of the thumb. Souques' phenomenon is not characteristic of a particular recovery stage (Brunnstrom, 1970).

The patient may attempt voluntary flexion and extension of the digits, with the arm in elevation, and if successful, in gradually lower positions, with support, manipulation or stimulation applied if necessary. A game of elevated draughts with large pieces, played from top to bottom, may utilize the phenomenon (Fig. 7.24). Whilst the movement is only semivoluntary the patient needs to be relaxed, and the upper limb may need external support.

Bobath (1978) stresses that patients need to learn to grasp and release, regardless of the position of the arm, and that in functional activities which include upper limb elevation, such as combing the hair, patients may be unable to maintain grip of objects because of Souques' phenomenon, and thus fail in the activity.

Johnstone (1978) suggests that if the patient is able to grasp but not release an object, upper limb weight bearing activities should be recommended.

Therapeutic rationale for grasp release activities:
• In the Twitchell (1951) study of recovery, those patients who attained grasp reflex progressed to normal hand skills. Grasp reflex differs from instinctive grasp reaction (Denny Brown, 1948), being elicited by deep pressure moving distally over the radial side of the palm from the wrist, the palmar surface of the fingers and medial palmar surface of the thumb, and consisting of weak contactions of flexor and adductor muscles. The grasp reaction is elicited by a stationary object in contact with the palm of the

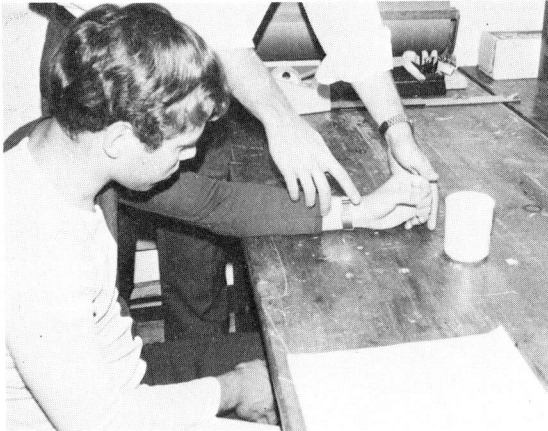

(a)

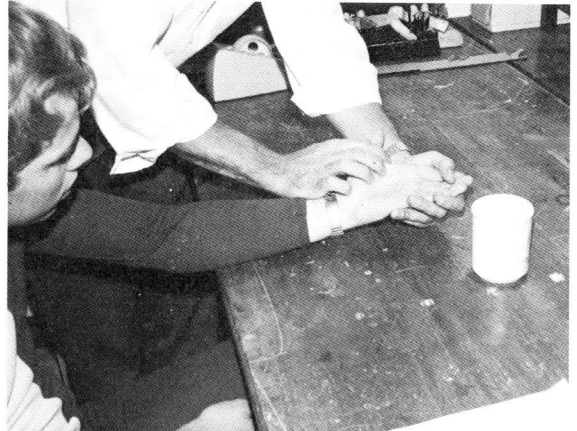

(b)

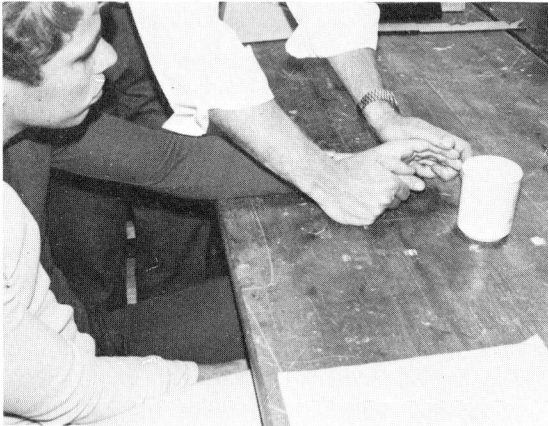

(c)

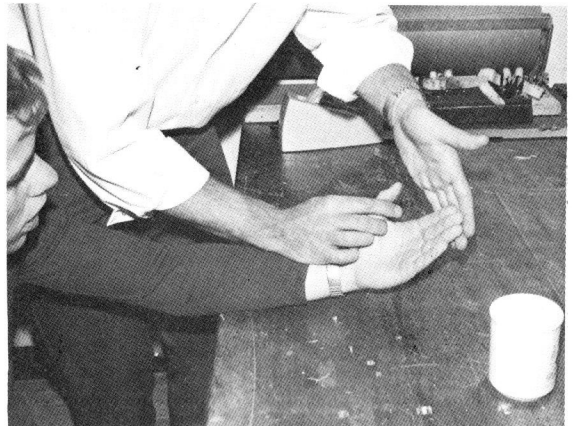

(d)

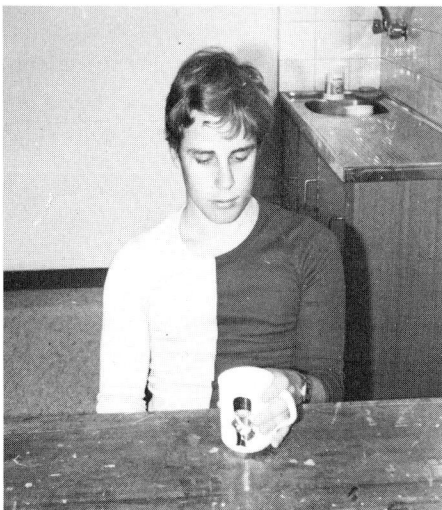

(e)

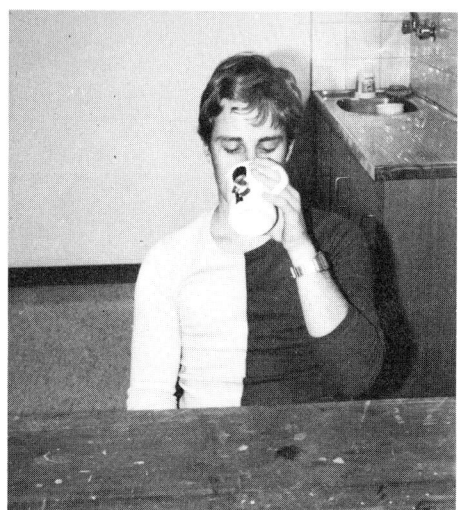

(f)

Fig. 7.21 Passive assisted extension alternates with active grasp during activity (Brunnstorm, 1970.) (a) Therapist taps thumb extensors. (b) Therapist pulls the thumb proximally outwards supinating the forearm. (c) Passive alternate forearm pronation and supination. (d) Rapid proximal to distal stroking over finger extensors. (e) Hand assisted to grasp a large cup. (f) Patient encouraged, assisted if necessary, to lift it to the mouth keeping the upper arm in contact with the trunk.

hand, causing involuntary fist closure, and inability to release.

- Developmentally, control of grasp release occurs before fine hand skills.
- Allows functional bilateral hand activity.
- Provides greater potential for independence.
- Promotes awareness of the hemiplegic upper limb.
- Promotes motivation and patient pleasure on achievement.

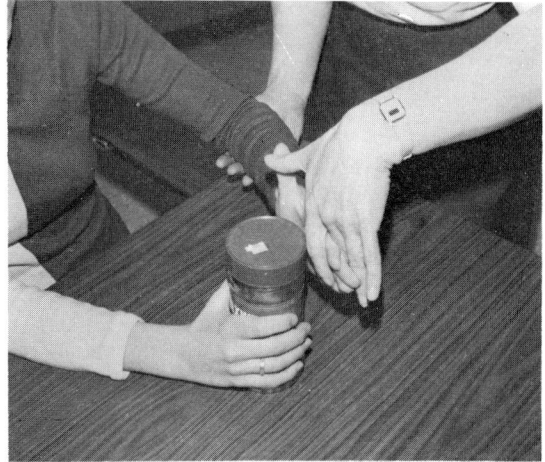

(a)

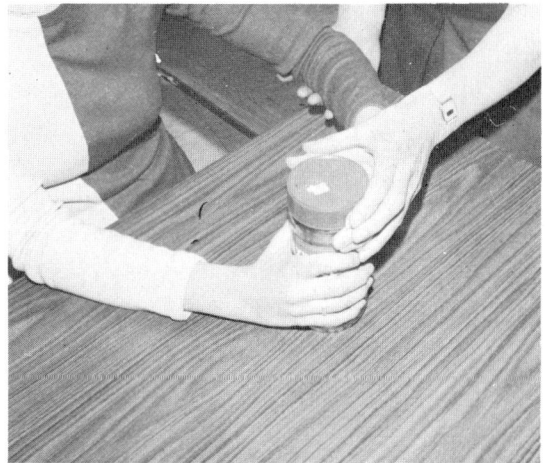

(a)

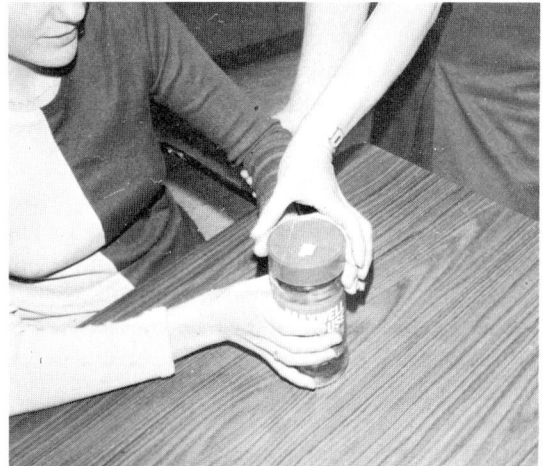

(b)

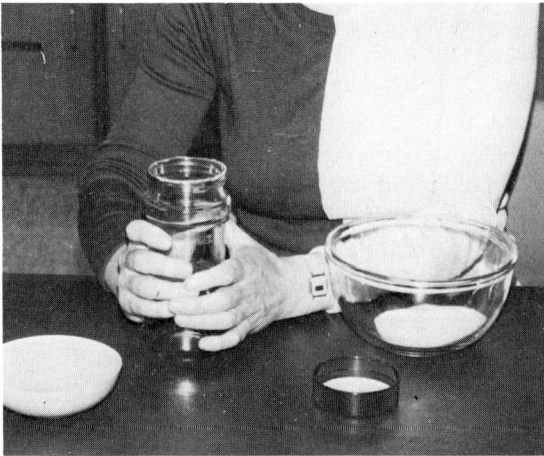

(b)

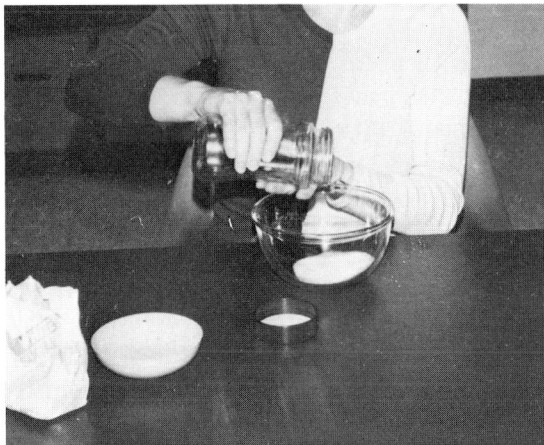

(c)

Fig. 7.22 Practice of forearm pronation and supination, with grasp and release in cooking activity, using a jar slightly larger in diameter at the base than the top.

Fig. 7.23 Bilateral asymmetrical activity, taking a lid off a jar to promote voluntary wrist movement.

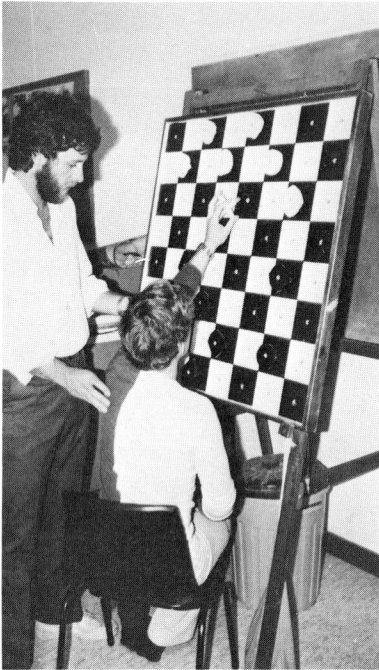

Fig. 7.24 Playing 'elevated draughts' from top to bottom, utilizing 'Souques' phenomenon to facilitate release of the pieces.

RE-EDUCATION OF SKILLED HAND MOVEMENT

Patients who experience good recovery, whether soon after stroke or following intensive rehabilitation, may find difficulty in using the hemiplegic hand for skilled manipulative tasks, despite ability to use it for gross grasp and release activities, and as a stabilizer or support.

Although spasticity may be slight and transient, and the patient able voluntarily to change abnormal positions when they occur, individual controlled movement of fingers and thumbs may be slow and difficult, particularly in the execution of functional activities rather than exercise.

Bobath (1978) suggests that in treatment to promote selective movement, it is important to practise inhibition to prevent movement at other joints. She further suggests that therapists should be aware of the developmental and recovery sequence of movement, so that practice during task performance may be graded from movements easier for the patient, to practising the same movements in more difficult positions, and then with more complex components. Many patients do not regain the use of skilled hand movement. Bobath states that opposition of the thumb and index finger is rarely achieved, and that although grasp and release using the whole hand may be possible, individual discrete finger movement for dexterous tasks is beyond the ability of most patients. She suggests, however, that movements such as wiping, scratching, raking, waving, pulling, pushing, patting, poking with the index finger, picking up small objects between thumb and index finger, throwing and releasing objects, which will be needed in complex combinations in functional tasks, be practised in preparation. She recommends that occupational therapists analyse particular activities, in order to recognise those components difficult for the patient, so that practice may be specific to each individual.

Brunnstrom (1970) makes use of hand movements resulting from synergies throughout treatment, so that the patient utilizes control over synergies in functional activity, and continues to act as a two-armed individual. For example, she suggests that hook grasp may be used for adjusting clothing or carrying objects, as shown in Figure 7.25, when the patient has control of fist closure, though not necessarily of opening, and is able to make a willed effort to maintain the hand position for a short time.

Carr and Shepherd (1982) suggest that movements of the hand should be stimulated early following stroke, and that as soon as isolated muscle action is elicited, it should be practised and extended into meaningful activity. All unnecessary muscle activity, gross movement patterns, abnormal synergic movements, and bilateral activity should be avoided, and the patient should be encouraged to consciously eliminate such movements. They suggest functional tasks as an integral part of the program, with the patient practising, with guidance, in as many ways and for as many different activities as possible, any movement that is difficult, or any component seen to be performed in an abnormal manner.

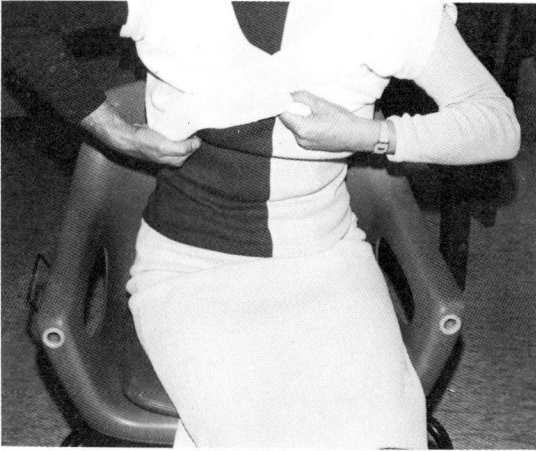

(a)

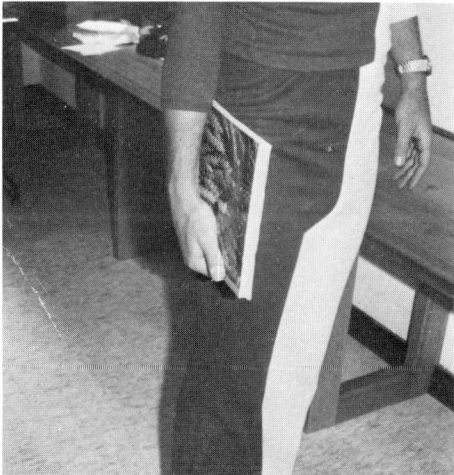

(b)

Fig. 7.25 Hook grasp used for; (a) Adjusting clothing, (b) Carrying a book.

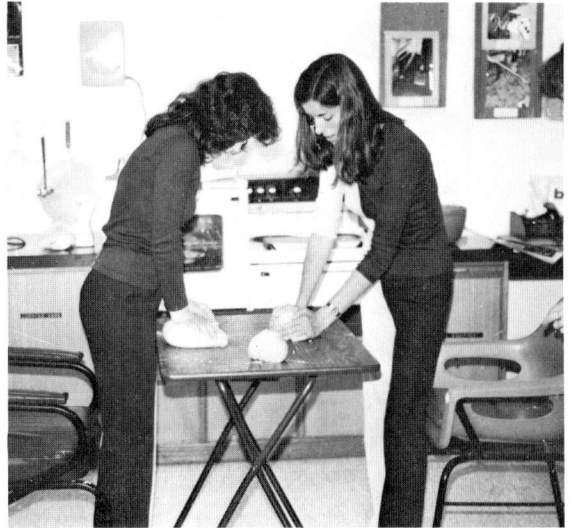

Fig. 7.26 Kneading warm bread dough to encourage bilateral symmetrical and asymmetrical co-ordinated activity of wrist and hand.

abduction of the fingers and wrist, opposition of thumb to fingers, and to strengthen individual intrinsic muscles. Clay or bread dough may be used similarly, with tangible results as an added bonus. Kneading warm dough may be a practical repetitive activity of great value, assisting bilateral, symmetrical and asymmetrical, co-ordinated activity of hands, extension of fingers and wrist, and upper limb weight bearing (Fig. 7.26).

Individual finger movements may be used in piecing strips for bread baskets, or modelling the dough into decorative forms (Fig. 7.27). The cooking process is useful in functional retraining of everyday skills.

Methods

1. Use of pliable modelling material

Some therapists recommend the use of theraplast (a soft, non-toxic, re-usable modelling material) for hand rehabilitation. Many patients appear to enjoy using it, even during their free time. Exercises to encourage particular movement, appropriate for each patient, should be given, taking care not to reinforce any undesirable or abnormal movement, such as hyperextension at the M.C.P. joints. It may be used to encourage extension and

2. Movement of thumb and index finger

Therapists should work towards the redevelopment of movement of thumb and index finger. Brunnstrom (1970) suggests that extension of the thumb is facilitated in upper limb elevation, particularly if the arm is supinated or if the thumb is flexed and allowed to rebound, extension of the index finger often reflecting the thumb movement. When mass release is possible, some semi-voluntary thumb abduction may occur and should be facilitated by cutaneous stimulation over the

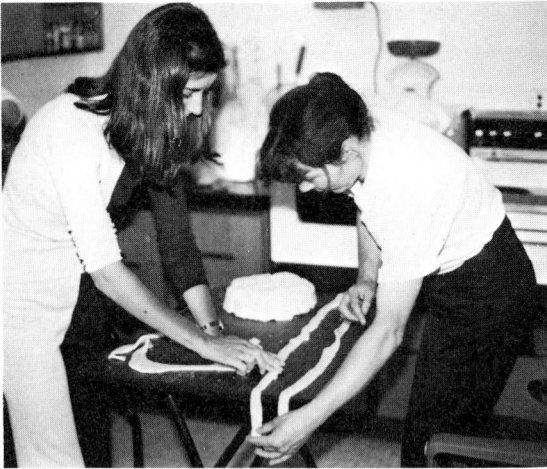

Fig. 7.27 Piecing strips of dough for a bread basket utilizes individual finger movements.

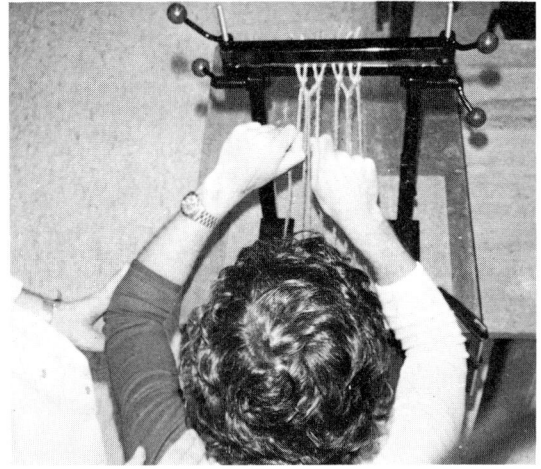

Fig. 7.28 Macrame project using lateral prehension.

tendons of abductor pollicis longus, and extensor pollicis brevis at the wrist. Patients may be instructed where and how to self-apply gentle tapping, particularly if the thumb movement enables lateral prehension, a functional grip which may be utilized in many activities when opposition between index and thumb is not achieved.

Lateral prehension is possible when the patients have only mass grasp and release, but are able to abduct and adduct the thumb. Objects may be held by maintained pressure against the radial side of the index finger. This grip may be used for clothing adjustment, holding a fork or spoon, when supination may need guiding initially, in card games, for carrying objects, or for recreational or craft activities (Fig. 7.28).

Because there is no contact with the palmar surface during lateral prehension, release is easy, but in order to facilitate functional use of other types of prehension, hours of practice in picking up and releasing objects which are in contact with the palmar surface may be necessary. Any activity of significance and interest to patients may be used for this purpose, as long as they do not become frustrated by their attempts. As improvement occurs, occupational therapists should make sure that daily functional activities such as dressing, personal care, eating and drinking, are upgraded to include new skills. This may not happen automatically.

3. Manipulative activities

Carr and Shepherd (1982) maintain that although functional manipulative activities are very complex, a patient's performance may be improved if the therapist can analyse, and work on, the major factor interfering with that performance. They suggest that when problem movements are identified, patients should practise similar movements before re-attempting the original activity.

Activities demanding rapid individual finger movement, such as typing, or playing a piano, are particularly difficult, as speed and timing are essential for success. Patients do not have time to concentrate on moving a finger or inhibiting another, and movement must be semi-automatic to result in a successful outcome. When attempting such activities abnormal movement such as hyperextension at the M.C.P. joint may be evident. Splints may be assistive, or inhibiting, in facilitating specific movements.

4. Splints

The use of splints, a controversial issue, may be advantageous when trying to promote or make use of digit movement. Therapists should not apply splints without first considering undesirable neural mechanisms which may be elicited. Nor should possible advantages be ignored. Basically, any splint used should have adynamic functional gain, should be engineered for individual patients, and the neurophysiological reactions following use of a splint observed, monitored, and recorded, so that decisions concerning adjustments, or continued and future use, are based on sound clinical evidence.

Carr and Shepherd (1980) state that if splints need to be considered, they must fulfil the objective of enabling muscles to regain function, by positioning joints to enhance relearning of certain movements.

In Figure 7.29(a), hyperextension of the meta-carpal phalangeal joints, and mass flexion of the interphalangeal joints can be clearly seen, as the patient attempts to play an organ. These move-ments are corrected by a dynamic knuckle-duster type splint, with individual finger abductors and an opponens bar (Fig. 7.29(b)). The patient reported better movement in her fingers for several days after wearing the splint for piano playing. She also reported more controlled use of her hand, when her arm was supported by sling or gutter. Without this support the effort required to main-tain the upper limb against gravity decreased func-tional use of the arm and hand, despite full return of function to shoulder and elbow.

Dorsal or palmar resting splints are sometimes advocated to decrease spasticity (Trombly, 1983), and some experiments have been reported using prolonged immobilization in full stretch (Brennan, 1959). If contractures occur, serial splinting may be useful, and cone shapes may be incorporated into splint designs.

Bobath (1978) recommends the use of a foam rubber 'finger spreader' to abduct fingers and thumb to facilitate extension, and reduce flexor spasticity during rest. This is simply made by punching holes for each finger and the thumb in thick foam rubber or plastazote.

COMPENSATORY APPROACHES

As recovery may plateau at any stage, many patients have to cope with living with residual loss or impaired function of the hemiplegic arm and hand.

If necessary and lifestyle significant activities are

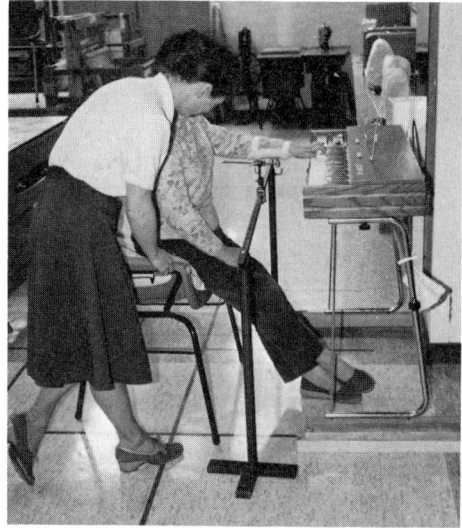

(a)

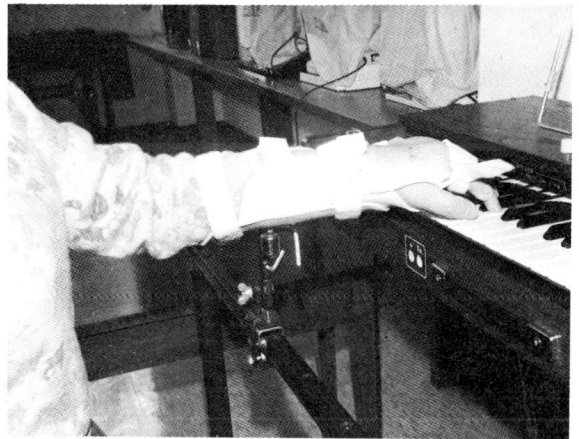

(b)

Fig. 7.29 (a) Hyperextension of the M.C.P. joints and mass flexion of the I.P. joints as the patient attempts to play an organ. (b) Abnormal movement is corrected by the 'knuckle duster' type splint which abducts individual fingers, and promotes thumb opposition.

used for treatment during all stages of recovery, when recovery ceases, patients will not have to start learning compensatory methods. They will instead only require reinforcement and practice of the highest level skills they have.

Methods

1. When flaccidity persists

If the upper limb remains totally flaccid, training

of the sound limb in one handed activity is required; however, the hemiplegic limb must be included in retraining, the sound hand positioning it to act as a stabilizer whenever possible, and safely at all times. This is to prevent further damage, and to ensure the patient retains awareness of both sides of the body.

2. When spasticity persists

If the arm has increased tone, and little or no function of the hand, compensatory methods should include anti-reflex positioning, which may be useful for stabilizing, and to prevent possible contractures of hand and elbow causing difficulties with self care and dressing tasks. Methods of self caring for the hemiplegic upper limb, to maintain awareness of bilaterality, and to prevent flexion contractures, should be included in retraining.

3. The sound upper limb

The sound upper limb, whether it be the dominant or non-dominant hand, will need training in maximizing manipulative skills and strength. Activities which the patient wishes to continue may require adaptation. As an example, one excellent woodwork aid is shown in Figure 7.30.

The need to train the dominant hand is often ignored, but not only is increased dexterity demanded when only one hand remains func-

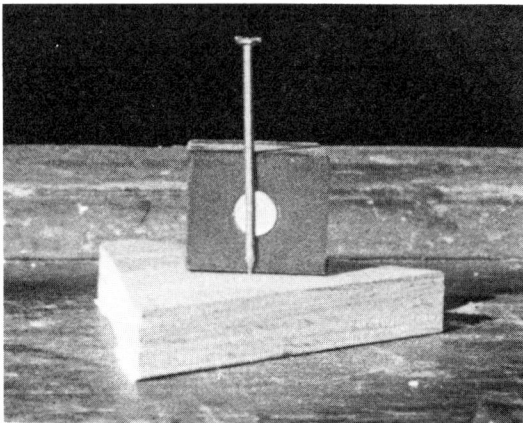

Fig. 7.30 A magnetic nail holder. A small magnet is set into a rubber block, which when placed on horizontal timber will hold a nail upright until 'started' in the wood. (Designed at Queen Elizabeth Hospital, Adelaide, South Australia).

tional, motor planning disturbances may affect former manipulative skills. In a study measuring hand skills, Bell et al (1976) reported severe disability in right dominant hand skills in left hemiplegics, compared to left non-dominant hand skills in right hemiplegics.

The need for training the non-dominant hand to be more dexterous is obvious, and in particular fine motor skills such as writing, if only a signature, may be of vital psychological importance to the patient. Patients will often take hold of a pen with no preparatory thought, and try to write, obtaining poor results. Although it may be difficult, the therapist should attempt to grade writing practice through abstract doodling, and large to small writing patterns, before cursive writing is approached. If patients can be 'educated' that this is the natural way of learning control and penmanship, they may be receptive to the approach, and spared frustration caused by poor writing. The therapist should certainly ensure the patient uses a light, flexible grip on the pen, has turned the paper so what is written can be seen, and that the paper will not slip because it has been stabilized with the hemiplegic hand, weights, clips or a non-slip surface.

Practice to increase sound upper limb dexterity and co-ordination should be graded in speed and accuracy (Trombly, 1983), and from simple to complex. Recreational and creative activities may be used as well as necessary functional tasks for this purpose, so that skill training is enjoyable and flexible.

Patients who have good function in other parts of the body, and are able to think adaptively, may be encouraged to consider other parts of the body for holding and stabilizing, such as teeth, knees or feet, which may not be useful all the time, but of help in times of difficulty. Choice of clothing to include pockets big enough for carrying objects may also be recommended.

4. One handed techniques

One handed techniques are well documented in publications such as *Help Yourselves: a Handbook for hemiplegics and their families* by Peggy Jay, and *The One Handers Book, a basic guide to Activities of Daily Living* by Veronica Washam. Occu-

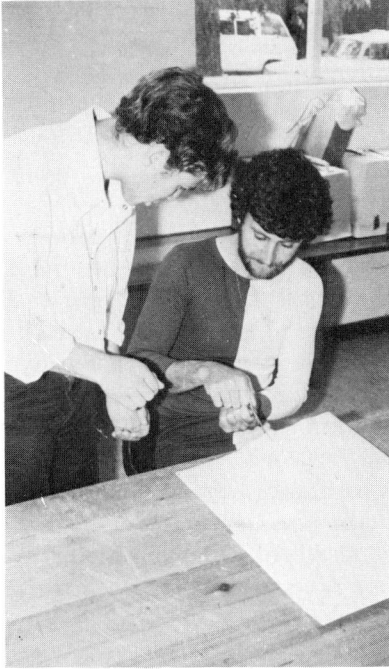
(a)

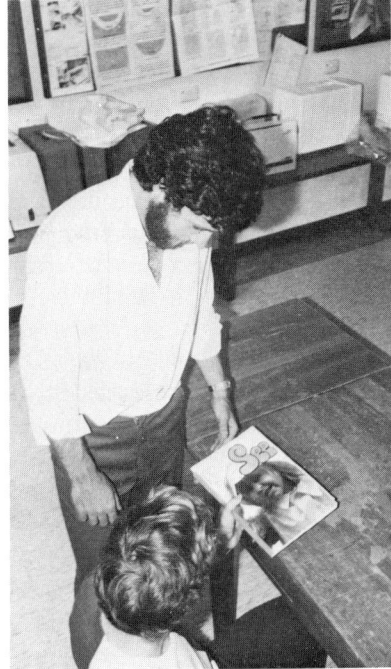
(b)

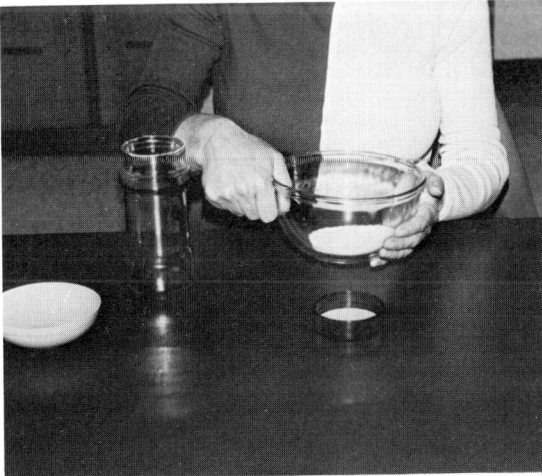
(c)

Fig. 7.31 Lateral prehension used for; (a) Manipulating scissors, (b) Holding and carrying a book, (c) Holding and manipulating a bowl during cooking.

pational therapists should teach patients how to achieve independence related to their future lifestyle: for example, dressing retraining should make use of clothes the patient wishes to wear and will feel comfortable in, despite a restricted life-style, and retraining in household tasks should reflect each patient's home needs. Equipment, tools and aids are constantly improving and the occupational therapist should keep up to date by visiting, with patients, specialist display centres, such as the Independent Living Centres in Australia, and the Disabled Living Foundation in the United Kingdom.

Sharing experiences and ideas with others in group discussion is often valuable, and therapists may structure groups so that work simplification, organization of work areas, choice of equipment, how to stabilize objects, and practical self-help ideas for usually bilateral tasks, are covered. Practice sessions may be programmed for those topics patients find most relevant.

5. Utilizing recovery of hemiplegic limb

If patients have regained some use of the hemiplegic hand, methods which incorporate such recovery should be explored and practised. This may facilitate further improvement, will maintain patient awareness of bilaterality, be safer, and usually helps patients to feel more in control of their environment. For example, hook grasp may be used for carrying light objects, or adjusting clothing, and lateral prehension may be developed for a range of activities, for example manipulating scissors, lifting, or carrying (Fig. 7.31). If used for carrying, the sound hand may need to assist.

Therapeutic rationale for an adaptive approach:

- Many patients have to cope with residual loss or impaired functions in hemiplegic arm and hand. The sooner practice starts post stroke, the greater the patient skill on discharge.
- Transfer of abstract skills learned is unnecessary as learning proceeds with treatment.
- Promotes and maintains self-esteem, and patients feel more independent and in control of their environment.
- If, as it should, the hemiplegic limb is considered during all aspects of compensatory procedures, bilateral awareness is promoted.

- Confidence in coping with lifestyle after discharge is enhanced if sound side skills are maximized and related to real needs.

SUMMARY

Despite the reality that many patients do not regain normal function of the hemiplegic upper limb, occupational therapists can offer re-education throughout treatment. For all patients, sensory input to increase awareness of bilaterality is essential for safety, and to trigger sensory and motor engrams. Therapists may assist patients to integrate skill development into function progressively, to maximize their potential, and to utilize rehabilitation time economically.

Studies to record and publish effects of intervention are necessary for approach appraisal and future direction.

REFERENCES

Bell E, Jurek K, Wilson T 1976 Hand skill measurement. A gauge for treatment. American Journal of Occupational Therapy 30 (2): 80–86
Bobath B 1978 Adult hemiplegia, evaluation and treatment, 2nd edn. Heinemann Medical books Ltd, London
Brennan J B 1959 Response to stretch of hypertonic muscle groups in hemiplegia. British Medical Journal 1(5136): 1504–1507
Brunnstrom S 1970 Movement therapy in hemiplegia, a neurophysiological approach. Harper and Row, New York
Cailliet R 1981 Neck and arm pain. F A Davis Co, Philadelphia
Carr J, Shepherd R 1982 A motor relearning programme for stroke. Heinemann Medical books Ltd, London
Dayhoff N 1975 Rethinking stroke, soft or hard devices to position hands? American Journal of Nursing 7: 1142–1144
Denny Brown 1948. In: Brunnstrom S 1970 Movement therapy in hemiplegia. Harper & Row, New York
Farber S D 1982 Neuro rehabilitation, a multi sensory approach. Saunders, Philadelphia
Jay P 1979 Help yourselves: a handbook for hemiplegics and their families, 3rd edn. Ian Henry publications, Essex
Johnstone M 1978 Restoration of motor function in the

stroke patient, a physiotherapists approach. Churchill Livingstone, Edinburgh
Johnstone M 1982 The stroke patient, principles of rehabilitation, 2nd edn. Churchill Livingstone, Edinburgh
Jones M S 1964 An approach to occupational therapy, 2nd edn. Butterworths, London
Matyas T A, Spicer S D 1980 Facilitation of the tonic vibration reflex (TVR) by cutaneous stimulation in hemiplegics. American Journal of Physical Medicine 59.6: 280–287
Marie P, Foix C 1916 In: Brunnstrom S 1970 Movement therapy in hemiplegia. Harper & Row, New York
Norton B J, Sahrmann S A 1978 Reflex and voluntary electromyographic activity in patients with hemiparesis. Physical Therapy, 58.8: 951–955
Pedretti L W 1981 Occupational therapy, practice skills for physical dysfunction. C V Mosby Co, St Louis, Mo, ch 13
Trombly C A 1983 Occupational therapy for physical dysfunction, 2nd edn. Williams and Wilkins, Baltimore
Twitchell T E 1951 The restoration of motor function following hemiplegia in man. Brain 74: 443–480.
Washam V 1973 The onehanders book, a basic guide to activities of daily living. John Day, New York

RECOMMENDED READING

Bobath B 1978 Adult hemiplegia, evaluation and treatment, 2nd edn. Heinemann Medical books Ltd, London, ch 4
Brunnstrom S 1970 Movement therapy in hemiplegia, a neurophysiological approach. Harper and Row, New York
Carr J, Shepherd R 1982 A motor relearning programme for stroke. Heinemann Medical books Ltd, London

Jay P 1977 Mary S Jones: An approach to occupational therapy, 3rd edn. Butterworths, London, ch 10
Scott A D 1983 Evaluation and treatment of sensation. In: Trombly C (ed) Occupational therapy for physical dysfunction, 2nd edn. Williams and Wilkins, Baltimore

8

When higher cortical functions are priorities

The importance of higher cortical functions in the redevelopment of motor abilities is becoming recognised. Trombly (1983) suggests that spasticity may not be *the* major problem it was considered in the past, and that careful consideration should be given to the effects of motor programming, learning, and perceptual problems.

Patients with motor impairment alone, can call on their intact higher cortical abilities to overcome dysfunction, because they are able to understand what has happened, remain aware of whole body image, and are able to personally implement treatment strategies.

Impairment of body awareness and visuo-spatial perception was found by Anderson and Choy (1970) to correlate highly with poor rehabilitation progress. They recommend training to improve perceptual abilities, prior to training in activities of daily living. Lorenze and Cancro (1962), in a study of the relationship of activities of daily living to visual perceptual dysfunction in left hemiplegics, found that patients who showed impaired performance in block design and object assembly, remained dependent in activities of daily living.

Patients with left (speech dominant) hemisphere lesions may have difficulty in receiving and understanding oral instructions, or in coping with analysis of ideas, logical thinking, concepts and symbolism, with or without an obvious disturbance of speech (Fordyce, 1971), and therefore have impaired ability to assimilate or retain rehabilitative procedures.

Integration of sensory-motor, perceptual and cognitive abilities is inherent in all voluntary programmed activity. It is therefore important for occupational therapists to analyse and grade all therapeutic and other regular activities, to maximize effect of all components, according to the individual impairment of patients. It is also important to remember that left or right hemispheres normally respond to different aspects of the same experience (Trombly, 1983), so different approaches will be necessary, depending on the side of the lesion.

Right hemiplegics usually respond best to demonstration, need frequent specific feedback and encouragement, and, as they tend to work slowly and methodically when made aware of a problem, need more time to complete an activity than normally.

Left hemiplegics usually respond best to verbal instruction but, as they tend to rush at tasks, or to omit or pay little attention to detail, they need to be encouraged to work slowly and methodically, and to concentrate on, and attend to the task.

As visual, auditory and attention skills are usually necessary for functional activity appropriate to sensory stimuli, retraining in practical skills will be applicable for retraining impairment of primary sensation, attention, perception and cognition.

Siev and Freishtat (1976) suggest that treatment for perceptual dysfunction may be approached in three ways, a sensory integrative approach, a transfer of training approach, and a functional approach. A similar method to identify treatment approaches for impaired higher cognitive skills generally, will be adopted, namely developmental approaches, transfer of training approaches, functional remedial approaches, and compensatory approaches.

DEVELOPMENTAL APPROACHES

Motor re-education techniques based on neuro-developmental sequencing, because of the multi-level linking of neural mechanisms within the central nervous system, will be stimulating to re-education of sensation, perception and cognition, as well as movement.

Therapists must be aware of sensory cognitive components during movement re-education, or motor responses during sensory-cognitive re-education, in order to enhance activity, and facilitate central nervous system integration to promote adaptive responses to the environment.

The neurodevelopmental physiological training regimes which emphasize bilaterality, or use of hemiplegic limbs, during balance retraining, inhibition and modification of abnormal movement, and facilitation of normal sensory-motor response, may be of use in retraining higher cortical functions. In order to do this sensory input should be increased, patient participation expected, and recognition of body parts demanded. The type, amount and timing of cutaneous, visual and audi-

tory input should be monitored, controlled and modified according to individual responses.

Those following developmental approaches suggest that awareness and understanding of the body redevelops sequentially, in the same way as it develops during infancy. It is almost certain that body awareness will be enhanced because of emphasis and use of the total body in the prescribed postures and activities. Whether the developmental approaches necessary lead to the development of refined higher cortical skills is not certain.

Siev and Freishtat (1976) describe a sensory integrative approach as a common occupational therapy approach for treating perceptual problems in children, based on the neurophysiological and development model suggested by Ayres (1972). They report a statement by Ayres that her approach may be impractical for adults because the time needed for treatment may be unrealistic, the extent of lesion or generalized cortical damage plus decreased flexibility may prevent re-integration, and because extensive motor activities may be inappropriate or dangerous for elderly patients with other medical conditions.

Some therapists (Farber, 1982) have modified Ayres' approach and found it useful in the treatment of higher cortical dysfunction in adult stroke patients, although little statistical evidence is yet available to support the claims. Certainly the rationale behind a multisensory-developmental approach to higher cortical dysfunction seems worthy of consideration and studies of findings, following use of such approaches, will be of interest to all therapists.

Method

The developmental approach described in the treatment of balance and gross mobility is seen as an integral part of retraining higher cortical function. It is used to increase basic skills in patients' awareness and control of their own body, through vestibular and tactile integration, control of posture and equilibrium, and encouraging use of both sides of the body in goal-directed, low level, activity. Figure 8.1 illustrates simple perceptual and cognitive activities being used in conjunction with low level postural tasks.

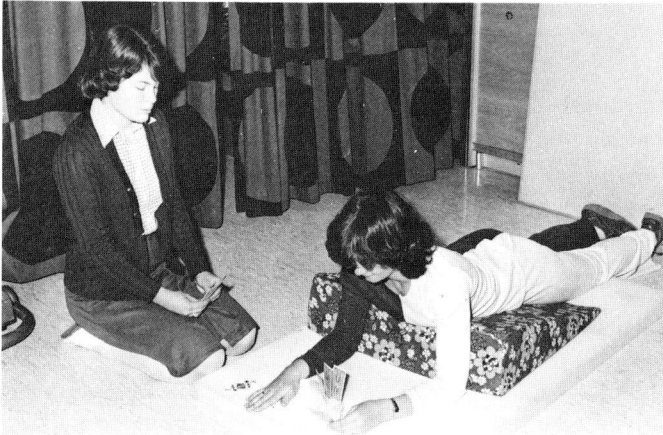

(a)

Fig. 8.1 Simple perceptual-motor tasks being used in conjunction with low level postural tasks.

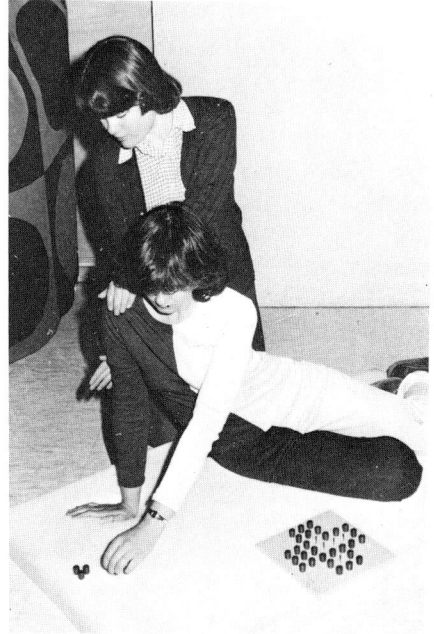

(b)

As integration of basic abilities improves, and posture, balance and mobility become controllable, tasks may be graded to encourage high level praxis, visuo-spatial, auditory and cognitive skills.

Therapeutic rationale

- In order to respond successfully to external stimuli, patients need to be aware of, and in control of, their own body.
- The approach considers the integrative functioning of the central nervous system, rather than localizing, and treating in isolation, a specific problem of higher cortical function.
- As sensory-motor skills develop inter-dependently, sensory-motor systems should be treated in unison.
- Motor and higher cortical skills are re-educated by the same approach, which is time and personnel efficient.

TRANSFER OF TRAINING APPROACH

This approach assumes that practice in tasks requiring specific cognitive and perceptual-motor skills will generalise, and lead to improved ability in other activities with similar cognitive-perceptual requirements.

Therapists select tasks for retraining because particular perceptual or cognitive skills are required for task completion, rather than because the activities are relevant to patients' lifestyle. Siev and Freishtat (1976) call this a 'transfer of training approach', because any gains made through repetition and practice in the selected tasks need to be abstractly transferred and integrated into the performance of functional activities. There has been little research into whether or not this occurs.

It seems reasonable to assume that improvement in skills which are impaired by the stroke, and apparent in the performance of one task, should make another task requiring the same skill, easier to perform. It is on this premise that therapists continue to follow this approach. There is some feeling, however, that skills may not generalise, and practice may only develop irrelevant splinter skills.

It is a commonly used approach, table games, tasks similar to those used for testing and educational task material frequently being the chosen treatment modalities. The position of task components and therapist in relation to patients, is aimed at encouraging visual scanning and auditory attention, as well as specific perceptual-cognitive skills. Cutaneous stimulation to direct and increase attention to the hemiplegic side is used in conjunction with tasks.

Tasks may be chosen because they are simple and allow those with gross dysfunction a chance to succeed, because they isolate particular perceptual or cognitive skills, or because they require cross modal matching and complex integration of higher cortical skills.

To make maximum use of this approach some planning needs to be done prior to treatment. Simply giving patients tasks to do haphazardly, to improve perception or cognition, is unlikely to maximise positive gains. There are no inbuilt guidelines in this approach to suggest order of progression, so order and sequence of approach requires consideration and planning.

Planning may be guided by results of evaluation which will have indicated major difficulties in higher cortical skills, patient interests and priorities, and level of understanding of impairments.

The previously suggested treatment progression of increasing body awareness and understanding, before demanding controlled use of objects unrelated to body requirements, and then generally extending treatment to assist patients to deal with an expanding environment, is relevant to retraining of higher cortical skills.

Methods

1. Involvement of the patient

It has been clinically observed that greater improvement appears to occur when patients understand why they are asked to undertake a specific task, can appreciate feedback on performance, and are helped to change or modify responses according to input. This means that the starting point of the program must be discussion with the patient on the suggested treatment plan. If short-term memory is impaired, this may need to be repeated regularly.

2. Working position

Before asking patients to participate in tasks demanding high concentration, they need to be stable, balanced, and comfortable, so that undue effort is not required to maintain posture and equilibrium. The instruction method needs to be suitable for the side of lesion.

3. Primary sensation

Treatment for primary sensation should be commenced before those of perception and intellect. This does not imply that sensory skills have to fully recover before progression, only that the patient should understand impairment, and have some basic sensory abilities before adding other aspects of treatment. For example, stereognosis is not possible if there is complete loss of tactile sensation, but once there is some return of function, stereognosis retraining may be used to some effect, in combination with other tactile treatments, to assist localisation and discrimination.

Scott (1983) reports tactile sensory retraining techniques, including:

(a) Vigorous rubbing of a limb with towelling before repetitive movement.
(b) Patient identification of objects or tactile stimuli without vision, followed immediately by the patient looking at, discussing and 'feeling' the tactile stimulus, for feedback, reinforcement, and to help cognitive awareness of tactile characteristics.

Similarly, programs to increase body awareness, and later, visuo-spatial abilities, will be enhanced if primary visual deficits are attended to before, or in conjunction with, perceptual retraining.

The ability to visually scan is extremely important. This does not only mean that patients can move eyes from one side to the other, but that they can control visual exploration of the environment, and can fixate on any given stimulus.

Although homonymous hemianopia may occur as a single entity, it is commonly associated with other deficits, particularly hemi-inattention, or contralateral neglect, as major complicating factors following lesions of the non-dominant hemisphere.

It may be that some patients automatically compensate for the visual defect, particularly those with lesions of the speech dominant hemisphere: however, defects may be hidden because:

(a) Some patients tend to behave as though there is no visual impairment (Gassel & Williams, 1963)

(b) The visual completion phenomenon disguises visual loss, by automatically utilizing visual memory (Poppelreuter, 1917).

(c) Western society routinely scans from left to right (Diller & Weinberg, 1977).

(d) Those with left hemisphere lesions tend to work slowly and methodically (McFie & Zangwill, 1960; Diller & Weinberg, 1977).

(e) Speech impairment makes assessment difficult (Batersby et al, 1956).

Scanning training should be included for both left and right hemiplegics, as many patients with speech dominant hemisphere lesions, clinically demonstrate an inability to fully visually explore the environment or stimuli unless prompted, or may be unable to do so in hurried or pressured situations. Speed and attention during scanning should be monitored, and feedback given to speed up or slow down performance.

When visual inattention is a complication, normal results may be obtained during formal testing, in contrast to functional situations when attention to the hemiplegic side is inconsistent depending on the degree of stimulus in the intact visual field (Mossman, 1976). Repetitive scanning retraining and patient awareness is essential for patients seen to demonstrate this problem.

To develop patient awareness it is important for therapists to approach from the sound side and initiate activity from there, before, in the same session demanding eye following to, and activity on, the hemianopic side.

Scanning training may be combined with rotation during balance retraining, therapists specifically structuring tasks by positioning activity parts on both sides of the body and grading outwards. Snooker, large floor, or table draughts, cards or video games may all be appropriate training modalities. Word, colour and picture matching or sequencing, visual cancellation tasks, and daily reading of a large-print newspaper are other useful activities.

Therapists should position themselves so that they may see both the patient's eye movements and the activity, to enable them to cue or change the situation if necessary, to gain an appropriate response.

4. Asomatognosia

Body awareness training should be an early treatment consideration, normally started before training in manipulation of extrapersonal objects, although these may be combined.

Before trying to improve body awareness, therapists may need to help the patient understand the nature of the problem. It has been clinically observed that patients often express the feeling that they may be going mad because of confusion caused by rejection or confabulation concerning their hemiplegic limbs. This is confirmed by Hewson (1982) in a personal account of disturbed body awareness. Often the simplest way to tackle this, is for the therapist to explain that patients often feel this way, and to reassure them that they are not 'going mad'. They should then be encouraged to locate, touch, look at, and talk about the hemiplegic side. Such discussion may need to be repeated often in a simple, yet adult, manner before it is truly understood.

Any activity which increases the patient's awareness of the hemiplegic side may be used as treatment for asomatognosia. Exercises in touching, naming body parts, and in copying positions, may be assisted by activities such as manikin assembly, drawing or outlining pictures of people, as in Figures 5.31 and 6.12, people and face jigsaw puzzles, or games such as 'people beetle' (Fig. 8.2(a)), or face matching (Fig. 8.2(b)).

The therapist may need to verbally and tactually cue, to facilitate task achievement. It has been clinically observed that if this type of task is used preliminarily to functional retraining, and related to it, there appears to be improvement in performance. Williams (1967) found a positive correlation between the patient who could reproduce simple drawings and the ability to dress independently.

Finger agnosia, which is often bilateral, may be treated by using cutaneous stimulation, bilateral activity, such as puzzles and games, exercises in finger identification, and activities which include finger identification, localisation, or specific use of

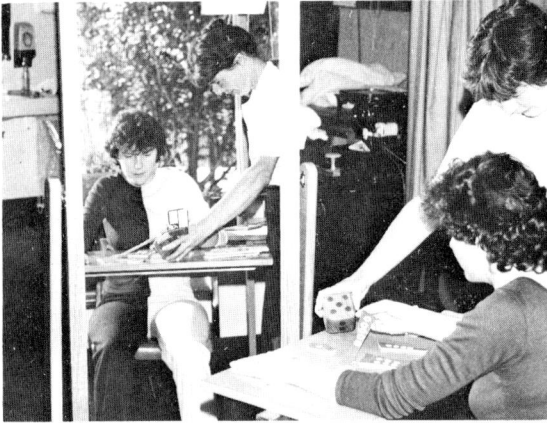

(a)

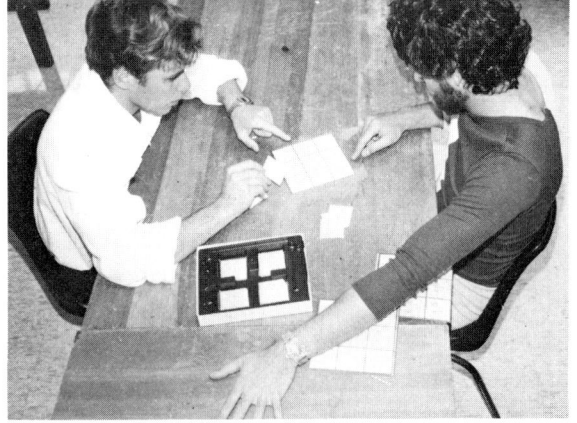

(b)

Fig. 8.2 (a) Using an adapted form of 'Beetle' with a manikin, to stimulate awareness of body parts and their inter-relationships. (b) Faces on individual cards are matched with those on a master board.

one or other finger or hand, such as typing or piano playing.

Fox (1964) recommends rubbing the extensor surface of forearm, hand, and fingers, and the palmar surface of the fingers with a rough cloth for a minimum of two minutes, and asking or assisting the patient to grip a cardboard cone shape for the same length of time. The two may be alternated for thirty seconds each. Therapists should be alert for withdrawal response or discomfort, and if seen should change the activity.

5. Apraxia

Little has been documented about the treatment of motor apraxia, and approaches that have been used, have yet to be substantiated. However, attempts at retraining should be commenced early, particularly if impairment of speech is compounded by impairment of secondary communication skills, such as gesture. Treatment may include manual contact and guidance of the upper limb by the therapist during tasks, and imitation of body postures. Simple sequential tasks may be devised in which the patient has to make small changes in action or direction, in order to overcome problems of hesitancy and perseveration. Feldt et al (1979) suggest the patient is asked to touch a series of coloured spots on the table, in a given sequence, in time to metronome. The spots are identified by letter or number. This activity is based on exer-

cises devised by Dr Heinrich Frenkel, a nineteenth century neurologist, to increase co-ordination.

Table games such as finger basketball (Fig. 8.3), also demand slight changes of movement. Players are required to press one of five buttons corresponding to the position of the ball in order to make a shot. The ball's starting position is random, being dependent on the bounce from the previous shot. Patients have to plan the slight movement change accordingly.

As patients become able to understand, and respond to verbal or non-verbal instruction, and can basically appreciate, even if not aware at all

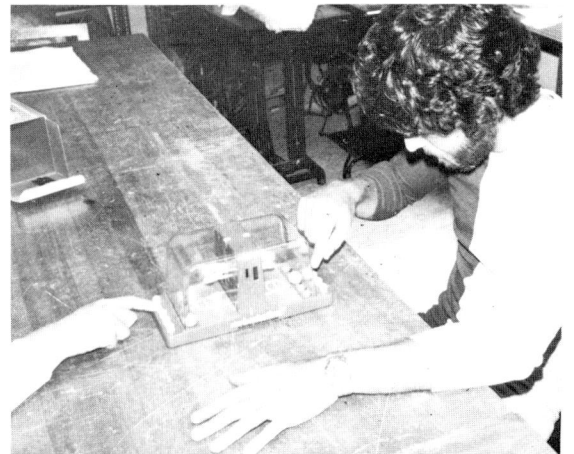

Fig. 8.3 Finger basketball demands slight changes in finger movements, and may be used for treating appraxic disorder.

times, their own bilaterality, increasingly complex movements and manipulation of objects in space may be introduced.

6. Astereognosis

Farber (1982) recommends that treatment for astereognosis should utilise visual input as a primary step, with patients watching the therapist move an object slowly through all planes then continuing to watch, as firstly their own sound hand, secondly both hands, and thirdly the affected hand handle the object. Visual input may be increased by the use of mirrors. Patients are then encouraged to handle the object in a similar way, but without watching. Following consistent identification of several objects, these may be hidden in a 'feely box' filled with split peas, rice or sand. If overstimulation is a danger, objects may be placed in an empty bag. The patient is asked to find specific objects. New objects may be added after consistent success.

Similarly, therapists may use pictures for patients to identify and tactually match, as shown in Figure 8.4. The inclusion of multi-sensory inputs, to increase the amount of available information to trigger neural circuits, may be useful to facilitate tactual identification.

Visual stimulation is useful because stereognosis probably combines cross-modal sensory memory, normal tactual identification prompting 3 dimen-

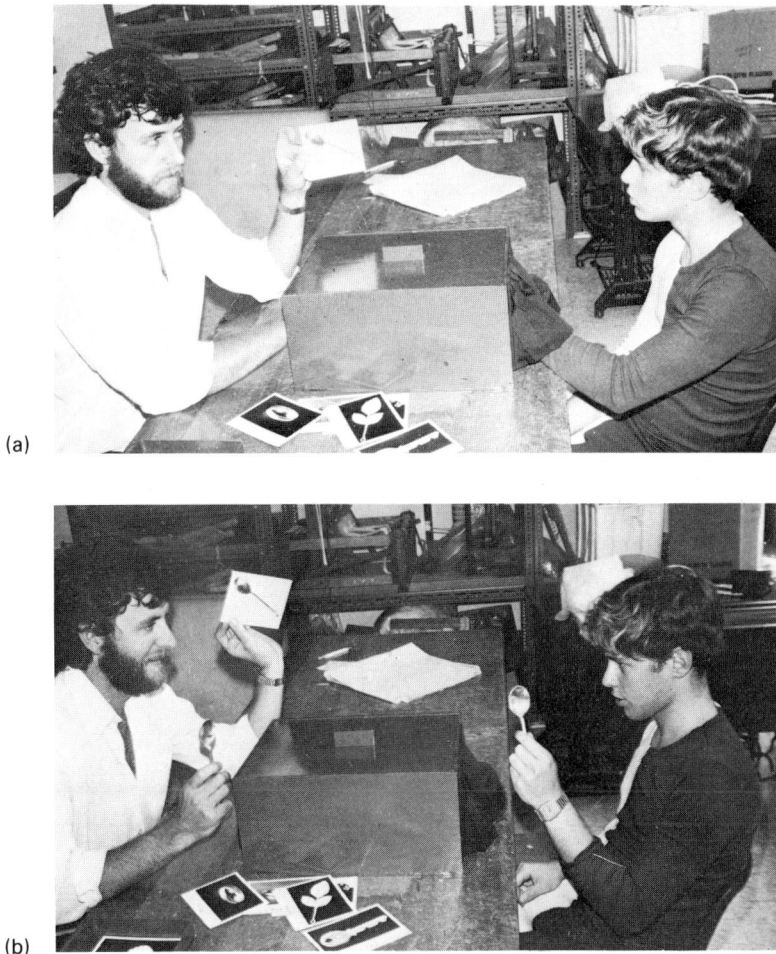

(a)

(b)

Fig. 8.4 Matching pictures and objects by feeling for the same object hidden in a box.

sional visual memory for the object. For some specific objects other sensory memories may be prompted, for example, taste and smell when feeling an orange.

As stereognosis combines cutaneous and spatial cues, peripheral stimulation, to increase tactual awareness and awareness of movement through space, may also be useful.

7. Visuo-spatial impairment

Impairment of visuo-spatial perceptual-motor skills is commonly treated by graded use of the activities the patient finds difficult. Therefore those activities discussed as evaluation tools may be used for treatment.

Therapists often use block construction, pegboard patterns, jigsaw puzzles, formboards, 2 and 3 dimensional figure ground puzzles, mazes and sorting tasks.

Other activities that occupational therapists have found useful are table games such as draughts, noughts and crosses, jigsaw puzzles, pencil and paper, educational and developmental games, and video games. Care is taken that whatever is used, is of adult content, or that the patient is able to use it in an adult fashion because they understand the purpose behind its use.

Therapists facilitate success in the carefully graded activities, by appropriate cueing, and cognitive reminders, usually starting with simple one-part activities, and progressing to complex multi-modal tasks.

Activities may be chosen because they incorporate several aspects of treatment. In a study by Weinberg et al (1979) on training sensory awareness and spatial organisation, it was found that combined multiple treatment was more effective than single purpose treatment, and that those with greater impairment improved more than those with mild impairment. The multiple treatment was conducted for one hour a day for four weeks, in addition to usual occupational and physiotherapy programs. It included visual scanning by cueing the starting position on the hemiplegic side and increasing the distances between targets, controlling speed to inhibit impulsivity, and feedback. The spatial organization task was to visually estimate the size of objects, and the sensory awareness component was a non-visual task, in which patients were touched on the back, and then had to touch a manikin in the same place.

This appears to imply that carefully chosen activities of a cross modal nature may trigger greater response and assist relearning. Examples of cross modal activity include:

(a) Copying a 2 dimensional plan to construct a 3 dimensional object, as in bead threading (Fig. 8.5). The activity calls for construction sequencing, discrimination between size, shape and colour, and fine co-ordinated motor activity. (Use tactile or auditory cues.)

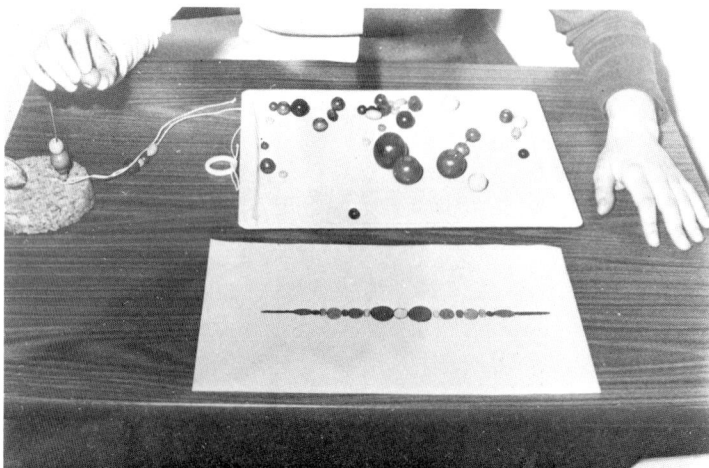

Fig. 8.5 Copying a plan to construct a bead necklace, using pre-organized, different sizes and colours.

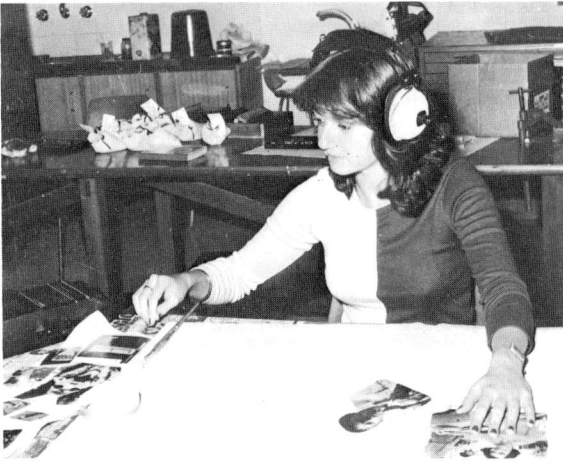

Fig. 8.6 Auditory information given through the ear pieces provides cues for visual selection of items for a collage.

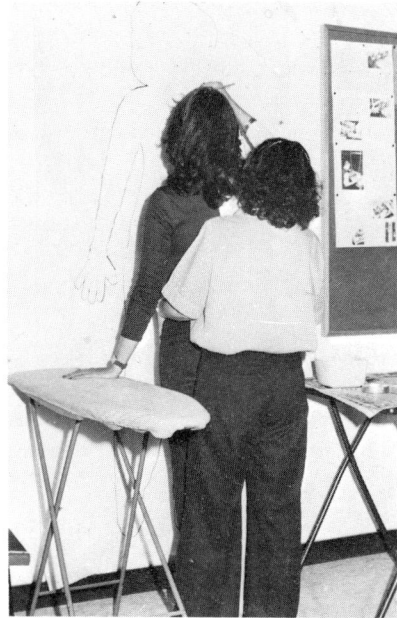

Fig. 8.7 Large scale figure drawing aimed at integrating body awareness, weight bearing, and balance activity.

(b) Stereognosis retraining which includes 2 and 3 dimensional visual information to assist tactile integration, reinforced by verbal cues, as shown in Figure 8.4.
(c) Auditory information providing cues for picking out pictures for a 'current affairs' collage (Fig. 8.6).
(d) A fun art activity aimed at integration of body awareness and extra-personal space. Large scale figure drawing may be combined with weight bearing and balance activity, tactile and verbal cues being provided by the therapist (Fig. 8.7).

games, puzzles, pencil and paper, educational and developmental games, used in an adult fashion.

Activities may need to be simplified, adapted, or have components modified, so that particular cognitive aspects are increased or decreased. This, once again, implies that accurate activity analysis is important. It may be necessary to adapt or

8. Cognitive impairment

As basic skills become established, more intellectual activities may be gradually introduced into treatment. Word games, such as the various forms of Scrabble (Fig. 8.8), can be simplified, adapted or used as designed, and may lead to puzzles and games requiring abstract reasoning and conceptualisation. Games requiring the use of numbers (Fig. 8.9) for progression may lead to re-development of number skills practised with 'Do it yourself' mathematics books. As with visuo-spatial impairment, other activities which occupational therapists have found useful are table and video

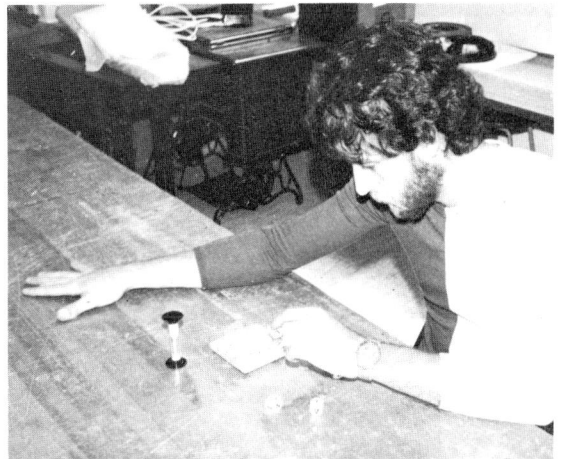

Fig. 8.8 Scrabble used to help abstract reasoning and conceptualization skills.

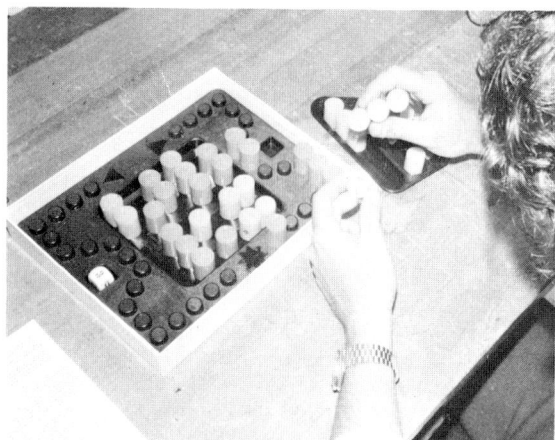

Fig. 8.9 Games requiring numbers — such as those needing action according to the number on a dice — may be used to redevelop number skills.

modify rules of chosen games during a treatment, to meet the changing needs of a patient.

The therapist does not always need to be a player in games used; careful choice of one or more other patients to participate may enable a therapist to combine sensory motor, perceptual or cognitive retraining for several patients, during what appears to be an enjoyable social situation. To fully utilize such a situation demands forethought, careful pre-planning, an ability to develop positive aspects of the situation as they materialize, and to inhibit any negative aspects should they occur.

Therapeutic rationale for transfer of training approach:

● Concentration of treatment on problem aspects of higher cortical dysfunction may lead to increased skill generally.
● Effort will be directed at specific problems

FUNCTIONAL REMEDIAL APPROACHES

Siev and Freishtat (1976) reports that therapists following a functional approach to the treatment of perceptual impairment do so because they feel it is more practical than other approaches, when treatment time is limited, and also because patients are able to understand it. Some therapists feel that patients often find a 'transfer of training approach'

childish, degrading, and not relevant to their problems.

A functional approach may be used for specific treatment of higher cortical abilities, when, instead of using prescribed positioning or abstract tasks, patients use those in which they need competence in their individual everyday lives.

Carr and Shepherd (1982) hypothesize that an early upright position, weight bearing, and emphasis on active movement of an adult nature, of hemiplegic limbs and body, reduces early perceptual dysfunction, and prevents the disuse of central nervous system mechanisms, compounding any cognitive problems.

Activities which need to be, or can be done frequently, without producing antipathy, are suitable tasks for retraining higher cortical functions, because repetition is important in acquiring skills, both motor and cognitive memory for activity being acquired cumulatively. However, repetition of an actual activity rather than an exercise, will usually include slight variations, making extra integrative and cognitive demands of the patient. If the patient is able to deal with the variations satisfactorily, the increased range of skills may facilitate volitional variations and adaptability to altered situations.

Methods

A functional approach, if started early, is likely to be appropriately biased to the achievement of personally related skills, before those of an extrapersonal nature, and before those demanding adaptive response to an expanded environment.

1. Body-related activity

In the discussion of the use of self-care tasks in the ward situation (Ch. 5), emphasis was put on the personal sensory aspects inherent in such activities. They are used in this way, not simply to improve independence in activities of daily living, although that may be an added bonus, but to assist patients from the earliest possible time to become aware of their body as a totally integrated unit and object in space, by the use of *meaningful* proprioceptive, kinesthetic, tactile, visual and verbal input.

Sensory treatment through personal care activities is not restricted to the first few days when the patient may be confined to the ward. They should be continued as long as necessary, with the patient being encouraged to take more responsibility for their planning, to take over the verbal and sensory cueing and input as they are able, and to build up independent motor skills, which involve more normal bilateral movement and equilibrium reactions.

Initially, emphasis should be on the components of the task which supply direct tactile sensory input, whilst postural stability is maintained, and graded, controlled, rotational movement is facilitated. Washing, showering, creaming and dressing should be used with patient awareness, and conscious thought directed towards the feel of the touch and movement of the hemiplegic side. Choice of soap, cream and powder may add pleasant olfactory stimulation and reminders. Soft, warm towels with a highly textured surface are recommended. Clothes should be easy to put on, allow patient movement, and not disguise body parts. Legs should be covered by 'slacks' rather than a rug.

Functional scanning to assist visual input may be initiated by verbal and tactile cues. Assistance may be given quietly, in the beginning, to aspects of the task which may be particularly difficult for those with apraxia or visuo-spatial impairment, such as positioning a garment, so it is easy to find an armhole or to put on. Increasing visual input by using a full length mirror is often useful, as long as the patient does not find this disturbing. Seeing oneself in a mirror, during such tasks, is how people usually see a total image of themselves.

When right/left discrimination is impaired, initial practice in bilateral skills should use visual, tactile or verbal cues other than right or left to promote achievement. As patients' abilities develop, the terms should be used as often as possible during the activities, with visual and tactile reinforcement. Activities should be chosen in which right and left may be stressed. Siev and Freishtat (1976) recommend giving extra tactile and proprioceptive stimulation consistently to one limb, for example, using a weighted cuff on one wrist to assist patient discrimination. An alternative suggestion may be the use of air pressure splints as recommended by Johnstone (1978). As body integrative skills improve, external visuospatial demands may be increased.

2. Visual impairment

To prevent anxiety and frustration, personal requirements should remain on the sound side until the patient understands the nature of the visual deficit and can begin to compensate.

After assisting the patient to become aware of the problem, and the patient is able to scan and locate stimuli to the affected side, activities should be used which demand looking to the left and right, such as reading, looking through a newspaper, or any activity of interest to the patient in which positioning of components to right and left facilitates rotation, recognition and manipulation of objects in the space on the hemiplegic side. Visual guides may be useful to assist the patient initially, such as a marker to the extreme left of a newspaper. Patients may need repetitive training to use the visual guides effectively.

Sitting and standing during activities of daily living, and at a window with a rail for support, provides appropriate opportunities for patients to visually scan and explore the environment. Structured groups or social opportunities, in the ward or department, should encourage natural scanning activity, although initially it may need prompting and reinforcement. If patients normally wear spectacles they should be found and worn.

Patients should be encouraged to think about and avoid dangerous situations which may occur during treatment sessions and in the ward, such as bumping into or falling over objects. Mobility retraining should include discussion of the environment, followed by visual location of obstacles and architectural features. This should occur before the patient is taken on walks to the bathroom, ward and between treatment departments, so that repetition promotes habituation and continued safe practice.

3. Apraxia

With appropriate support, activities of a fairly gross nature should not pose many problems for patients with apraxia: however, activities such as combing hair, cleaning teeth and handling cutlery may do.

Apraxia is often difficult to treat but certain techniques do seem to be accepted as useful by many clinicians, and these include:

(a) Using simple one part activity, or breaking down activity into individual components; teaching these to the patient and grading them into a whole as achievement becomes possible. Forward or backward chaining are examples of a useful method of breaking down activities.
(b) Guiding limbs through the movements demanded by the task.
(c) Using simple, one part sentences to direct the patient.
(d) Practice and repetition of difficult tasks.
(e) Reinforcing brief, verbal instructions with tactual and proprioceptive cues, such as manual pressure and approximation.
(f) Using demonstration and visual cues as an alternative to verbal command.

As apraxia commonly affects fine motor skills of face and upper limbs, particularly hands, rather than those of the trunk and lower extremities, patients should be encouraged to participate in, and succeed in, gross mobility activities, so that frustration may be tempered by achievement.

If patients are experiencing particular difficulties with A.D.L., such as eating, dressing, or hygiene tasks, the therapist should either attempt to plan treatment programs so that individual retraining times coincide with ward schedules for these activities, or teach others how to assist in the most useful way, at the appropriate times.

Solet (1974), when discussing treatment implications for apraxia, suggests that most apraxic patients will experience less difficulty if using real objects and activities, rather than practice objects or activities. She suggests that the not uncommon practice of the therapist asking patients to try using eating utensils with plasticine instead of food, or practise lifting an empty glass, especially if the patient is not thirsty, may confound the apraxic patient who functions at a very concrete level. This suggests training in real tasks should take place as and when they occur naturally.

Because apraxia is most usually associated with left hemisphere lesions, approach by demonstration is recommended, the therapist positioned to the side of the patient, rather than in front, to avoid left/right confusion (another left hemisphere function). The hemiplegic side may be most suitable when patients respond to manual guidance; however, directions and demonstrations need to be presented to 'intact' auditory and visual fields.

Although simplification of activity including the breaking down of tasks into small parts is often recommended, some patients may reveal during evaluation that they are able to respond better to total body instructions than to those specific to upper limb and face. Therapists in this case may find general instruction easier for the patient to follow than those of a simpler, more specific nature. Grading should be adjusted accordingly.

4. Visuo-spatial activity

The therapist should gradually increase activities demanding selection and goal-directed manipulation of objects, perhaps having started early in rehabilitation by making use of private, then social eating situations, or using a patient's own 2 or 3 dimensional possessions for scanning and fixation, object recognition, figure ground and spatial relationship retraining. Letters, photographs, get well cards, newspapers, magazines and personal toiletries may all be utilised effectively by the thinking therapist in simple or complex cross modal activity. Stereognosis training may be incorporated, by activities such as coin matching, recognition and addition, followed by searching for the coins in trouser pockets, or purse, without vision.

Treatment should expand to include visuo-spatial use of the environment, for example retraining of judgment of door size and position of handles, as illustrated in Figure 8.10, finding a route from the ward to the bathroom or the occupational therapy department, and visually exploring the floor and surroundings for hazards, before walking practice.

Activities which will be part of the patient's future, that is home, vocational or avocational activities should be used for higher cortical retraining. These may be graded from simple components to gradually include more modalities and complexities.

Therapists need to analyse the activities that a

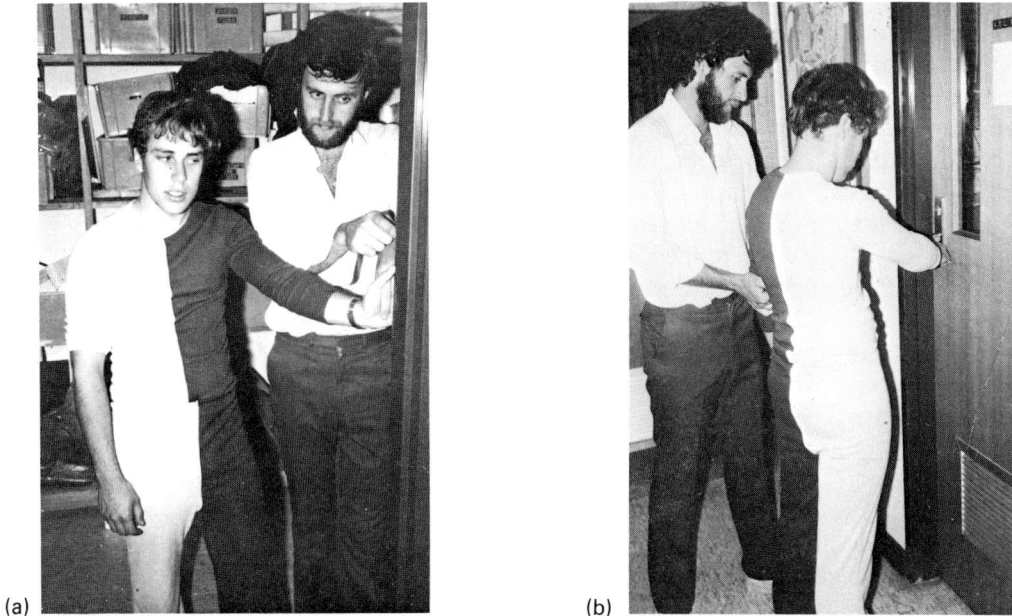

Fig. 8.10 (a) Retraining in judging door size. (b) Retraining in finding the position of handles.

patient needs or wishes to do, for the visuo-spatial components, and either encourage the patient to practise these small components repetitively until achievement is possible, or attempt the activity as a whole, with sensory input and/or assistance increased at the points of greatest difficulty, so that achievement is possible. Input is reduced as improvement occurs. Simple, step-by-step verbal input is likely to be more effective than demonstration, and it is sometimes helpful to guide movement and to give tactual cues. Therapists may need to use sensory, perceptual or cognitive skills which remain intact to facilitate patient achievement. Routine, repetition and reinforcement are essential to this approach. Awareness of, and attention to, level of functioning prior to stroke, is important for patient motivation, and as a guide to recovery.

5. Auditory disorders

Should the patient have a particular auditory perceptual impairment, practice in identifying and locating relevant sounds should be included in the program. This should incorporate, if possible, practice in their own environment.

6. Communication disorders

The psychological impact of lost speech and habitual methods of communication is devastating, and it may be that reading and writing skills and understanding of symbols is also impaired. Loss of verbal ability is often seen by the patient and others as a reflection of loss of intellect. People tend to shout, use baby talk, prompt, guess, and talk about, rather than to, the dysphasic patient.

Occupational therapists must co-operate with speech pathologists so that particular aspects of treatment being undertaken in speech therapy may be included in other aspects of retraining, when appropriate.

When communicating with dysphasic patients in treatment, attention should be attracted by the use of their name. Short, simple, one part sentences should be used with a slow, even, but adult tone. Patients should be able to see clearly the people talking with them, so that facial expression and gesture may give them clues as to what is being said.

Plenty of time for response should be allowed, and patients should not be interrupted except when they are perseverating. Perfect pronunciation is unnecessary unless it is a specific part of the retraining program, and if the patient swears, he or she should not be laughed at or rebuked.

Demonstration of activity may assist if verbal understanding is impaired, as might suggesting to patients that they use gesture to communicate, when verbal expression is difficult.

A realistic, honest approach is essential if patients are to recognise and accept their disorder, so it is unwise to comfort stressed patients by telling them that they will be speaking soon, or to pretend understanding.

It is important to observe the effect of the environment on patients and adapt it if necessary. Initially, more than one or two people in the room may confuse patients, particularly if there is a lot of conversation. Extraneous noise may also distract. As it may be tiring for patients to follow and understand the language around them, and to respond appropriately, rapid conversation, and changes of topic, are contraindicated. It helps if people around patients are relaxed.

Fluctuations in ability will occur if patients become fatigued or upset. Fatigue will also reduce attention span, so therapists must watch for indications of tiring and allow for rest periods.

Patients should not be talked about as if they were not there, but included in the conversation. Social singing, particularly of older, well-known songs may be appropriate in group situations, as the patient may be able to participate and derive the benefit of using words, which may not otherwise be possible.

Patients with lesions of either hemisphere may be somewhat impaired in appreciating humour, but those with left hemisphere lesions will be more impaired when humour is basically verbal, and those with right hemisphere lesions will be more impaired if humour is basically visual (Gardner et al, 1976).

Clinicians report some success using computers and video games to motivate and interest patients with speech impairment. This indicates an area for research and evaluation.

7. Cognitive disorders

Creative, domestic, recreational or vocational activities may be judiciously graded for cognitive factors, from simple to complex.

Suggested functional activity which may be useful in developing practical skills of a cognitive nature include:

(a) Cooking and housekeeping tasks, such as planning and organizing meals, budgeting and marketing.
(b) Garden and home handyperson tasks such as following directions for spraying and planting, or cleaning and maintaining household and garden equipment.
(c) Map reading and orienteering.
(d) Simple recreational activities, such as reading, watching television, or listening to the radio, when understanding and retention of content are important.
(e) Individually relevant recreational activities, such as knitting, crochet, or sewing when patterns need to be followed, woodwork or building tasks when measurement and order of tasks are necessary.
(f) Vocational tasks for those likely to return to work.

If there are differences between attention abilities in visual or verbal activities, the use of one may be included with the other, to improve the impaired modality. For example, if a patient is unable to attend to verbal instructions, demonstration with only limited verbal input may command attention. As improvement occurs, one or two steps may be described verbally, the therapist upgrading until the whole process may be completed with verbal input alone.

Distractability may require that early treatment take place in a distraction-free environment, which is gradually modified to simulate likely future demands.

If a patient has need to develop complex conceptual tracking skills, this should be pursued gradually, with the patient understanding and wishing to participate in a graded program which makes increasing demands upon their attention. Examples of such programs include a housewife having to prepare and set out a three course meal for a family, including courses or ingredients which may spoil if not attended to; or a business man practising writing a report, answering enquiries and the telephone, during a pre-specified time period. Eventually, patients for whom it is appropriate should be involved in the planning of each rehabilitation day and week, so that they may be able to better plan duties when they are discharged.

For those with interest in more intellectual pursuits, discrete cognitive skills may need redeveloping. This should not be considered unnecessary, as perhaps without this type of retraining, patients with such interests may become utterly frustrated and depressed after return to home, despite having learned to cope with activities of daily living independently.

Upgrading activity to maximize planning, memory, attention, and problem-solving skills as patients improve is essential. Use of word and number concepts in abstract ways, associated with real life, and initiation of ideas, may be of importance to patients who have had mainly intellectual interests prior to the stroke. For such patients, functional retraining may include involvement of friends and colleagues in suitable discussion and activity.

COMPENSATORY APPROACHES

If, as patient recovery ceases or plateaus, higher cortical skills are not fully redeveloped, compensatory methods for resultant dysfunction will have to be taught.

Methods

1. Patient awareness

In order for patients to be able to compensate they must become aware of problems, and choose to use an alternative method of function. Patient education is an important aspect of retraining, and when therapists evaluate each patient, they should discover strengths as well as impairment, so they are able to advise on possible alternatives. For example, patients may be able, with repetitive practice, to 'talk themselves' into clothes, using concepts of right and left and verbal memory, if visuo-spatial disorders prevent them 'seeing' the

way to dress. Or they may need to practise repetitively head turning to the hemiplegic side, to compensate for unilateral spatial neglect, or homonymous hemianopia.

2. Changes to environment

The physical environment may be altered by positioning chairs or beds, so that the patient can see and respond to what is going on. It may be uncluttered to make mobility safer, or objects easier to find, for patients with figure ground impairment. Objects may be chosen for use because they can be easily seen: for example, use of different coloured bedding may assist bed making. Objects should be positioned so that patients may see them from regular resting spots.

3. Changes of technique

Techniques may be changed to assist compensation: for example, patients may be taught to turn their plates during meals, or to position them to the sound side to ensure all food can be seen. Order of putting on clothes may be organised so that one part of the body is dressed before another, or according to rehearsed sequence. Methods of transfer and mobility may need to emphasise the sound side for safety.

Visual cues may be added to objects or environment to reinforce a technique, for example a brightly coloured book mark may be placed to the extreme left or right of a book or paper, to assist reading a full line; different coloured tags may be attached to arm holes of garments, to assist recognition and facilitate dressing procedures; an easily seen chair may be placed by the bathroom door to cue topographical orientation. Some therapists have used proprioceptive cues, such as a wrist weight to help awareness of the hemiplegic side and to remind patients to include it in activity.

4. Practice

Teaching patients, by repetitive practice, how to verbally and tactually cue themselves may be assistive for some, or teaching those they live with how to do this, may be appropriate. Patients may be helped to talk through a learned sequence as they perform daily tasks; or objects may be described aloud and thought through cognitively so recognition is possible. Methods may be taught where one step cues the next.

Repetitive practice in touching and caring for the hemiplegic side is essential for safety and hygiene, and because it may continue to increase awareness of neglected body parts, or space, to the hemiplegic side.

5. Memory impairment

Treatment to redevelop comprehensive memory skills following impairment, has proved difficult. The most effective functional methods appear to be compensatory approaches: for example, should a patient display poor verbal memory, practice to improve visual, motor or tactual memory may be more successful than concentrating on verbal memory, and vice versa.

Because memory traces are built up cumulatively, any retraining must include repetition and consistency of input. It is particularly important in cases of memory impairment that all the treatment team use consistent retraining approaches.

It is important for therapists to assist patients to be selective in what they try to remember. Patients should be encouraged to nominate potential priority memories, be assisted with the development of internal and external cueing to help recall, and be reminded of the event frequently, within the time limit of their short-term memory. To try to have the patient remember everything is to clutter the system with unnecessary trivia which may prevent wanted recall from occurring.

If external aids such as diaries are used, patients will probably require repetitive prompts to remember to record, or look up, information.

6. Communication

Some patients with language disorders may find communication charts helpful, but often practice with mime or gesture is more useful, unless the patient is apraxic. Mime or gesture is not restricted to objects on a chart, does not rely on ability to interpret symbols, and uses probably intact, visual-spatial abilities.

When right/left disorientation is a problem, reduction or elimination of the terms, when instructing the patient or helping the relatives to use pointing or touching in communications with the patient, will lessen confusion.

If difficulties are still being experienced on discharge, and treatment is not to be continued, relatives or nursing home personnel should be advised to approach and address the patient from the sound side.

Whatever compensatory or adaptive procedure is used, repetitive practice and reinforcement is essential if it is to be of functional use to the patient.

Therapeutic rationale for compensatory approaches:

- Despite residual dysfunction, allows patients to function appropriately within a limited environment.
- Teaches the patient to make use of residual abilities to overcome lifestyle difficulties.
- Helps those who live with the patient to understand the nature of higher cortical dysfunction, and to respond appropriately to altered behaviour.
- May assist continued awareness of bilaterality.

SUMMARY

Any of the approaches, by demanding active participation of the patient in thinking about, and executing sequential planned activity, should assist in cognitive and perceptual processes, if indeed it is demands made on it that develop the central nervous system. However, the demands should be appropriate, and achievement possible, or learning may be retarded by a negative affective response. Therapists need to be constantly monitoring the sensory, motor and cognitive experience and patient responses, changing input if response is undesirable. Findings should be recorded in an ordered and useful fashion.

REFERENCES

Anderson E, Choy E 1970 Parietal lobe syndromes in hemiplegia, a program for treatment. American Journal of Occupational Therapy 24.1: 13–18

Ayres J A 1972 Sensory integration and learning disorders. Western Psychological Services, Los Angeles

Batersby W S, Bender M B, Pollack M 1956 Unilateral spatial agnosia (inattention) in patients with cerebral lesions. Brain 79: 68–93

Carr J, Shepherd R 1982 A motor relearning programme for stroke. Heinemann Medical books Ltd, London

Diller L, Weinberg J 1977 Hemi-inattention in rehabilitation: The evolution of a rational remedial program. Advances in Neurology 18: 63–82

Farber S D 1982 Neurorehabilitation, a multi sensory approach. Saunders, Philadelphia

Feldt R, Holzberg C, Hren M, McKenzie J 1979 Perceptual training manual. Ontario Society of Occupational Therapists study group on the brain damaged adult

Fordyce W 1971 Psychological assessment and management. In: Krusen F H, Kottke F J, Ellwood P M (eds) Handbook of physical medicine and rehabilitation, 2nd edn. W B Saunders, Philadelphia

Fox J 1964 Cutaneous stimulation: effects on selected tests of perception. American Journal of Occupational therapy 18(2): 53–55

Gardner H, Ling P K, Flamm L, Silverman J 1976 Comprehension and appreciation of humorous material following brain damage. Brain 98: 399–412

Gassel M M, Williams D 1963 Visual function in patients with homonymous hemianopia. Brain 175, 86: 229–260

Hewson L 1982 When half is whole. Dove communications, Blackburn, Victoria

Johnstone M 1978 Restoration of motor function in the stroke patient, a physiotherapist's approach. Churchill Livingstone, Edinburgh

Lorenze E J, Cancro R 1962 Dysfunction in visual perception with hemiplegia: its relation to activities of daily living. Archives of Physical Medicine and rehabilitation 43: 514–517

McFie J, Zangwill O L 1960 Visual constructive disabilities associated with lesions of the left cerebral hemisphere. Brain 83: 243–260

Mossman P L 1976 A problem oriented approach to stroke rehabilitation. Charles A Thomas, Springfield

Poppelreuter W 1917 Die Psychischen schadigungen durch kopfschuss im Kriege 1914–1916. Voss, Leipzig

Scott A D 1983 Evaluation and treatment of sensation. In: Trombly C A (ed) Occupational therapy for physical dysfunction, 2nd edn. Williams & Wilkins, Baltimore

Siev E, Freishtat B 1976 Perceptual dysfunction in the adult stroke patient, a manual for evaluation and treatment. Charles B Slack, Inc, USA

Solet J M 1974 Solet test for apraxia. Thesis, Boston University

Trombly C 1983 (ed) Occupational therapy for physical dysfunction, 2nd edn. Williams & Wilkins, Baltimore

Weinberg J, Diller L, Wayne A, Gerstman L J, Lieberman A, Lakin P, Hodges G, Ezrachi O 1979 Training sensory awareness and spatial organisation in people with (R) brain damage. Archives of Physical Medicine and rehabilitation 60 (Nov): 491–496

Williams N 1967 Correlations between copying ability and dressing activities in hemiplegia. American Journal of Physical Medicine 46: 1332–1340

RECOMMENDED READING

Hewson L 1982 When half is whole. Dove communications, Blackburn, Victoria

Kolb B, Whishaw I Q 1980 Fundamentals of human neuropsychology. W H Freeman, San Francisco, ch. 10, 12–16

Siev E, Freishtat B 1976 Perceptual dysfunction in the adult stroke patient, a manual for evaluation and treatment. Charles B Slack, Inc, USA

9

When social and affective problems are priorities

AFFECTIVE RESPONSES

The sudden nature of C.V.A. and the many and varied ways in which function can be affected is extremely distressing and confusing to patients. Coping with their own feelings, and relating them to their previous self-concepts, must be devastating. They are powerless to change the situation, dependent and unable to control their own lives by using former coping mechanisms. It is unlikely that the confused thoughts and emotions they may experience initially are able to be shown or shared, particularly when language disorders disrupt, or unilateral neglect and denial impair abstract thought processes.

It is likely that the patient's abstract understanding of their own identity is complicated by approaches made by hospital personnel who, as strangers, communicate with the present reality, and not in a manner with which the patient is familiar and had come to expect when meeting new people.

Therapists should be extremely aware of how the patient may be feeling, particularly when they make their initial approaches, and try to lessen confusion by applying judiciously acquired information about previous lifestyle, interests, and personality traits, so that differences of approach between past and present are reduced.

As patients become more aware of the effects of the stroke and possible future lifestyle restrictions, it is important for the occupational therapist to offer empathetic support and encouragement to aid the patient's adjustment to disability and to hospitalization. An understanding of the normal adjustment processes to loss of function, will allow the therapist to be understanding and responsive to the patient's feelings of denial, pre-occupation with loss, anxiety and depression during the rehabilitation process. Some patients may not feel able to participate wholeheartedly in treatment programs for weeks or months, whilst others may dwell on the possibility of full recovery, and be unable to accept the possibility of residual dysfunction (Pedretti, 1981).

These factors may mean that patients are unable to gain maximally from the program offered at the time it is offered, and indicate that there may be a need for ongoing review of all patients' progress and attitudes for at least one year after stroke, so that programs may be made available, when patients are most motivated to participate, and likely to make most use of treatment offered.

The changing nature of affective responses to disability and lifestyle should be under constant review so that approaches are appropriate to the patient's psychological state. Therapists should be aware that patients will be most susceptible to fluctuations in affect when major change in the ongoing program occurs, such as transfer to another unit, or change of therapist.

Possible differences between right and left affective reactions should be considered early, the therapist making positive approaches to prevent either catastrophic depression or denial becoming overriding symptoms, by an empathetic, realistic manner from the time of initial contact, and by offering realistic, mature, achievable activities as treatment modalities as rehabilitation progresses.

SOCIAL CONSIDERATIONS

Patients' social situations may alter dramatically as a result of stroke. They may be unable to return to their former role, or even to their former environment. For many, life skills will have to be adapted or modified in order to be possible; life roles and relationships with others will be changed, and status within the community will be affected, even if they do return home. For those unable to return home because of gross dysfunction or inadequate support, learning to cope with dependence, either in an alternative domestic situation or dependent care agency, is likely to be a depressing and difficult adjustment.

From the earliest possible date, the patient's social future should be considered and reflected in the occupational therapy programs, so that negative affective responses, such as depression and anxiety, are lessened by positive problem-solving approaches. The program should allow time for private discussion, family education and participation, patient group problem solving, and improvement of practical skills.

Patient's social priorities and goals should be encouraged, and relatives' responses, and future roles, considered and co-ordinated with the

patients where possible. For example, although physical independence in self-care activities may be a worthy goal, they may be so time consuming and fatiguing that other interests are impossible. Encouraging a partner to assist in energy consuming activity so that other interests may be pursued, may result in a richer shared lifestyle, interdependence being an acceptable alternative to frustrating independence.

Patients' personalities are usually reflected in work and leisure interests, and also in the various roles they assumed pre-stroke, such as their role in the community, at work, at home, and as a friend. The relationships shared with others reinforced their individuality, growth and change being effected by normal social response. For those close to stroke patients, alterations in role and relationships will be necessary and difficult. For those less close, such as work or community colleagues, after an initial shock, roles are likely to be re-organised. This re-organisation may cause difficulties for colleagues in continued contact with the patient during hospitalisation, and in patient reintegration into their previous life situation when they return home. The occupational therapy program should provide situations where the patient may work through some of these problems.

LABILITY

When lability is a problem, patients are likely to be concerned by the apparent lack of control they have over their emotions, which may compound the lack of control they are experiencing over their bodies and personal independence, leading to withdrawal and isolation. Embarrassment may lead to loss of self-esteem, uncomfortable relationships between patients and relatives, and in the treatment situation, which may cause them not to want visitors or to attend treatment.

In many cases lability decreases with time, but for some patients the impairment may continue for years. In such cases the need to look at the effect of lability on treatment personnel, relatives and friends is vital if embarrassment and withdrawal are not to lead to depression.

Some therapists feel that the most useful

approach is to ignore labile behaviour, others that some intervention may be indicated.

Methods

(a) Early discussion with the patient, relatives and friends about the nature of the impairment, the likelihood that it will gradually decrease, and the measures that will be used by therapists when outbursts occur, and which may be helpful for others.

(b) Turner (1981) suggests that therapists neither ignore, or make a fuss, but allow patients to cry and to recompose themselves. Therapists may pause and give brief comfort verbally or tactually, or simply pause for a moment before continuing to talk, whilst the patient regains composure.

(c) Relaxation techniques, such as deep breathing, may be used by the patient when they are about to, or do, lose control. Carr and Shepherd (1982) suggest . that whenever patients look as if they are about to cry, they should be instructed to take a deep breath, then to breathe quietly through the nose. If they are crying and have lost control, they should be instructed to take a deep breath and stop crying, with a positive reinforcer 'Good' after control is regained.

(d) Expressive techniques may be used sometimes, to provide a time when patients may appropriately express emotion. This may enable the patient to be more controlled at other times.

Therapists should choose activities that patients enjoy and may succeed in, so that frustration is minimized and social withdrawal is less likely. The choice of other patients to share activity, or to whom the patient is close in a social or group situation, may be critical, as they may need to understand the nature of lability and remain relaxed when an outburst occurs. Therapists should attempt to become aware of how the patient may react or feel about situations or conversations, so they may intervene, if necessary, and grade the treatment process so that patients may learn to control their emotions in many different circumstances.

METHODS TO HANDLE AFFECTIVE AND SOCIAL PROBLEMS

Private discussion

(a) Counselling and advising

Private discussion allows therapists the opportunity to counsel or give advice and information. Counselling helps patients to explore problems, clarify issues and alternative methods of intervention so that they may decide what course of action to choose (Fransella, 1982). The therapist does not hand out solutions to problems, but assists the patient to discover intact resource skills, so they may look for their own answers to current and future problems. Teaching, giving advice, and information, is necessary when the therapist has expert knowledge that will help the patient to problem solve. The giving of information and counselling may occur concurrently.

(b) When and how discussion may be promoted

Discussion with the patient usually takes place during treatment or retraining, for example, whilst helping the patient to improve physical or perceptual skills, or during practice of activities of daily living. Discussion of personal problems will occur when a patient feels trust, liking, and respect for the therapist, and if the situation is suitable for the sharing of confidences.

A regular time for quiet, individual, one to one treatment will be helpful for patients wishing to share a problem. Depending on the activity the therapist is using with the patient, it is probably better if they are not face to face, so that flexibility of eye contact is possible. The therapist should be close enough to touch, but not overwhelming or invasive of the patient's personal space. Sharing is assisted if heads are level, and the therapist assumes an attending, listening attitude (Nelson–Jones, 1983). The activity may continue, often providing patients or therapists the opportunity to pause, or terminate discussion, if this is desirable. Therapists may wish to suggest that patients talk with other treatment staff if they are known to have greater expertise in problem areas.

However, the patient's wishes about who they talk with, must be considered.

(c) Reminiscence

Often, prior to, or as part of sharing current problems, patients may reminisce about past roles, relationships and skills. This should be attended to and facilitated, as it may be considered part of the grieving process which needs to be experienced, before adaptation and new role modelling may begin; it may be a way patients can share self-concepts, establishing a positive identity on which to base personal revelations; and it may also test the therapist's attitudes, prejudices, beliefs, values and biases.

(d) Sexuality

One of the topics which patients may need to discuss is sexuality. All members of the treatment team need to anticipate sexual concerns, and be prepared to assist the patient to discuss anxieties and to adapt to any necessary change in role, relationships and sexual expression.

Hewson (1982) suggests, from personal experience, that after the initial crisis of stroke, patients often experience great urgency to renew sexual relationships with their partner, to be reassured that they are still loved, despite disablement.

Provision of a place where patients and partners can have private discussion, may enable sharing of feelings and sexual expression, promoting and maintaining the patient's self-confidence and positive sexual identity. Weinberg (1982) suggests that one of the greatest deterrents to sexual expression of patients in hospital is lack of privacy, and points out that the patient's partner is also often left without chance of sexual expression.

Patients may have difficulty expressing their sexual needs, particularly if they feel dependent, unsure of their identity, unable to communicate with their partner, or because of cultural differences. This may be helped by therapists encouraging sexual awareness and responsibility, as part of activities of daily living, having patients practise grooming and dressing skills which help them to feel attractive (Hopkins & Smith, 1978), and

initiating discussion of practical sexual expression as part of the regular rehabilitation program, using interpreters if necessary. When aphasia is a major complication the speech pathologist may be the counsellor of choice.

There may be fears or anxiety by patient or partner about sexual activity causing another stroke, and these concerns should be referred to the physician in charge of the patient's medical program. Impaired mobility, sensation, or body awareness, plus alterations in tone may cause positioning problems during sexual activity. Possible difficulties should be included in discussion with the patient, and with the partner, who may have to take a more active, or different role, to previously. If patients find difficulty in talking about their sexuality with others, they may be referred to books dealing with the subject, with the understanding that they may ask for further advice or clarification should it be required.

Therapists should be aware that they may cause a sexual response, particularly during treatment procedures of a personal nature, such as bathing or dressing, and should not over-react, verbally, or non-verbally, as patients may be embarrassed by the response. A commonsense approach to the subject is necessary, appearing to patients as open, sincere, sensitive and concerned.

(e) Other issues

Other important discussion subjects may include whether, and how, they can cope with property, financial concerns, health worries, and with relatives who feel the patient can no longer cope and are suggesting dependent care.

Attention should be given as to whether catastrophic depression or denial is affecting decision-making about the future. Such affective responses should be primary treatment issues, treatment modalities being chosen which allow positive achievement and satisfaction, and promote self-concepts

Therapeutic rationale for private discussion:
- Patients are assisted to work through concerns as they occur.
- Risk of introverted worries and fears causing secondary affective disorders is reduced.

- Positive, practical programs can be developed to meet patients' requirements as they see them.

2. Family education and participation

After the initial crisis of stroke, when family members may fear the death of the patient, they are often left with feelings of anxiety and a sense of powerlessness (Lambert & Lambert, 1979). They may be unable to communicate naturally with the patient and may not understand what to do, what to say, where to stand, how to react, and so on. An early chance to help families understand the nature and extent of the stroke, and to provide some practical suggestions of how they may best approach the patient, is likely to be helpful.

(a) Roles

Getting to know the family will help therapists to appreciate the family dynamics, the former roles, relationships, possible resources, or difficulties which may need to be considered in future planning.

When possible, families should be included in treatment, taught how to handle hemiplegic limbs, how to communicate most effectively, how to cope with emotional lability, how to assist transfers and daily living activities, how to provide appropriate sensory input, and understand perceptual impairment. With this degree of involvement, both family and patient will be learning from the start role modification. Strongmann (1979) suggests that roles are not taught but acquired through practice, problem solving, and observation of others in the role. Practical learning of this nature may be combined with formal and informal giving of information.

Occupational therapists may initially be shy of having an 'audience' and family participation may not be appropriate or convenient at all sessions, as their presence may inhibit the patient's performance or distract attention away from treatment. However, the overall gains from participation of relatives in the program, is likely to assist the patient's transition to home.

(b) Patient activity

When others are not present, the patient should sometimes be encouraged and assisted in activity which will receive praise from the family, such as preparation of a special meal to be shared by family members, or making something for a birthday present, so that positive aspects of abilities are emphasised in a pleasurable experience. Treatment emphasis needs to be on intact as well as impaired skills, to decrease risk of secondary affective disorder.

(c) Counselling

The therapist may use counselling skills to help family members formulate future plans, using the same process as with individual patients, initially building rapport through an empathetic approach, showing respect for individual values and concerns. This will assist the family in feeling understood and valued members of the treatment team, facilitating their willingness to talk and explore the problems they face, and how they feel. The therapist should help the family to explore and clarify options and alternatives, so they may problem solve, plan objectives, action and strategies. The therapist should take care not to try to solve the problem for the family and patient, but to help them do it for themselves (Fransella, 1982). This role may be shared with others in the treatment team and a co-ordinated approach should be determined.

Therapeutic rationale for relative participation:
- Gives relatives a positive role in the patient's rehabilitation, providing a practical approach to communication.
- Both family and patient experience role modification as an ongoing process, to ease transition from hospital to home.
- Assists family understanding of patient's intact as well as impaired abilities, so that maximum potential is encouraged after discharge.
- Promotes reinforcement of retraining techniques.
- Provides an empathetic environment for families to share worries and concerns about the future.

3. Group problem solving

In most rehabilitation settings there are a number of stroke patients being treated at the same time, and many find the sharing of problems and feelings with others who have experienced the same illness, helpful.

(a) Social groups

Groups may be unstructured or structured, the former happening when several patients are grouped together around a table, for example, at individual or common tasks, for a meal, or rest between treatment sessions. The therapist, by careful choice of who sits next to whom, may promote useful low level social sharing of experience. This is a valuable technique to promote acceptance and mutual trust slowly, so that structured groups with the same patients may proceed more smoothly, and without the need for several trust building sessions. What people learn in groups is affected by its cohesiveness, which is based on mutual objectives, liking and trust between group members.

(b) Structured groups

In structured groups the issues presented for problem solving may initially be quite simple, and deal with day to day problems such as how to stabilize a nail brush or get a good night's sleep. It is likely that patients will also discuss issues such as how stroke happened to them, and theories of cause and effect. This may cause emotive reactions for some patients, and therapists should guide the discussion away from such patients whilst they regain composure, providing them with reassurance and support, perhaps by touch or brief verbal caring comment.

Patients should be provided with correct information about the causes of stroke, and discussion of possible changes to lifestyle which may retard further deterioration of the circulatory system, should be initiated.

(c) Practical problem solving

Discussion of nutrition, and suggestions for diet modification should lead to practical sessions trying out recipes that appeal to patients. Therapists will find recipe books such as *Guide to Healthy Eating* published by The National Heart Foundation of Australia (1982) extremely useful for such sessions.

Because stroke results in so many different aspects of dysfunction, easy communication is unlikely. Concepts and practical ideas resulting from group discussion may only be assimilated slowly, repetition and practice being necessary reinforcers.

The inclusion of both out and in patients in groups will facilitate discussion of problems that may be encountered after discharge, providing therapists and patients with an opportunity to develop practical problem-solving programs to reduce difficulties on discharge. Issues that may be covered in this situation range from specific problems in activities of daily living, family and community attitudes, role and status changes, vocational and recreational difficulties.

Group situations offer support and encouragement to patients' problem solving, and if guided so that possible major issues are considered, undesirable affective reactions, following discharge, may be reduced.

All patients should be encouraged to participate, even if only to nod agreement to a solution. If the same group of patients continue for some time, it is likely that the group will form some kind of structure of its own, the structure being influenced by the role and status each patient begins to assume (Strongmann, 1979). This will influence the problems the group is willing to discuss, and therapists may need to promote those issues of importance which the group is unwilling to pursue. Therapists should also help patients to initiate topics of concern if they find it difficult to do this for themselves, and guide interaction so that some positive ideas are formulated at each session. To be effective at group guidance, therapists need to be good listeners, who are able to express their concern for both individuals and the group, without dominating the group process. Patients who are labile may be gradually introduced into group situations, the other participants being helped to understand and respond in an appropriate manner to labile behaviour.

Therapeutic rationale for group problem solving:

- Patients are often helped by discussing problems with others who have had similar trauma.

- Group members offer support and encouragement to problem solving.
- Facilitates expression of feelings to reduce stress, possibly decreasing the risk of secondary affective disorders.
- Promotes exploration of a range of practical solutions to problems experienced.
- Promotes continuance of patients' social skills and expression of self.

4. Relaxation techniques

Relaxation techniques may be of value in helping patients to overcome anxiety and frustration, and because of the simple nature of most techniques, may also be of value in helping patients to feel in control of some activity suggested to them (Hewson, 1982). Techniques may be taught individually or in group sessions, and careful choice of time when these are programmed in relation to other parts of the rehabilitation schedule, may increase their usefulness.

Relaxation may be seen as a technique useful at the time of doing, but also as a modality for patients to use at other times, to decrease stress or tension.

There are many different techniques to assist relaxation, and not all will be effective with an individual. Patient participation and some understanding of the need to reduce tension is required before specific relaxation formulae can be designed or evaluated. An effective program should take into consideration the patient's physical and emotional condition, diet, work load and total rehabilitation schedule, and so should be formulated in consultation with the treatment team. If effective methods of relaxation can be found whilst patients are in hospital, they are more likely to continue using them after discharge, particularly if future circumstances are discussed in relaxation sessions. Techniques which may be useful include:

(a) *Progressive relaxation* (Jacobson, 1939, 1957, 1964). A comfortable, symmetrical position is assumed such as lying in supine, or sitting in bed or chair. The patient is asked to think about, contract, and slowly relax the muscles in a body part, starting with the toes and progressing proximally, throughout the body. This may be done in conjunction with deep breathing.

(b) *Deep breathing* (Farber 1982). A comfortable, symmetrical position is assumed. Palms may be placed on the abdomen. The patient should inhale through the nose to an even, rhythmical count of four, expanding abdomen, chest, and elevating shoulders, before exhaling to a count of four. Fantasy thoughts may be encouraged during deep breathing, and may be facilitated by music or visual stimuli. This is contraindicated if the patient is impaired in reality orientation.

(c) *Meditation* (Benson et al, 1976). This may be used with deep breathing and involves patients repeating silently a word they have chosen, as they exhale. The word may have meaning, or be meaningless. Patients allow themselves to relax, maintaining the process for about twenty minutes. This is also contraindicated for those with impaired reality orientation. The process of digestion appears to interfere with meditation, so it is best not done within two hours of eating.

(d) *Yoga* (Hewson, 1982). This may be useful for some patients utilizing, as it does, deep breathing, meditation and physiological control, though not all exercises will be suitable for stroke patients. An experienced yoga teacher is recommended.

(e) *Differential relaxation* (Farber 1982). During activity patients are encouraged to become aware of, and to differentiate between, muscular tensions that are necessary and those not required. Hemiplegic patients may use comparison between sides, in order to assist this process. Patients are then encouraged to consciously relax unwanted tension as they continue the activity. Bio-feedback may be used to help with accurate differentiation.

(f) *Activity*. This may be used as a direct method of relaxation, or to complement other relaxation techniques. Activities of a creative nature, those to do with the earth or animals, or of a rhythmical nature, such as movement to music, have been found to be relaxing for some people. Activities including warmth and slow stroking may also be of use. Tasks which make achievable physical demands may be used to promote satisfied fatigue, conducive to relaxation, by meditation or deep breathing.

Therapeutic rationale for relaxation:
- May be used by patients when frustrated, and in times of stress.

- May encourage awareness of bilaterality.
- May encourage awareness of individual muscles, and help patients to cognitively control undesirable tone.
- Encourages increased intake of oxygen.

5. Improvement in practical skills

Practice of skills necessary, or desirable for future life, will have started from early treatment intervention. To make these significant to individuals, they should be planned and graded, according to improvement of physical and higher cortical skills, with the patient being encouraged to suggest and initiate relevant areas of practice.

Following initial emphasis on body awareness and control, with maximum use of personal care skills as treatment modalities, those activities which the patient pursues at home may be seen by the patient as next in importance. Sometimes affective response, such as depression or denial, will make patients unenthusiastic about tackling tasks related to real life, as the activities may bring the patient face to face with the reality of change. Therapists must understand the reason for any reluctance and help patients to work through their feelings, combining practical activity with an empathetic approach, discussion and counselling.

Practice should include the activities the patient is likely to pursue on discharge, so consideration of whether the patient lives alone, with a partner or family, and whether no, a little, or a lot of support may be expected, is important.

Activities and practice should be discussed both with the patient and relatives. The availability of local helping agencies may also affect the choice of tasks each patient requires to practise. Activities may include food preparation, perhaps trying out recipes suggested as nutritionally sensible, simple to complex housekeeping tasks, home handyperson activities, gardening, budgeting, marketing,

and practice using relevant transport. Any task which needs modification, either of a physical or cognitive nature, will require constant practice before patients may be expected to retain the new skill.

Regular groups to consider, practice, or share recreational skills are recommended, and may be as varied as the patients themselves. Probably the most regular avocational activities requiring practice are use of television, reading, knitting, crochet, sewing, card games, bowls, golf, snooker, gardening and photography. Patients from different cultural backgrounds should be encouraged to share any different recreational activity with others in the patient group, as appropriate. New hobbies or interests may be introduced for specific treatment gains, and to extend the patients' repertoire of possible future activities.

Therapeutic rationale for improving practical skills:
- Practice in required skills will promote patient independence.
- Cognitive, perceptual, and physical improvement is linked with real life requirements.
- Patients' self-concepts are reinforced by positive skills.
- Future plans may be based on acquired skills.
- Time for introspection is reduced.
- Positive achievement is promoted to enhance self concepts.

SUMMARY

Consideration of the affective and social problems which may follow stroke should be ongoing with treatment of other impairments. Opportunities should be structured to assist patients and relatives cope more effectively with problems that they face in the acute stages of recovery, and following discharge.

REFERENCES

Benson H, Bleary J F, Carol M P 1976 The relaxation responses. In: White J, Fadiman J (eds) Relax. Dell, New York

Carr J, Shepherd R 1982 A motor retraining programme for stroke. Heinemann Medical books Ltd, London

Farber S D 1982 Neurorehabilitation, a multi sensory approach. W B Saunders, Philadelphia

Fransella F 1982 Psychology for occupational therapists. The British Psychological Society and the Macmillan Press Ltd, London

Heart Foundation Cookbook 1982 Guide to healthy eating. The National Heart Foundation of Australia

Hewson L 1982 When half is whole. Dove communications, Blackburn, Vic

Hopkins H L, Smith H D 1978 Willard & Spackman's Occupational therapy, 5th edn. J B Lippincott Co, Philadelphia.

Jacobson E 1939 Progressive relaxation. University of Chicago Press, Chicago

Jacobson E 1957 You must relax. McGraw Hill, New York

Jacobson E 1964 Anxiety and tension control. J B Lippincott & Co, Philadelphia

Lambert V A, Lambert C E 1979 Impacts of physical illness on related health concepts. Prentice-Hall Inc, Englewood Cliffs, New Jersey

Nelson-Jones R 1983 Practical counselling skills. Holt, Rinehart and Winston, London

Pedretti L W 1981 Occupational therapy, practice skills for physical dysfunctions. C V Mosby Co, St Louis

Strongmann K T 1979 Psychology for the paramedical professions. Croom Helm, London

Turner A (ed) 1981 The practice of occupational therapy. Churchill Livingstone, Edinburgh

Weinberg J S 1982 Sexuality, human needs and nursing practice. W B Saunders Co, Philadelphia

RECOMMENDED READING

Farber S D 1982 Neurorehabilitation, a multi sensory approach. W B Saunders, Philadelphia, ch 6

Fransella F 1982 Psychology for occupational therapists. The British Psychological Society and the Macmillan Press Ltd, London

Hewson L 1982 When half is whole. Dove communications, Blackburn, Vic

Weinberg J S 1982 Sexuality, human needs and nursing practice. W B Saunders Co, Philadelphia, ch 12

Approaches to extended rehabilitation

10

Long term care

CHOICE AND TIMING OF DISCHARGE TO LONG-TERM CARE

There is no standard criterion for the discharge of acute stroke patients to long-term care institutions between treatment agencies (Wilcock & Hall, 1982). To some extent discharge may be dependent upon the policy of the agency administering acute care; whether there is a shortage of beds; whether selection for rehabilitation is based on patient need or potential; whether social judgments influence rehabilitation selection; and, in the case of some private hospitals, whether rehabilitation services are offered at all. From clinical experience it often appears that the timing of discharge to dependent care and the selection of a suitable institution for each patient, is an unevaluated decision, based on the fact that a 'bed' is available 'somewhere'.

Spontaneous recovery progresses for months, and sometimes years, following the period of cerebral shock. With patients experiencing massive insult to cerebral tissue, the period of shock is likely to be lengthy. The larger the lesion, the greater amount of oedema may be expected, patients initially having gross dysfunction, the extent of which may not be evaluated fully until oedema subsides. Patients may be discharged to dependent care before any recovery occurs, or before recovery potential may be fully evaluated. If adequate stimulation and appropriate techniques are not employed to harness improvement as recovery commences, patients may remain extremely dysfunctional.

For patients with gross impairment, slowly progressing programs maximizing potential are essential, if this group of patients have the same right as others to expect some rehabilitation and future quality of life. The need to be active, out of bed, as independent as possible, and taking some responsibility for their own life is as true of this group of stroke patients as the others; yet, frequently, systems prevent or hinder the achievement of such goals—for example, dependent care agencies may actually be financially advantaged by keeping patients in bed. In Australia, patients classified as requiring intensive care are additionally subsidised by the Government.

GENERAL CONSIDERATIONS FOR PROGRAMS

1. Prevention of sensory deprivation

When patients are discharged to dependent care agencies it is likely that they will remain in these establishments for the remainder of their lives. Physical care alone will be insufficient to meet the many and varied life needs of individuals, which would normally include work, leisure, pleasure, relaxation, problem solving, and both private and social times. Whilst occupational therapists will be concerned with encouraging maximum return of function, they need also to consider the enhancement of intact abilities, and the total quality of the environment. They should promote the establishment of a 'mini' society which meets the psychological, emotional, and social needs of patients, and prevents sensory deprivation, which may cause secondary deficits and undesirable behavioural changes. Sensory deprivation experiments on normal young volunteers (Corso, 1967) produced changes in their behaviour, including difficulties in abstract reasoning, word finding, thought, concentration and perception, and sometimes led to hallucinations.

Programs in dependent care agencies often lack sensory stimulation, the daily rituals being a monotonous continuum of sleep in bed, regular routine hygiene activities, meals of depressing similarity, and sleep in chairs. Many of the symptoms of stroke, such as visual field defect, impairment of cutaneous sensation and movement, or memory deficits impose a decrease in sensory input, so that any additional deprivation may lead to general deterioration and confusion.

Holden and Woods (1982) suggest that a change of input is necessary for sensory stimulation, and point to a number of studies showing that daily programs which include activities of daily living, recreational and social activity, and psychological and environmental stimulation, have facilitated improved behaviour in patients with senile dementia.

Such studies indicate that programs offering more than simple physical care, which centres patients' existence around being washed, fed and rested, should be provided. The establishment of an environment which promotes and encourages normal social behaviour, to maintain skills patients had prior to admission, is suggested (Holden & Woods, 1982). This may be difficult to implement unless patients are actively involved in planning programs because, as Strongmann (1979) points out, institutions (generally) tend to desocialize by cutting people off from previous roles, and attempting to build up new roles. Only patients have sufficient information about themselves and their priorities to successfully combine old and new.

2. Relationships between staff and patients

An informal study (O'Toole, 1980) of a frail aged day centre population indicated that two-way personal communication between those caring for, and those being cared for, was seen by patients as more important than the actual activities within the program, and that they saw loving, respecting, understanding, and being treated as an equal, as necessary to successful programs. The need to discuss spiritual issues, and death and dying, was also highlighted.

Dependent care is a 24 hour a day situation and any patient–staff interaction may be significant in facilitating improved patient functioning. Communication between staff and patients provides ongoing opportunity to reinforce patients' self-awareness, orientation, appropriate social behaviour and physical improvement. Therapists need to show respect and concern, be willing to share two-way communication, listen to what the patient says, and be responsive to non-verbal expression of how patients feel.

3. Opportunities for pleasure and fun

Opportunities for pleasure and fun with others may be very limited, and consideration of how best to provide occasions for enjoyment and laughter should be paramount from the time of each patient's admission to dependent care. Personal interests and skills should be maintained, encouraged and shared.

4. Sexuality

The sexual needs of the elderly in dependent care also need to be considered in program development. Moran (1977) suggests that nursing homes are frequently responsible for neutering the elderly, as it is common practice to separate sexes, even married couples who enter a nursing home together, and there is often lack of privacy and opportunity for sexual expression.

Sexual overtures to staff members may be met with disgust, and developing relationships between patients discouraged and ridiculed (Weinberg, 1982). Activity programs may not sufficiently consider male and female preferences and to some may appear juvenile. Care should be taken to maintain mature attitudes, and respect, for each patient's sexual identity. The provision of, or respect of, use of a private place should be promoted, even if it only be a knock on a patient's door and a pause for their response before entering the room.

5. Physical exercise

The inclusion of light physical exercise of a structured nature in programs is also recommended as it is thought to produce positive cognitive changes (Diesfeldt & Diesfeldt-Groendijk, 1977). This is possible because of attention demands, or the effect of exercise on the nature of breathing, which may increase the amount of oxygen to cerebral tissue.

6. Community and family contact

In an unpublished student paper, Bates (1983) found that stroke patients in institutions considered community and family contact, and transport to facilitate such contact, of prime importance to their quality of life. Programs should promote maintenance of community interests, and relative contact, with regular opportunity to take part in 'outside' occasions.

7. Physical environment

The physical environment in which programs take place should be considered as an important adjunct

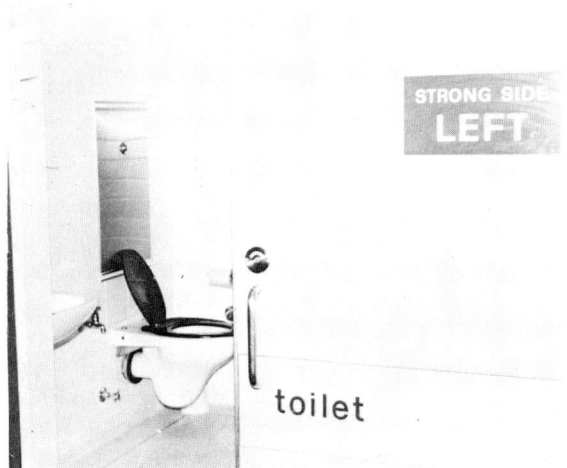

Fig. 10.1 Clear marking on the lavatory doorway indicates suitability for patient use according to side of hemiplegia. (Hampstead Centre, Adelaide, South Australia.)

to the therapeutic process. Topographical information should be provided and discussed with patients, such as colour coding of floor level or rooms, visual or cognitive clues made prominent, without being childish, for example door frames painted to contrast with walls so they can be easily seen, bells to summon help made decoratively obvious, and rooms clearly named to denote their purpose, as in Figure 10.1

Day rooms should be pleasant places in which to sit, with good light and ventilation, interesting views, and not smelling of urine or disinfectant. Furniture should be chosen for height, stability, comfort and appearance, and arranged socially rather than in the inevitable rows around the walls. The floors should not be slippery or madly patterned, so that falls are not caused by polish, wet mops, or tripping over obstacles undistinguished from the 'busy' pattern of the carpet.

Television, radio, or recorders should be available, but not compulsory; patients should select programs, and ear pieces should be available if not all want to listen. Newspapers and magazines should be available, up to date, and relevant to patient interests. Adult games should also be provided and encouraged, and facilities for making a social drink or occasional snack should be adjacent; toilet facilities should be close by. The physical environment in which the patient lives, and the staff who support them, should promote choice and self-responsibility.

8. Relationships between patients

The other patients within the dependent care agency will also influence the behaviour and responses of each patient. It has been found that large groups may be inhibitory to participating (Townsend & Kimbele, 1975), and that effective group interaction is best promoted with between 8–10 patients. They should be grouped so that interaction between them is comfortable; for example, when seated at 45° to each other, and 2 to 4 feet apart, each patient has a reasonable area of personal space, and pauses or silences may occur with little embarrassment. When patients are grouped so that social interaction is possible, shared interest or activity will promote the development of group feeling. For example, when treatment for some specific difficulty is shared, particularly in a small treatment room, the gains made by one patient may act as a spur to others. Sometimes other patients appear to experience satisfaction equal to the one showing improvement. As group feeling grows, less able patients appear to be supported and encouraged by the others, so interaction and sensory stimulation continue when therapists and other staff are elsewhere.

Sometimes patients will be worried and distressed by those less able, or grossly dysfunctional, and feel unable to cope with regular or even occasional contact. Staff should be aware of, and responsive to, such attitudes. Care should be taken about social grouping of patients in the ward during the day, or for meals, and attention given to bed proximity.

9. Time for solitude

Each patient will also require some time to themselves for private thoughts and reflections, and attention should be given to whether the environment can cater for this need. Patients with limited mobility may be given the opportunity for a quiet sit in the garden, for example, when they feel like it.

10. Maintenance of patient dignity and self-esteem

Occurrences which are detrimental to self-image and dignity, and embarrassing for patient if public, should be avoided, so that the 'niceties of society' are preserved. Examples of situations injurious to dignity are: assisting walking by hanging on to the back of pajama pants, a very unsafe procedure without neurophysiological benefit; tieing a baby blue ribbon in an old lady's hair, without asking first if she would like it; or sitting patients on a commode or toilet, and leaving them in semi-public view with clothes disarranged and revealing.

11. Contact with animals

Consideration should be given to the part animals may play in promoting patient pleasure, relaxation, awareness, action and interaction. In one excellent Adelaide elderly citizens' complex, a dog and a cat are 'on staff'. The animals 'staff appointment' followed an informal study of the apparent benefits of patient interaction with them. A chicken coop is situated in the small, domestic-style garden leading from the day room, to promote a feeling of 'home' rather than institution.

12. Suitable activities for daily programs

Suggestions for suitable activities include:
- music programs, chosen by the patients
- simple craft activity for gifts or community projects
- gardening, pot plant care, and ward flowers
- adult games such as whist, chess, scrabble, carpet bowls, snooker, bingo
- cooking morning or afternoon snacks, making beer or wines.
- seasonal cooking tasks, such as hot-cross buns or preserves
- entertaining—lunches, special occasion dinners, or barbeques for external guests
- some form of participation in special community occasions, such as local agricultural shows, elections, test matches, international games
- daily keep-fit and relaxation at an appropriate physical level

- object discussion, to trigger recollections
- showing movies or videotapes of special programs on television for selected audiences.

SPECIFIC REMEDIAL APPROACHES

Simple, repetitive procedures may be required over a long period of time for achievement of sometimes quite minimal goals. In studies of patients with impairment or absence of short-term memory, motor ability has improved with repetitive motor activity, despite patients having no recollection of the activity (Kolb & Whishaw, 1980). This indicates that even when patients have gross intellectual deficits, motor learning will occur if movement is simple and practised many times.

A functionally oriented program is suggested so that patients will be able to perform some personal independence skills from an early date, to decrease the risks of undesirable affective response occurring. Some neurophysiological and neuropsychological treatment approaches may be used in conjunction with functional retraining to promote maximum sensory-motor ability. A motor developmental approach, using ontogenetic sequence, is rarely suitable for this group of patients, because the positions are frequently difficult for those with gross dysfunction, and patients may not understand that the procedures relate to problems, particularly as recovery may be slow.

Methods

1. Awareness of body

Early treatment procedures should include activity directly relating to understanding and control of the body as, until this is achieved in some measure, patients will be unable to respond appropriately to external stimuli and their new environment. Practice of bed mobility, transfers, showering, bathing, toileting, skin care, and dressing, should be initial priorities, with effort being made to enable each patient to make use of intact sensory abilities during the activities, awareness of body parts, and position, being enhanced by sensory input, as described in earlier chapters.

2. Repetition and reinforcement

Using the same procedures which are part of different activities, or modifying activity so that the same procedures can be used, will facilitate learning by reinforcing newly acquired memory traces.

The approach described as the 'Newcastle Method' (Mort, 1976) of managing hemiplegia in the elderly, mentioned in Chapter 1, incorporates this idea by using modest goals, repetition, and continuity of procedures which are based on the analysis of skills required for mobility. Tasks required as part of the daily routine are treatment modalities, and all staff members are trained to use the same approach. This avoids confusion caused by conflicting directions and helps patient safety and progress. The basic movements used at the beginning of treatment continue throughout, new components being added as the patient improves. The approach is simple, based on patients using intact limbs to stand and move, weight being taken initially on the sound leg, positioned centrally, and through the sound arm and hand to push up or lean on a four point stick. Equipment is well chosen, stable furniture, of a height which allows feet to be firm on the floor, and which will not topple over when weight is applied to one side only. The height of the four point sticks encourage a slight lean to the sound side.

Those with gross impairment are able to learn safe transfers without the necessity for staff to be involved in heavy lifting, because the patient balances on the sound side, safety taking precedence over postural refinements. This approach, which has generally been disregarded in recent years, is appropriate when simple, basic, repetitive training is required, and especially when stroke is complicated by other physical and psychological problems associated with ageing.

Despite concern that an asymmetrical approach may inhibit patient recovery, or cause uncontrollable abnormal tone, there is no evidence that spasticity is greater in the long term, or that symmetrical independent walking is prevented if the patient reaches that stage of recovery.

3. Sensory stimulation

Depending on the degree of recovery, one-sided

methods of transfer, bathing and dressing may be a long-term necessity, but this does not imply that the hemiplegic side should be neglected. Inherent in the suggestion that treatment should include activity relating to the understanding and control of the body, is the need to provide sensory input, and cues of a proprioceptive, kinesthetic, tactile, verbal, visual and olfactory nature, which are used to improve neuromuscular activity at peripheral and cortical level, body awareness, and visuospatial perception. Stimulation needs to be controlled and used at a fairly simple level, because bombardment may confuse and inhibit neural response.

4. Sensory-motor re-education

Reflex-inhibiting posture and patterns of movement, modification of reflex synergies, or mass movement patterns may be included as part of treatment, and normal balance and postural mechanisms facilitated in positions in which the patient feels and is safe, such as when standing holding the bed end or rail, or when seated safely in a stable chair for dressing practice.

Those methods described in Chapter 5 to retrain bed mobility, transfers and dressing when the therapist assists the hemiplegic side, are appropriate for dependent care patients, and may incorporate the Newcastle Method of a slight lean to the sound side, sound leg centrally placed, and sound arm used for pushing down on, to promote safety, a feeling of security, and early independent mobility. It may be necessary to have a person positioned on both sides during mobility practice, not necessarily to assist patients to move, but so they are aware of help, because the presence of the therapist and any tactual or verbal cues given on the hemiplegic side may be totally ignored. Assistance to the side, rather than from the front, is recommended because the therapist can be more in control of (particularly heavy) patients leaning or falling to the hemiplegic side. Relatives are safer and more comfortable using a side approach, and it lessens confusion if everyone uses the same method; and most importantly, the therapist will not occlude the patient's vision, or inhibit visual location and fixation, will not invade personal space, or prevent normal forward sequence of movement in transfers. Any intact sensory skills should be fully utilized.

5. Toilet mobility and adapted clothing

In some agencies patients are encouraged to remain in bed from a very early tea time until after breakfast the following morning, so many may need to use a bed pan. Bed mobility exercises should include rolling and bridging practice, and training in how to manage clothing. Adapted clothing may be useful for those who need to use a bed pan regularly. In Figure 10.2 the patient's nightdress has been divided down the back for this purpose. The patient is assisted to roll to the sound side to release one back flap, and then to the hemiplegic side to release the other. Legs are bent up, and the patient is encouraged to keep knees slightly apart to help micturition, and then to bridge symmetrically to allow the bed pan to be inserted. A nightdress adapted in this way will stay modestly in place without getting wet during bed pan use. As mobility skills improve with repetitive practice, less assistance will be required.

Adapted clothing will also be useful if patients are wheeled to the lavatory on a toilet chair. If patients are sitting out of bed, they may be transferred to a toilet chair using 'end of bed' exercise. When standing, adapted clothing may be adjusted before the patient sits on the toilet chair. This is particularly useful for those patients who have difficulty transferring to the lavatory and adjusting clothing in a confined space, as they can be simply wheeled into position over the lavatory, the difficult balance activity having been done in a more suitable place and dignified manner.

Nightdresses and pyjamas may be modified to facilitate adjustment of clothing for toilet purposes such as is illustrated in Figures 10.3 and 10.4. Any exposed body parts should be covered during transport to the lavatory.

Sometimes, most regrettably, patients are left sitting on the lavatory for considerable periods, so clothing should be chosen or adapted so that if this occurs patients will not suffer loss of dignity, be embarrassed, or catch cold. A wrap-around skirt may be suitable for female day wear, with the

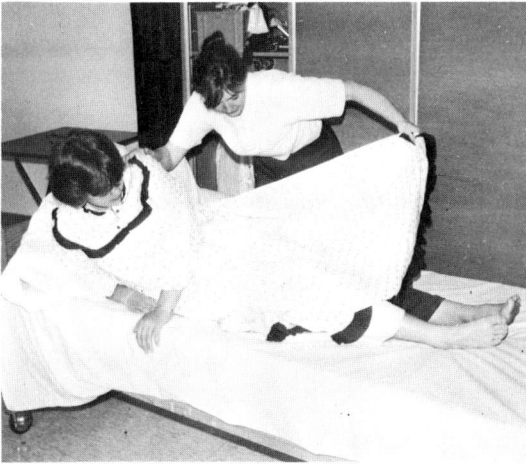

(a)

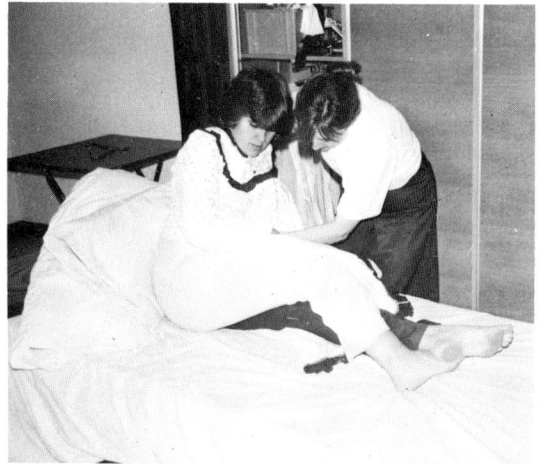

(b)

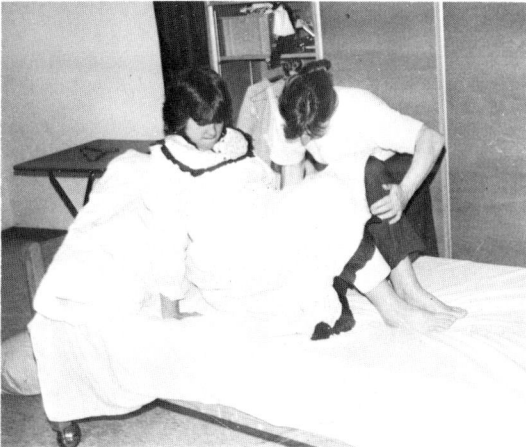

(c)

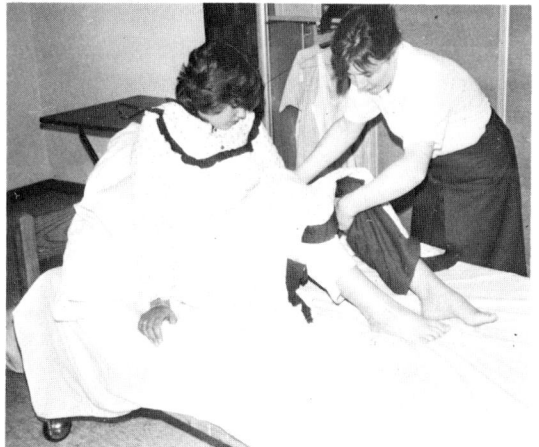

(d)

Fig. 10.2 Nightdress has been divided down the back to assist modest use of a bed pan. The patient is taught to roll to release back flaps, and then to bridge.

opening to the back, which will fall naturally to cover nakedness when the patient sits on the lavatory (Fig. 10.5).

Practice in putting on, taking off, and handling such clothing will be necessary, as demonstrated in Figure 10.6.

When patients are able to transfer from bed to chair independently and safely, a bedside commode may offer an acceptable alternative to bed pans, toilet chairs, or long walks to the lavatory. If commodes are used, attention should be given to matching the height of bed and commode seat and to ensuring that the commode is placed to the side of the bed which allows patients to sit on the bed with the sound side to the pillow. Commodes should have arms for pushing up on, not tip when pressure is applied unilaterally, and be of a height which allows patients' feet to be placed firmly on the floor. Male patients may manage adequately at night with a urinal. However, they should be taught to position it within their intact visual field if necessary, and always in the same place.

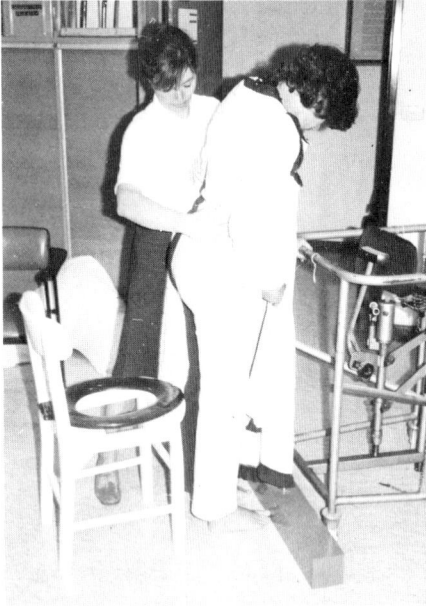

Fig. 10.3 Modified nightdress allows adjustment before transfer to a (simulated) toilet chair.

If patients are incontinent, therapists may need to be involved in 'timed' toileting during the day, should look for non-verbal signs which may indicate imminent bladder or bowel action so that accidents may be avoided, and may recommend special clothing to ensure comfort and dryness, and decrease embarrassment when incontinence occurs.

6. Personal care and dressing

The advantage of using personal care and dressing tasks to increase body awareness has already been indicated. For those with contralateral neglect, therapists should use regular bathing or showering activity as prime treatment time if this can be arranged. For other patients, therapists need to ensure their continued improvement towards independent personal care. Aids and equipment for bath or shower will be useful, such as a bathboard with a handle to the wall side, an armed shower chair, a hose type shower fitted to the taps, a non-slip mat, soap on a rope or in a pocketed towelling

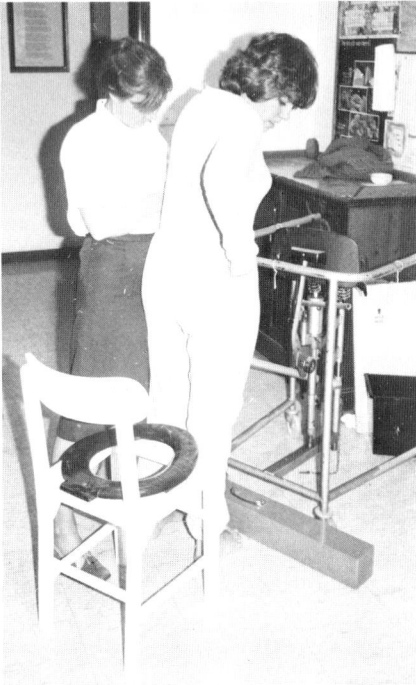

(a)

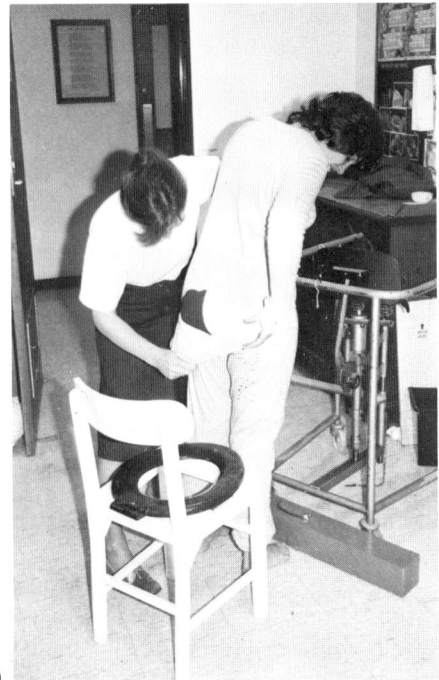

(b)

Fig. 10.4 Pyjamas modified with a back flap allows adjustment before transfer to a (simulated) toilet chair.

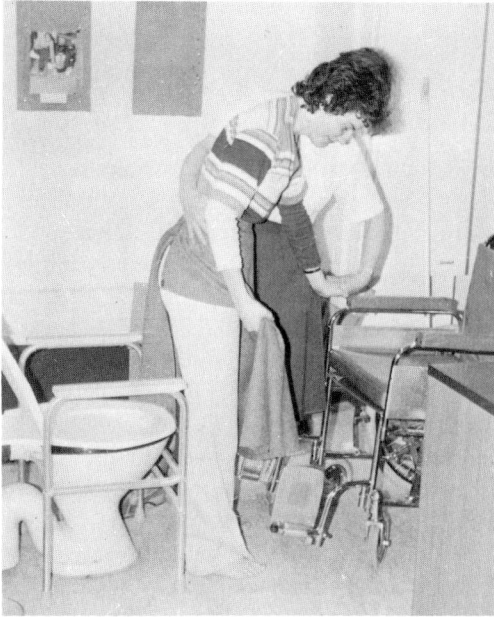

(a)

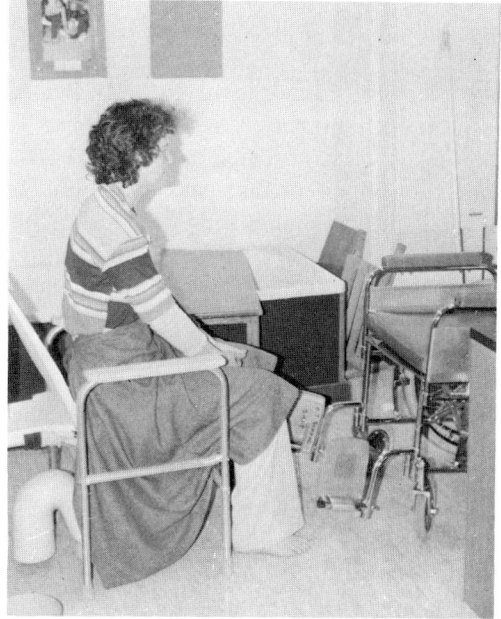

(b)

Fig. 10.5 A wrap around skirt makes clothing adjustment for lavatory use easier and prevents exposure of buttocks.

mitten. Procedures should include helping patients with balance, rotation, and location of body parts, encouraging their soaping and rubbing, particularly of the hemiplegic side, whilst looking at and talking about what they are doing. Abnormal movement and tone should be inhibited.

Using routine hygiene tasks for remediation is less common in dependent care agencies than during acute care, but the value of such activity should not be ignored, and opportunities should be taken to use them whenever possible.

Repetitive practice of dressing techniques will

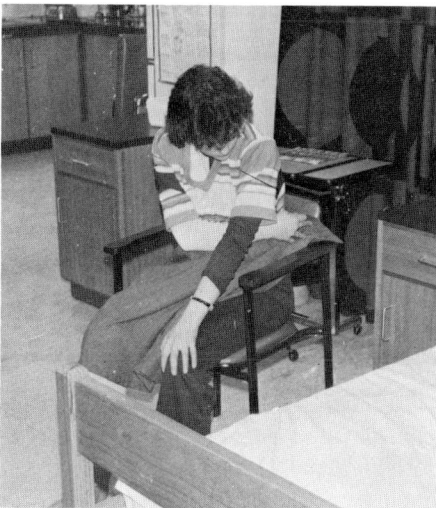

(a)

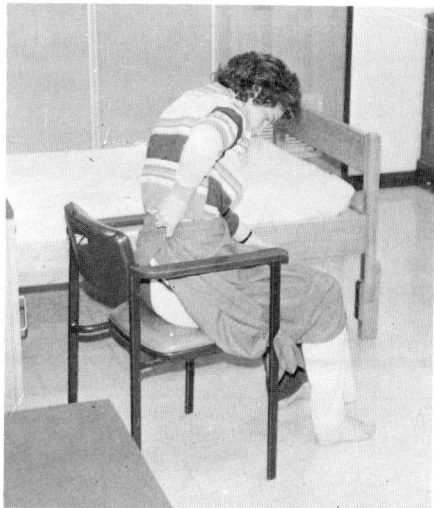

(b)

Fig. 10.6 Practice in putting on a wrap-around skirt.

be required daily. Choice of clothes may be limited by the amount and type of storage space available, and whether patients are able at first to learn only one or two basic methods, such as putting clothes over head, and over feet, being unable to cope with front or back fastening garments as well. It is especially important that patients choose, from suitable garments, clothes they would like to have with them, as they may have to wear them more often than they would have done previously. Therapists may need to discuss clothing choice with patients and relatives, the issues being very similar to those described in Chapter 5, and including such aspects as fabric characteristics, for example stretch, texture and ease of maintenance, as well as suitability for retraining methods and comfort. If clothing requires adaptation, the patient should be consulted and given information about the advantages of modification. If any special equipment, such as calipers or other foot control aids are used, dressing practice should include their application. Special consideration may need to be given to choice of footwear. Mort (1976) recommends laced shoes, firm around the heels, with a high cut front, leather soles and broad, low heels; and boots opening to the toes for patients with special problems such as recurrent oedema, poor ankle control, or those requiring foot dressings.

Retraining of memory, attention, sequencing and planning abilities may also be included in the simple tasks of daily life, by using techniques of forward or backward chaining, grading the amount of cueing or assistance given in tasks, and asking for participation in choice and decision making.

7. Eating

One handed eating techniques and equipment may be necessary, but therapists should also check if visual field defects or inattention, visuo-spatial agnosia, apraxia or cognitive impairment affect the patient's ability to cope with a meal. If so, tray or table settings should be simplified, distraction limited by initially helping the patient in a quiet place by himself, and sensory motor assistance provided. If dysphagia persists as a problem at this stage, programs to help patients with swallow should be continued (refer to Ch. 5).

8. Patient interaction

Patients should be encouraged to joint other residents as soon as possible, so that social unease due to unfamiliarity is decreased, and positive responses to their future life situation is enhanced. Initially they may need fairly constant attention in social situations, especially if body awareness and control, or communication is still grossly impaired, so that appropriate responses to other patients may be facilitated.

Gradually, simple, achievable activities, possibly of a creative or recreational nature, may be introduced to promote awareness and control of objects. This may include practice in activities that may be later shared with others, such as group games, making a snack, watching television, listening to music, or sharing an exercise group. Therapists should pay particular attention to choice of activity, so that it provides enjoyment to each patient, promotes sensory motor and cognitive improvement, and provides experience to promote a feeling of 'belonging' and 'home'.

9. Standard of work

Sometimes, a patient's work is undone and redone by staff so that a better 'end product' results. Patients may be aware of the standard of their work, through they may say nothing to indicate this. Therefore to find work redone without comment is likely to be detrimental to staff/patient relationships, as it implies lack of intellectual, as well as manipulative ability. If patients are unable to achieve to a reasonable standard, then the choice of activity is probably wrong.

10. Object appreciation

When patients are able to appreciate and enjoy objects it may be a suitable time to encourage their selection of personal treasures to keep by them permanently, although they may have had some photographs or personal things with them since acute hospitalization.

11. Lower limb mobility practice

Early weight bearing in standing is thought to increase tone in flaccid limbs, assist functional balance re-education and promote continence, so activity in standing is indicated as early as possible. To promote safe standing and weight bearing through both legs a back slab may be bandaged to support the knee in extension (Mort, 1976; Carr & Shepherd, 1982), or an air pressure splint may be used (Johnstone, 1978). A figure of eight bandage may be applied to the foot over a shoe if a flaccid ankle, or inversion or eversion of the foot requires control. The bandage should be applied so that it pulls the foot into a satisfactory position, opposite to that abnormally assumed, in the same way that a T strap on a caliper pulls the foot into normal alignment by fitting closely to the ankle with lax musculature, and fastening around the rod on the opposite side.

Some therapists make use of a standing box or buttock harness fitted to a high work table to support patients whilst they are standing during activity. The weight bearing becomes dynamic if the activity requires side to side or rotational movement (Fig. 10.7).

As patient's awareness and response to their environment increases, the program should be expanded to incorporate developing skills. Walking or wheelchair excursions around the agency, both inside and out, with visual and verbal cues being given, increase patient memory and orientation. Special topographical information should be given, and reinforced by repetition, such as any colour coding to indicate floor levels or rooms, number or name indicators, shape and direction of wards, corridors, day rooms, changes in floor surfaces, how to reach the garden, the positions of bell, or light switches. Information should be given in an adult, unpatronizing manner which may require practice. Students may find it helpful to listen to their tone and language on an audio-tape. Excursions into the community should also expand each patient's topographical orientation.

Therapeutic rationale for remedial approaches for dependent care patients:

- Promotes maximum sensory motor improvement and personal independence through functional retraining procedures.

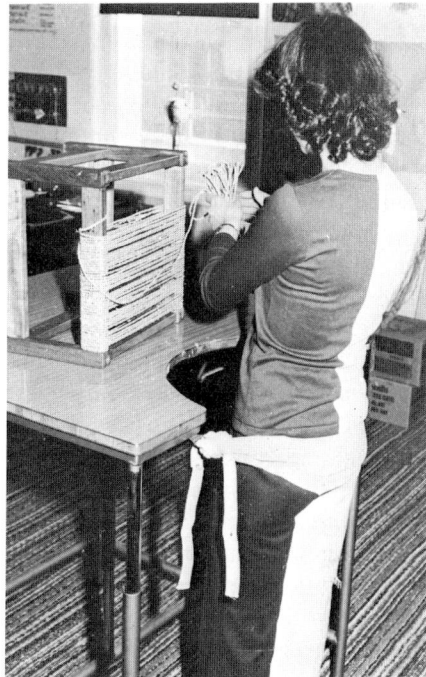

Fig. 10.7 A buttock harness attached to a high work table provides control for standing activity.

- Lessens likelihood of undesirable behavioural changes by requiring active participation and choice.
- Promotes cognitive, communication and perceptual abilities by grading rehabilitative and social activities.
- Maintains and improves self-esteem and quality of life through graded achievement and continuity of appropriate personal interests.

SECONDARY IMPAIRMENT

Patients may be admitted to dependent care with impairment secondary to stroke, namely contractures or decubitus ulcers (pressure sores). These are preventable by early and continuous emphasis on positioning, movement and sensory stimulus. From clinical experience it seems that patients who, for whatever reason, have contractures or pressure sores, are also likely to have sensory loss or asomatognosia as major symptoms.

For either contractures or pressure sores, sensory stimulation to the hemiplegic side is necessary, to increase patient awareness of the need to locate and position limbs constantly, and to change sitting or lying postures regularly.

Patients with contractures need encouragement, and usually manual assistance, to move within a pain free range to the extent of movement; highly motivating activities to encourage them to use any movement actively and often; serial splinting to try to extend the range of movement; and assessment to evaluate whether surgical intervention may be beneficial.

If serial splinting is used, therapists should be prepared to evaluate regularly, and change the splint as often as required. This may be more than once a day in some cases, or never in others. If several new splints are necessary this may prove expensive of thermo-plastics, and plaster of paris splints may be more appropriate. If trying to correct a totally flexed wrist and hand, it may be easier to initially tackle fingers, thumb and wrist separately. For example, the first splint may extend the interphalangeal joints of the thumb and the fingers as far as possible, with the wrist and M.C.P. joints remaining flexed. In succeeding splints, the fingers may be further extended with the M.C.P. joint maintained at 45°, then the wrist may be gradually extended, until finally a splint for total extension of fingers, hand, thumb and wrist is achieved.

Surgical intervention may appear necessary for any increase in range of movement, but before therapists recommend this, it is suggested that patients should have increased awareness of their hemiplegic limbs, and be highly motivated to participate in post-surgical rehabilitation to maximize gains.

Patients with decubitus ulcers will be constantly being turned and positioned by nursing staff. These positions should also be reflex inhibiting to prevent contractures. Motivating activity to encourage movement and circulation is suggested in order to speed recovery of the sore, to maintain normal tone in the rest of the body, and to lessen the time available for introspection, anxiety and undesirable affective response.

SUMMARY

In many dependent care agencies the intervention by occupational therapists is limited to provision of an activity program to maintain patient interest, and provide some measure of stimulation. Whilst these programs are extremely useful and should be continued, other benefits may be gained by expanding the program to include many of the treatment procedures found useful in acute care.

REFERENCES

Bates J 1983 A comparative study of the quality of life of elderly people following cerebrovascular accidents. A final year student paper. O.T. SAIT, Adelaide.
Carr J, Shepherd R 1982 A motor retraining programme for stroke. Heinemann Medical Books Ltd, London
Corso J F 1967 The experimental psychology of sensory behavior. Holt, Rinehart and Winston, New York
Diesfeldt H F A, Diesfeldt-Groendijk H 1977 Improving cognitive performance in psychogeriatric patients—the influence of physical exercise. Age and Ageing 6.1: 58–64
Holden U P, Woods R T 1982 Reality orientation, psychological approaches to the confused elderly. Churchill Livingstone, Edinburgh
Johnstone M 1978 Restoration of motor function in the stroke patient, a physiotherapist's approach. Churchill Livingstone, Edinburgh
Kolb B, Whishaw IQ 1980 Fundamentals of human neuropsychology. W H Freeman and Co, San Francisco

Moran J 1977 Sexuality after sixty. Association of rehabilitation nurses Journal 2(4): 19–21
Mort M 1976 The Newcastle method of managing hemiplegia in the elderly, a handbook to supplement the film of the same title. William Lyne Patients Community Service fund, Newcastle, NSW
O'Toole G 1980 Rapport from the elderly persons point of view. Paper presented at XIth biennial congress of AAOT, Hobart
Strongman K T 1978 Psychology for the paramedical professions. Croom Helm, London
Townsend J, Kimbele M 1975 Caring regimes in elderly persons' homes, Health and Social Services Journal 85 (11 October): 2286
Weinberg J S 1982 Sexuality, human needs and nursing practice. W B Saunders, Philadelphia
Wilcock A, Hall R E 1982 Disposal of postacute CVA patients, discussion of a statistical comparative study. Australian Occupational Therapy Journal 29, 4: 161–177

RECOMMENDED READING

Holden U P, Woods R T 1982 Reality Orientation,
Psychological approaches to the confused elderly. Churchill
Livingstone, Edinburgh
Mort M 1976 The Newcastle Method of Managing
hemiplegia in the elderly, a handbook to supplement the
film of the same title. William Lyne Patients Community
Service fund, Newcastle, NSW
Strongman K T 1979 Psychology for the paramedical
professions. Croom Helm, London

11

Home

Some patients may be discharged home very soon after stroke without intensive rehabilitation, the day to day caring being performed by families, with support, advice and expertise supplied by domiciliary rehabilitation services.

In such cases it is the role of therapists attending the patient's home to give relatives information and training about rehabilitation procedures they should incorporate into their day-to-day caring, and to assist the patient to understand how best to proceed with daily life to promote recovery (Johnstone, 1980).

Techniques which patient and family can learn easily and without heavy lifting will be most suitable. These should also be used by the therapist so that learning is reinforced by repetition. Retraining should be incorporated into necessary functional activity (such as hygiene and dressing tasks), and activity in which the patient is interested (such as hobbies), so that families do not have the burden of 'exercise time' in addition to the heavy load of caring for the patient's physical and psychological needs.

Treatment in the home has the advantage of providing realistic retraining related to the patient's future life, but the necessary intensity of treatment, on which may hinge success or failure of recovery, may be a problem if families and patients are unable to understand or follow techniques that are recommended. Therapists need to develop skills in teaching treatment procedures to people with no theoretical background.

Other patients may be discharged home after lengthy rehabilitation; even so retraining often needs extending into the home situation, or the gains made during rehabilitation may not be carried over into everyday life.

1. ATTITUDES

The need to escape to the security of one's own home at times of trauma is strong. Patients, following stroke, are likely to experience the strong desire to 'go home' and will work towards achieving this goal. However, many seem to deny the advent of dysfunction, feeling that 'all will be right' when they get home. Patients may experience depression and loss of motivation to continue when the reality of home is so different from their expectations. The need to extend treatment and retraining into the home is recognised, and it is probable that continued achievement of real goals will help prevent some undesirable affective response from occurring.

(a) Therapist's status

When therapists attend patients in their own home, they should do so with an awareness of reversal of status. In hospital therapists are in the nature of hosts, the patient and relatives, guests. At home the therapist must assume status as guest, extending courtesy and respect to patients and families as hosts. Being aware of and respecting property ownership will be important if changes are to be recommended. Therapists need to know if the patient or other family members own or rent the home, tact and sensitivity being necessary in discussion and practical intervention. Family members may not know the therapist and may be cautious, apologetic, over anxious or, occasionally, aggressive towards a stranger appearing to assume control over property and procedures.

(b) When suggesting changes

Therapists should be aware that patients may have just as strong an opinion of what they like and dislike, as therapists themselves, and of the personal importance of possessions which may have accumulated over many years, some having been chosen or given to mark a special occasion, and some to give visual pleasure or to express personality.

Suggestions for change should be made in a manner which allows for discussion and alternative suggestions. If families or patients offer workable solutions to problems, they are much more likely to be implemented than those which the therapist alone thinks a good idea.

Brickner (1978) considers that the highest level of professional maturity is evidenced by the ability to understand and put a patient's interests and prerogatives first.

If furniture or effects need changing for safety or function, the family needs to feel comfortable about how the changes fit into their own way of life, and be able to adjust to them, as well as to accept them because they will make life safer and easier for the patient.

(c) Family attitudes

If the patient's future home is with families in a dependent, cared for situation, they may be 'unwelcome' or 'just tolerated' additions to the nuclear family (Brickner, 1978). In such cases opportunities for patients to have alternative contact of a pleasant, welcoming nature is essential if they are not to respond to their home situation by feeling useless, unwanted and isolated. It is also important for family members to have respite from caring tasks and the 'permanent' presence of the patient.

Families may, on the other hand, care deeply, but because of the patient's age and stroke, may see them as different and treat them as separate from the rest of the family, doing things for them rather than allowing them to participate as valued family members.

Not all stroke patients will achieve independence, despite retraining. Sandler (1971) suggests there are three alternatives to tasks which are impossible for the patient, firstly that all tasks may not need to be done; secondly that family members will need to do them; and thirdly, that they may be done by an external agency. These points should be considered in discussions with the family. Information about local helping agencies should be provided.

Families should be given plenty of opportunity to share, discuss and solve problems, and feel comfortable and confident in the therapist's judgment, to seek ongoing help when necessary for problems of a physical or psychological and relationship nature.

2. ASSESSMENT OF SPECIFIC HOME REQUIREMENTS AND ROLES

It is easier to assess specific home and role requirements when in a patient's home, whether it be hostel accommodation, flat, town house, or country property, because these will differ according to the architecture and nature of the home. Problems particular to each case may become apparent when faced with the real home situation, so that questions may be asked about who did what, and how they feel about what they did. Evaluation of roles will include such practical considerations as:

- who prepared meals, how, and what did they prepare
- who marketed, budgetted, banked, or paid bills
- who cleaned the house, washed up, did the laundry and how
- who fed, and cared for, pets, chickens, or livestock

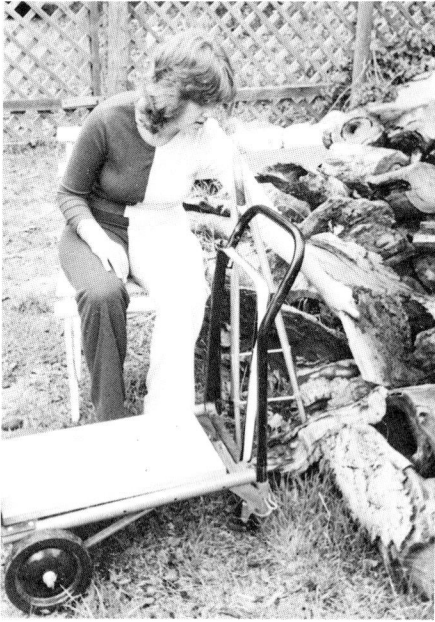

(a)

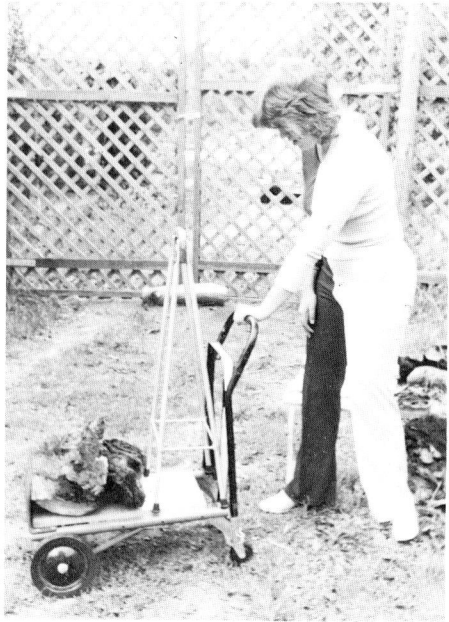

(c)

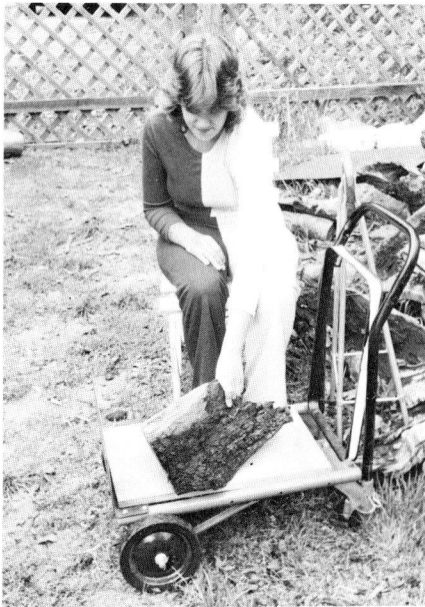

(b)

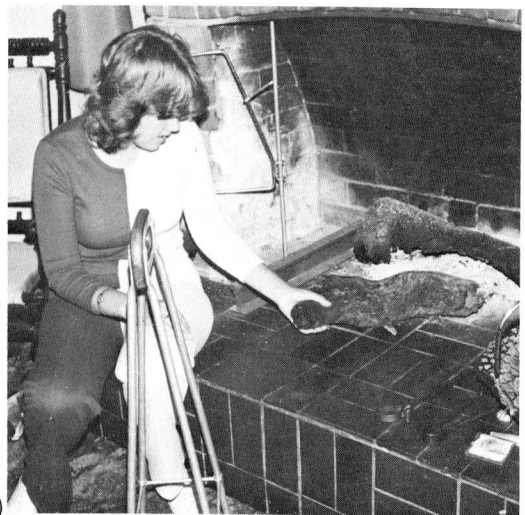

(d)

Fig. 11.1 Home heating may be dependent on an open fire. If patients live alone, adapted procedures such as use of a trolley to carry fuel may be necessary.

- who watered and weeded the garden, mowed the lawns and tended strubs
- who organized and tended home heating (Fig. 11.1), and cooling
- who put out the garbage, changed tap washers, fuses or light globes etc.

Discussion with all concerned may enable a redistribution of practical work roles, so that patients may participate to their maximum capacity, maintain progress and continue to re-develop required skills.

3. SIMPLIFICATION TECHNIQUES

Methods to simplify or enable a patient to carry out necessary or desirable activities may be worked out and practised.

The following steps may be a useful guide to work simplification:

(a) *Select household tasks* which the patient finds difficult, and define the problem; for example making the beds (Fig. 11.2) takes two hours; it exhausts the patient who requires rest before tackling other activities; time is reduced for other necessary or pleasurable tasks; frustration and fatigue cause undesirable emotional response to others.

(b) *Observe the method* used by breaking it down into basic elements, recording the time taken for each element, the level of difficulty of carrying out each element, and whether rest or pause is required between components of the activity; for example vacuum cleaning a carpet (Fig. 11.3) involves removing the equipment from storage, assembly, plugging it into power points, moving furniture, walking and manipulating the cleaner, emptying the dust bag, putting away the equip-ment. All or any of these may present difficulties and fatigue.

(c) *Analyse the method* by examining the purpose and need for the activity, how and why it is performed that way, where and when it is carried out and why there and then, how dysfunction has affected performance, whether equipment or materials could be improved, how the patient feels about the task and whether feelings about the task have changed since stroke; for example, washing clothes (Fig. 11.4) is a necessary, regular task being done in a bathroom wash basin, kitchen sink, outside copper, laundry tub or washing machine, because of habit and facilities available, in the place designated for such use by the plumbing or outside because of lack of plumbing and/or electricity, being done daily or weekly because of amount of washing or habit. Poor

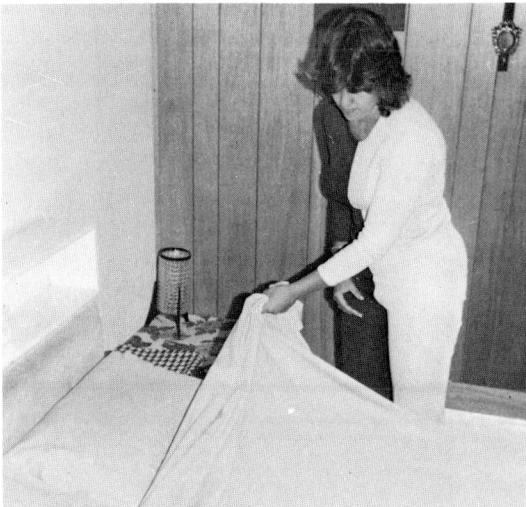

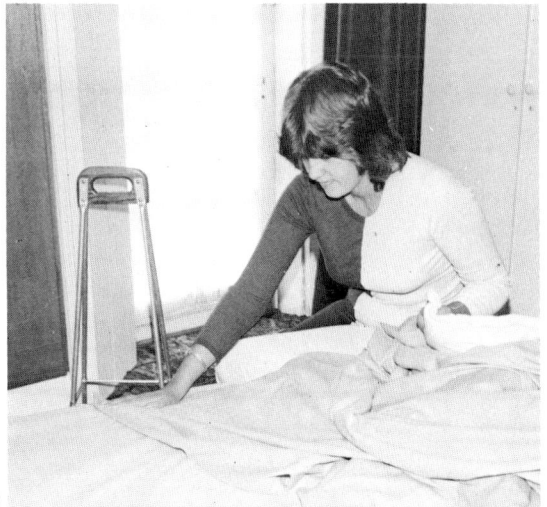

(a)   (b)

Fig. 11.2 (a) Bed making may be time consuming, requiring the patient to walk around the bed many times to straighten bedding, if balance is a problem and if only one hand is functional. (b) Putting on a quilt cover is difficult with one hand, and may be impossible for a patient with visuo-spatial impairment.

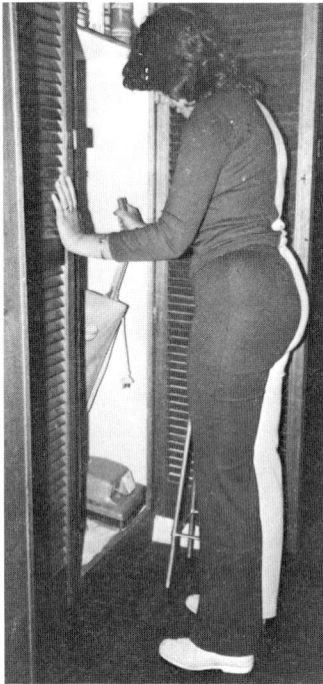
(a)

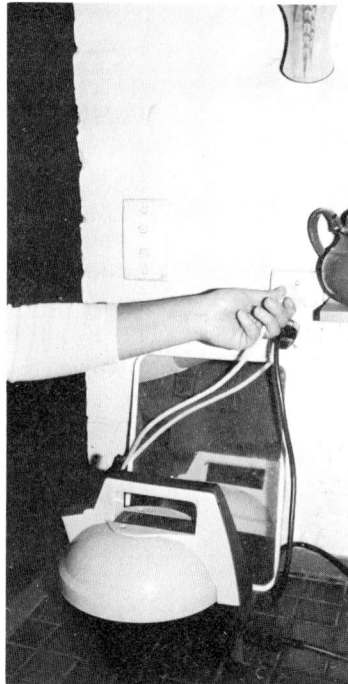
(b)

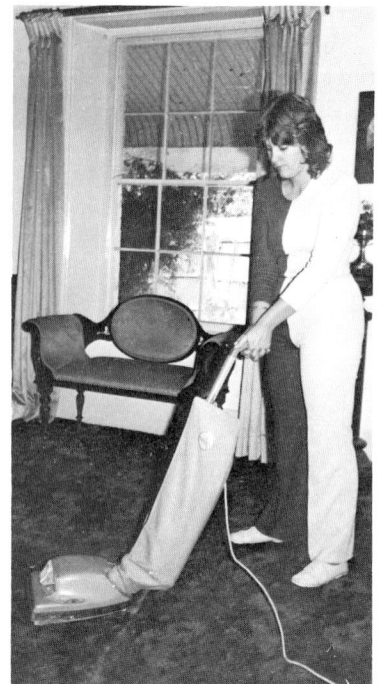
(c)

Fig. 11.3 Vacuum cleaning the carpet requires many different processes, any of which may prevent patients from coping with independent housekeeping.

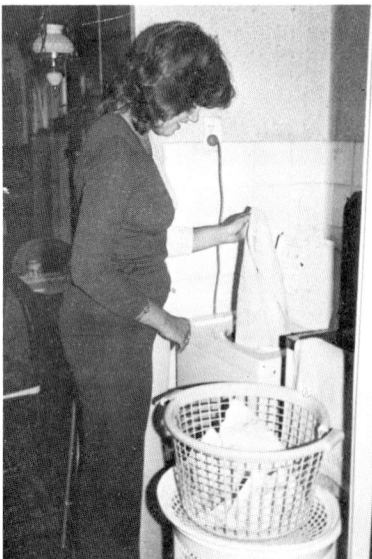
(a)

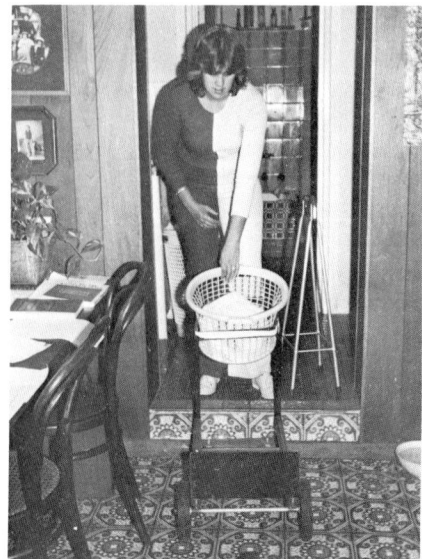
(b)

Fig. 11.4 Even with a washing machine, doing the laundry may require a careful analysis of the step-by-step processes required in each patient's home.

Table 11.1 Improve the method: Example: Shopping for food supplies

	Present procedure	Alternatives	Solutions
PLACE	Corner shop	1. Corner shop 2. Supermarket 3. Bulk store	Supermarket
TIME	Daily	1. Daily 2. Weekly 3. Monthly	Weekly
PERSON	Patient/homemaker	1. Patient 2. Relatives/friends 3. Deliver	Deliver
METHOD	On foot/basket	1. By 'phone 2. By taxi 3. By public transport	1. By 'phone 2. Increased planning 3. Increased storage
WHY	1. Can't drive 2. Limited carrying capacity 3. Limited storage	Increase storage	1. Physical effort decreased 2. Daily trips eliminated

balance and mobility may make standing or bending to the task difficult; impaired perception may make sorting and clothing manipulation difficult; one handed function may make untangling clothes, soaping, or hanging on the line difficult. Patients may feel frustrated by the extra time the task may take and problems they experience, taking little pleasure in the clean, fresh smell of the laundered clothes.

(d) Improve the method

(1) The method may be improved: by charting the breakdown of tasks and alternatives to difficulties, thus clarifying issues and simplifying solution finding.

Example: Shopping (Table 11.1)

(2) The method may be improved by analysis and rationalization of work place, equipment, materials, and physical movement patterns.

Example: Food preparation.

(i) *Workplace*—the kitchen. Should be designed so that patients sit rather than stand, and storage and work heights reduce the need for mobility, and keep bending and stretching to a minimum; unnecessary equipment and materials are discarded or stored elsewhere; the most regular tasks may be performed sequentially because of kitchen layout and position of storage and equipment; good light and ad-

equate ventilation is ensured to enhance visual acuity and reduce fatigue; power sockets and light switches plentiful, and in easy reach.

(ii) *Equipment* should be checked to ensure the patient can use it safely and independently. Anything the patient cannot handle should be put away unless there are other users. Any aids or adapted equipment should be positioned so they may be used in an integrated way. Equipment and aids should be well designed so that faults or unsafe handling are unlikely to occur, and so that assembly and cleaning is easy.

(iii) *Materials*, in this case food and ingredients, need assessment for ease of handling, perhaps speed of preparation, and suitability of cooking methods required. Also of consideration are nutritional aspects relevant to the health and lifestyle of patients and others for whom food is prepared.

(iv) *Movement patterning* should consider balance and postural ability, independence or dependence in transfers and walking, hand dominance, whether one-or two-handed activity is possible, the effects of gravity, pre-stroke movement habits, and whether limb movements naturally follow a curve or arc, rather than a straight line. Kitchen and equipment layout should be planned with any limitations in mind.

(e) *Practise the method* and the use of aids, equipment, and materials.

(f) *Evaluation* should be continuous so that further adjustment to workplace, equipment, materials, and movement patterning is possible when ongoing problems occur.

Whether the patient's role in the home is that of principal homemaker or assistant, emotional behaviour, interpersonal responses, planning, motivation and initiative are likely to be as important as physical work skills. It is necessary for therapists to try to gain insights into the patient's previous lifestyle and behaviour, so that they may help facilitate the same or similar emotional outlets and satisfaction. If, because of impairment, this is impossible, alternative behaviours to meet psychological needs of belonging and participation in family need to be developed.

4. ACCESS, ARCHITECTURE, FURNITURE AND FITTINGS

The physical characteristics of a home will influence patients' capacity to be independent, and therapists must consider details of architecture, access and fittings to determine those factors which will prove limiting.

Evaluation should be made of how patients can manage front and back doors (Fig. 11.5); steps and stairs inside or out (Fig. 11.6); changing floor surfaces and outside paths (Fig. 11.7); room, cupboard, storage, garage or toolshed doors; gates, windows, and light and appliance switches.

The proximity of rooms, such as bedroom, bathroom and lavatory, and whether the arrangement of furniture allows ease of access between rooms should be observed and discussed. Furniture such as the patient's favourite chair, and the bed, may need particular attention, as these may be unsuitable for the physical status of the patient (Fig. 11.8), or may be unsuitably positioned within the home. Modifying the favourite chair may be preferable to the patient to changing it for a more suitable one.

Bathroom fittings and kitchen layout require careful evaluation if patients are to use these safely and independently, as are appliances in frequent use, or those likely to be so in the future.

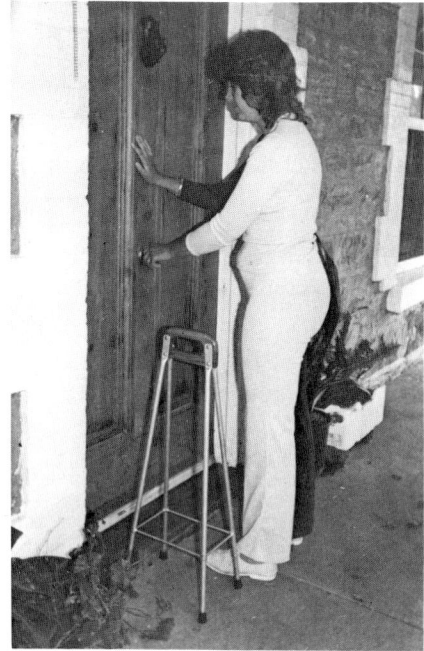

Fig. 11.5 Access into the house requires evaluation, not only of steps, but also door furniture and fittings.

Any adjustments or changes recommended must meet each patient's current ability and potential and should not be based solely on physical skills. Any problem remaining should be considered in conjunction with the physical features and role requirements of the patient's home. For example, should the patient have a residual visuo-spatial problem of figure-ground, particular attention may need to be given to changes in floor surfaces or heights, to colour differential between carpet and furniture, or light switches and door frames against walls.

Any equipment or aids suggested to overcome difficulties should also be considered in conjunction with any other remaining impairment; for example, a microwave oven may be seen as safer than a conventional model when there is tactile sensory loss and fear of burn injury; however, it will be unsuitable if the patient is unable to grasp the concepts of the difference between conventional and microwave cooking, and the need to use other than metal containers.

The most usual aids to be supplied are those which facilitate mobility, balance and safety such as fourpoint sticks, bathboards, shower seats, non-

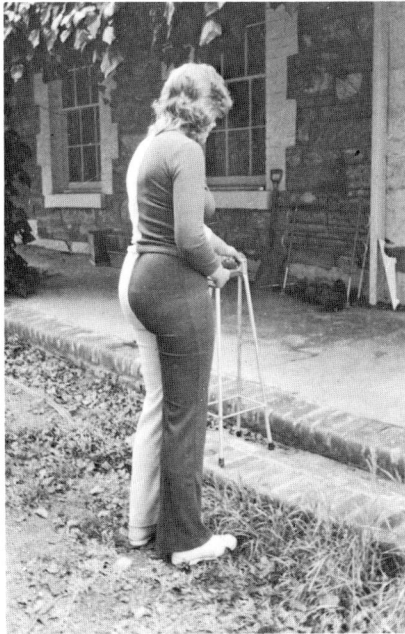
(a)

Fig. 11.6 Access inside and out should be evaluated for steps and stairs.

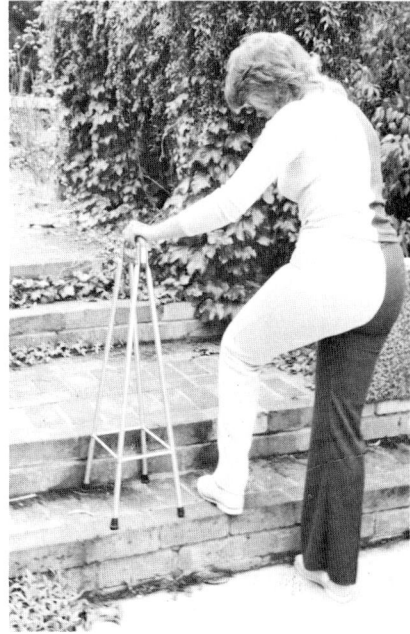
(b)

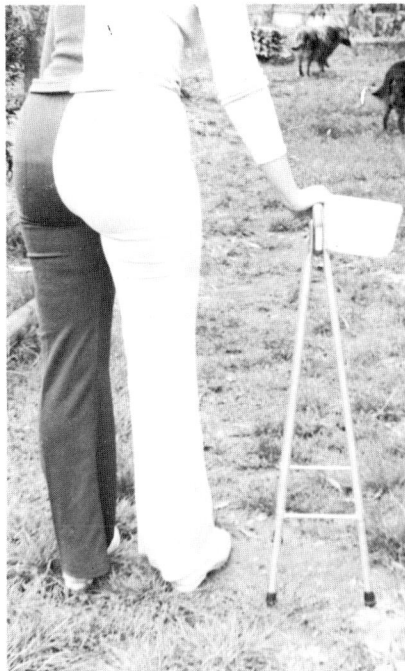

Fig. 11.7 Outside pathways are important for patients to make use of their total environment.

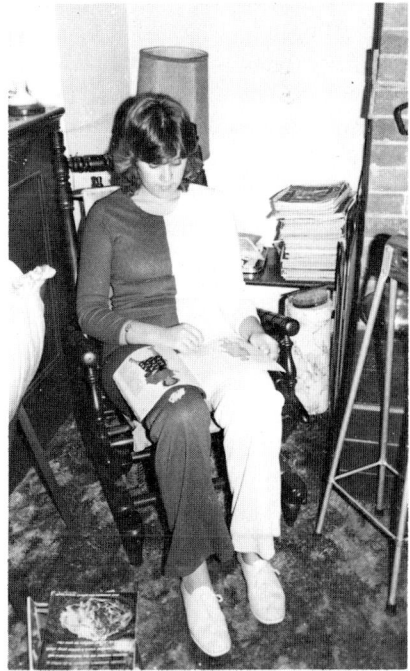

Fig. 11.8 Attention should be given to any difficulties caused by the patient's favourite chair.

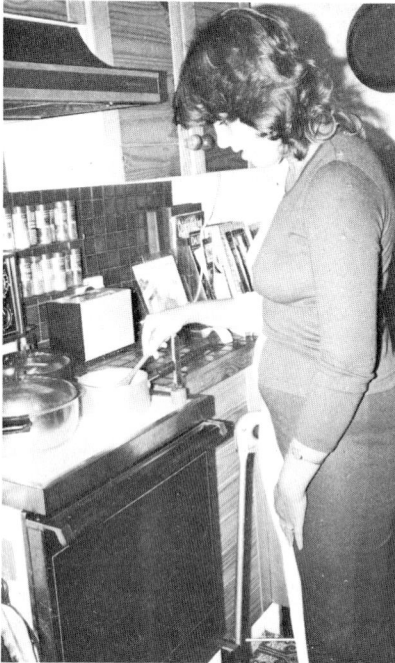

Fig. 11.9 Pan handle holders may be useful during cooking.

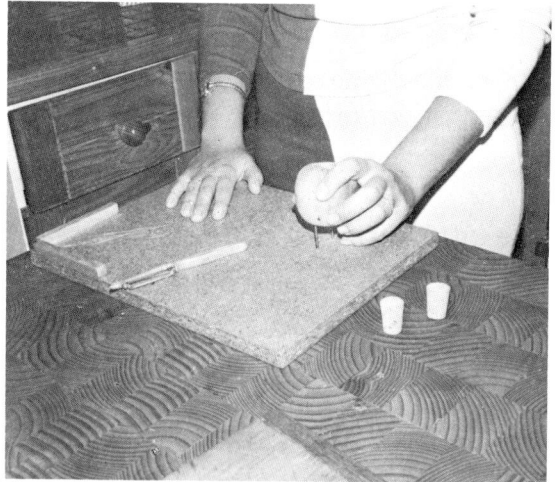

(a)

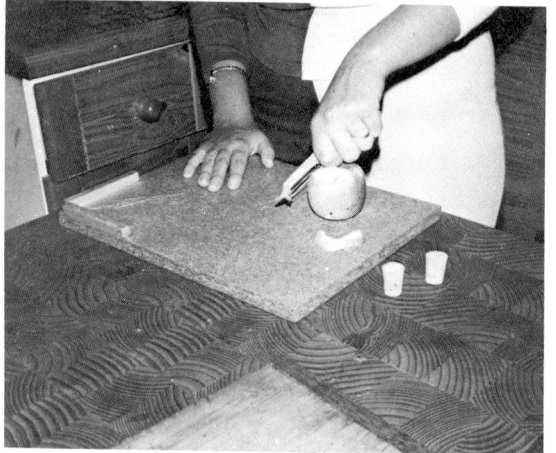

(b)

slip bath mats, raised lavatory seats with arms, furniture raisers, and rails in the bathroom and by steps and stairs; and those which stabilise objects so that tasks are possible one handed, such as bowl holders, pan handle holders (Fig. 11.9), spike boards (Fig. 11.10), and suction cups or non-slip mats (Fig. 11.11).

If adjustments are made or aids are supplied, both patients and families should feel they are useful, and be familiar with how best to adapt to the change or use the aid.

5. CONTINUITY

Because of the need for most patients going home to change ways of doing things, it is best if there is continuity of therapist throughout treatment, as repetition of training and continuity of methods facilitate new learning, and patient skills (once established) may be improved upon. Rapport and trust through working together will promote ongoing acceptance, understanding and motivation, which will not be broken by changes of treatment personnel.

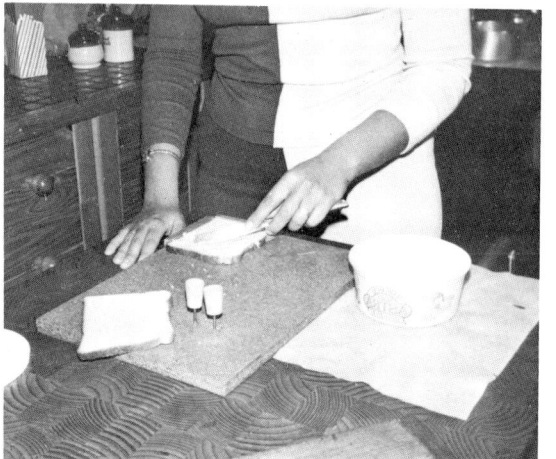

(c)

Fig. 11.10 A food preparation board with spikes to hold food during peeling and chopping, and bread whilst buttering, may be a necessary aid.

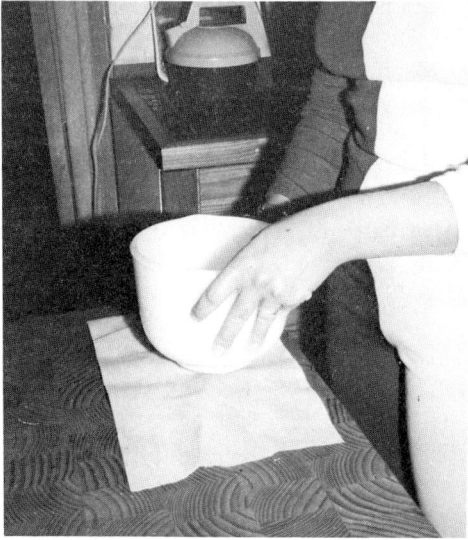

Fig. 11.11 Non-slip mats may allow patients to continue many housekeeping tasks which would otherwise be frustrating and difficult.

If hospital and domiciliary services are separate this may not be possible and in such cases a close liaison between services should be established, with the home therapist visiting the patient during treatment in the hospital if possible, so that learning may be continued smoothly during the transition from hospital to home, and from therapist to therapist.

Patients are likely to feel uncomfortable using new methods in the family situation where other ways have been used habitually. Newly acquired patterns of behaviour have to compete with the habits of years, which are likely to be reinforced by the behaviours of any others living with the patient, and the layout of the home.

Lack of reinforcement of recently acquired methods is probably a major reason for failure of patients to transfer techniques learned in hospital to the home situation. Without practical help, the cognitive and emotional demands of change and attempts to transfer ideas learned in hospital to home, may be impossible.

This will be easier if the hospital retraining unit, for example the kitchen, is mobile and adjustable, so that physical layout can assimilate the shape and pattern of a patient's kitchen, and new patterns of movement that can be continued in the home may be established as soon as possible, with oppor-

tunity for frequent practice to enhance cumulative motor memory. Such facilities and practice will realistically assist intellectual, perceptual and emotional adjustment, as well as sensory motor ability. Confusion will be reduced, as any remaining memory traces are used and built on throughout treatment, rather than manifesting as a complication when patients return home with different motor patterns having been freshly established.

6. INITIAL HOME TRAINING

Many Domiciliary Care Services provide occupational therapists to discuss problems, demonstrate techniques and recommend and/or supply aids, but these may be fairly short visits, possibly followed up weekly. This may be insufficient for patients who find the transition from hospital to a new way of home life difficult, for whatever reason. After weeks or months spent in retraining, patients may be unable to utilise what they have learnt because initially insufficient time is given by the occupational therapist to establishing the patient's use of newly learnt techniques in the home. At least one week of continuous attention should be given—perhaps each morning spent with the patient, going through the daily routine, supporting and reinforcing skills. This will show families the patient's real potential, help to establish sensory motor patterns and reinforce modified activity memory. In the long term such intervention may be seen as cost efficient, as lengthy retraining will not be wasted, and less frequent follow-up visits may be required.

Practical visits of this nature will also help to reduce depression and undesirable affective responses which are likely to occur when the patient first arrives home and finds everything is different.

7. COMMUNITY INVOLVEMENT

Regular visits to support, maintain and promote improvement will probably be necessary for some time.

It is important that therapists should consider

whether patients or their families are confined to home, and are unable to join in community pursuits or follow previous interests. It is probable that for some weeks the re-establishment of security and pleasure in their home may be a priority for many patients. However, some may feel frustrated by a restricted or different lifestyle and need change and opportunity to enjoy activity away from the home from a very early date post discharge. Those who live with, or help care for the patient, may need respite and a 'breathing space' for their own interests or simply for time to themselves.

The occupational therapist should encourage the re-establishment of previous or the development of new recreational and community interests wherever possible. Patients may need encouragement and support to help them face acquaintances when they are impaired and feel different. They may require assistance to communicate with others or to establish a basis for how they wish others to deal with them. Tactful, sensitive information-sharing with those coming into regular contact with the patient may enable a more comfortable re-establishment of contact than if the patient has to face others by themselves. Simply giving others the opportunity to observe how therapist and patient communicate with each other in a mature way may give them an example to follow.

There may be practical problems of access to community resources, or difficulties of carrying out former activities because of impairment. Discussion with those responsible for improvements to property may be appropriate, to suggest ramps, rails, parking or lavatory facilities for the disabled generally, and the patient in particular. If no permanent changes are possible, temporary or mobile aids may need to be devised. Having other members of a community group participate in problem solving is likely to be beneficial to all concerned, including helping the patient to feel wanted and important to the others.

If patients are unable to follow previous interests, the need for activity and involvement outside the home may be met by use of special agencies such as day activity centres. Attendance at such agencies will provide a routine respite for both patient and families. It is essential that the patient experiences enjoyment and social satisfaction from participation in programs offered, to maintain morale, self-esteem and higher cortical skills which may be damaged by frustrations of day-to-day life. Occupational therapists need to recognise the importance of emphasizing positive intact skills rather than concentrating solely on impairment (which is common practice) so that negative aspects of patients' current lifestyle are not being constantly reinforced.

8. FOLLOW UP

Establishing a means to 'follow up' the progress of patients once intense treatment and retraining has ceased is important, particularly if the patient lives alone or with an elderly partner who may fail to realise the significance of any change.

Patients may experience further recovery which may be enhanced by a period of intense treatment. If contact has ceased, opportunities for further treatment will be missed. On the other hand patients may experience deterioration in their physical or psychological state, which reduces their ability to be independent. Prompt attention to any such deterioration may enable patients to remain in their own home, and prevent hospitalization or dependent care becoming necessary. Brickner (1979) comments that any small change in health which restricts activity in the elderly living alone, may cause major deterioration in physical and psychological functioning, affecting quality of life including the basic needs of nutrition, cleanliness, and safety.

SUMMARY

Relevance and success of rehabilitation procedures may only be measured by the patient's ability to function maximally in the post-discharge environment. Because for many patients this will be in their own home, or with relatives, the need to be able to carry over relearned personal and domestic skills from hospital is paramount. Whenever possible, occupational therapists should extend services into each patient's home to reinforce learning, reduce undesirable affective response and promote an enjoyable future lifestyle. To do this the physical characteristics of each patient's home should be considered from early in rehabilitation, simulation of layout facilitating the patient's learning experiences. Patients' life roles and interests should be considered and promoted when possible. When impairment prevents this, alternatives should be sought.

The attitudes, feelings, responses and problems experienced by relatives and patients will be important in successful home settlement, and therapists should be uncritical, empathetic and practical with their support and encouragement.

REFERENCES

Brickner P W 1978 Home health care for the aged. Appleton-Century-Crofts, New York
Johnstone M 1980 Home care for the stroke patient—living in a pattern. Churchill Livingstone, Edinburgh
Sandler B 1971 Training in homemaking activities. In: Krusen F H, Kottke F J, Ellwood P M (eds) Handbook of physical medicine and rehabilitation. W B Saunders Co, Philadelphia

RECOMMENDED READING

Grandjean E 1973 Ergonomics of the home. Taylor and Francis, London
Jay P 1979 Help yourselves, a handbook for hemiplegics and their families, 3rd ed. Ian Henry Pubs, Hornchurch, Essex
Johnstone M 1980 Home care for the stroke patient—living in a pattern. Churchill Livingstone, Edinburgh

Work

Only a small proportion of stroke patients return to the work force because many are beyond working age and have already retired, and others have residual impairment which prevents them returning to a previous field of employment.

Rusk (1964) suggests that successful placement is dependent upon analysing patient and job which should be optimally matched. Analysis may need to include the patient's problems, the attitudes of employers, and community prejudices, fears and misinformation.

Those who do recover sufficiently to return to a job, may benefit if the therapeutic retraining program is geared primarily towards work-related activities. The Alabama Rehabilitation Media Service (1971) suggest that progress towards work goals or therapy goals may be interchangeable, both objectives being achieved by the same methods and modalities, the difference being a matter of emphasis on one or the other.

ASSESSMENT

An occupational therapist's approach to vocational retraining begins with a realistic assessment of the patient's abilities and future potential. This should include:

1. Prevocational evaluation

(a) Physical impairment such as paralysis or weakness; tactile, visual, auditory or other sensory changes and deficits; clumsiness, slowness, lack of precise or dexterous movement; mobility, balance and postural difficulties, or fatigue.

(b) Perceptual impairment of gross or minimal nature, such as decreased awareness of body parts; visuo-spatial, tactile or auditory agnosias; or dyspraxia.

(c) Cognitive, intellectual or language impairment, such as limited concentration and attention; short-term memory loss; inability to comprehend, retain or follow instructions; difficulty in reasoning logically and abstractly, making decisions, taking initiative, or problem solving; dysarthria, dysphasia, and difficulty in reading, writing or calculating.

(d) Behaviour such as affective response to tasks, situations and people, ability to relate effectively with others, appropriateness of dress and appearance, punctuality, motivation and dependability.

Kester (1983) described this type of assessment as 'prevocational evaluation'. She suggests that as well as physical capacities and deficits, evaluation should include activities of daily living and educational abilities. The information collected will then form part of an interdisciplinary vocational assessment which includes medical, psychological, educational, social, environmental, cultural and vocational factors. The latter are assessed through use of real or simulated work situations.

2. Real or work simulated activities

Robb (1975) describes procedures for work rehabilitation at the Australian Department of Social Security Rehabilitation Centre, 'Mt. Wilga', N.S.W., where patients are assessed by means of a series of tasks which are timed and administered with standardized instructions. Retraining is subsequently carried out in a variety of workshops, which provides ongoing evaluation, using structured work samples and simulated industrial operations.

Information collected during real or simulation work retraining should be precise, and should also include factors such as interpersonal relationships with co-workers and supervisors, motivation, work behaviour and readiness. In addition Kester (1983) suggests that knowledge of the patient's interests, health, transport problems and family concerns is important. The total evaluation findings should be shared with the patient, as work retraining may fail if patients are not sufficiently aware of their abilities, handicaps and potential.

There are a number of commercially available vocational evaluation systems, such as the 'Tower System', the 'Valpar Component Work Sample Series', 'McCarron-Dial Work Evaluation System' and 'Hester Evaluation System'. These vary in the amount of time required, test–retest reliability, validity, manner and place of administration, and whether testing is formal or uses real or simulated work situations (Bottersbusch & Sax, 1980). Availability may be limited by the expense of the systems. Some tests may be administered only by a registered psychologist, and therapists should check whether systems selected for purchase have restricted usage.

Many patients being evaluated for work potential will be returning to a previously held job, or to one similar with the same employer. The evaluation tool should be specifically designed to meet the individual case, involving appropriate and increasingly definitive work modalities and work tolerance (Kester, 1983).

SKILL DEVELOPMENT

Ross (1982) suggests that positive intensive rehabilitation and work assessment should be concurrent, because such an approach may reduce or prevent the frustration and loss of work habits experienced by many disabled persons discharged home to wait for recovery, and should simulate normal work hours although allowing for rest periods when necessary.

Intact and impaired abilities should be related to vocational requirements of each patient, that is those of the patient's job before the stroke, the same job modified, or a different type of employment which seems possible and is geographically viable. Treatment should be programmed to maintain intact work skills and to improve those that are difficult.

1. Use of routine office procedures

Hodges and Schwarz (1976) suggest that a retraining program in routine office procedures may be used to develop:

(a) Good sitting or standing posture and tolerance, by grading time spent on jobs requiring sitting and standing.
(b) Ability to cope with disability, for example, by teaching the patient positioning of upper limb to prevent subluxation and shoulder pain.
(c) Use of unaffected hand, especially when dominance needs to be changed in both general and manipulative activities, and specific tasks such as writing.
(d) Ability to comprehend and retain instructions by appropriate use of repetition and utilization of intact skills such as auditory or visual memory.

(e) Increased concentration span by frequent verbal stimulation, appropriate choice of position and timing of tasks.

(f) Ability to relate appropriately to staff and peers, and to modify undesirable behaviours by use of a firm but friendly approach.

2. Use of industrial workshop settings

Robb (1975) suggests that industrial workshop settings may be used remedially for increasing movement, speed and co-ordination, memory, concentration, endurance, and work habits, and for maintenance of intact abilities. Use of sub-contract jobs also allows for development in interpersonal relationships, self-esteem, good work habits, dependability, and appropriate work behaviour.

3. Use of general occupational therapy activities

Not all occupational therapy departments will have the full range of facilities which are available to vocational rehabilitation centres. However, many job skills are inherent in a variety of workshop, clerical, domestic, creative and gardening activities, which may be used for the redevelopment of specific vocational requirements.

4. Use of other hospital departments

Other departments in the hospital may also be willing to have patients take part in their work schedule as volunteers, so that they may redevelop particular skills, or be realistically evaluated in work tasks. Hospital departments which have co-operated in such retraining schemes have included reception areas, maintenance departments, medical supply units, laundries, kitchens, lifts, and various departments requiring telephone answering. Reasons for having the patients participate in such programs must be clearly understood by the patient, relatives, hospital personnel, and union officials.

5. Associated work skills

Required skills are not only those of the job itself, or those required by the employer, such as re-liability, punctuality or safe work practice, but are also those of coping with the actual work environment, such as tolerating noise or temperature, managing personal care tasks such as getting to and from toilet facilities in reasonable time, social skills for relating with other workers, safe use of mobility aids for negotiating the work environment, transport to and from work, and managing to tolerate the daily time involved which includes work, preparation for work, and travelling time.

6. Technical and professional jobs

Rusk (1964) indicates that stroke patients previously employed in technical and professional jobs have a more favourable prognosis for vocational rehabilitation, but points out the importance of sensory, perceptual and psychological abilities for employment of this type.

Occupational therapists may have patients practise repetitively tasks such as mathematics, writing, abstract and practical problem solving, and use of such modalities as electronic games to speed up reactions, but it may be impossible to judge whether patients are able to resume their former responsibilities, especially if they are in dynamic and demanding positions.

7. Specific skill training

Specific skill training may include:

(a) Practice in the type of mobility required by the job, including sitting, standing, negotiating obstacles, steps and furniture; reaching or rotating to select materials or use equipment; walking required distances, such as between job components, or to the toilet and back.

(b) Redeveloping stamina, fatigue tolerance, attention and concentration to slightly above the level required by the job, by upgrading the time, complexity and relevance of treatment activities so that any unexpected or additional demands may be handled without undue stress.

(c) Practice in communication towards acceptable job requirements, including speech, answering the telephone, writing, typing, using word processors, computers, or other pertinent machinery.

(d) Redeveloping manual dexterity either bilaterally or unilaterally, eye/hand co-ordination, speed and accuracy by upgrading activities of interest to the patient and similar to those required by the job, or by simulated or actual work tasks.

(e) Practice in the use of special tools or equipment, adapted, if necessary, to the skill and speed required to be economically viable in the work situation.

(f) Redeveloping sensory skills such as visual scanning and fixation, appropriate attention to auditory or olfactory cues, and tactile discrimination as required by the job.

(g) Practice in intellectual pursuits to redevelop abstract reasoning, logical thinking, memory and complex conceptual tracking towards the level required by the job, by use of reading and discussion, puzzles, table and computer games, and mathematical problems.

Time spent in vocational retraining should not be limited to half-hour treatment sessions, which is completely unrealistic, but gradually upgraded as work tolerance and skills improve, to simulate a normal working day.

ACCESS

1. Transport to work

(a) Driving a car will need careful assessment as ability may not only be affected by a decrease in sensory motor skills, but by visual or auditory impairment of a primary sensory or perceptual nature, by neglect or inattention to one side, by cognitive impairment such as inability to understand signs or signals, poor concentration, decreased reasoning ability, and by behavioural responses such as decreased frustration levels or lack of emotional control. In most countries an application to renew a driving licence requires the applicant to declare certain impairments, which if answered in the affirmative may require a special test be taken. It is then at the discretion of the relevant authority whether or not a licence is issued. Occupational therapists should ensure that any person who has suffered stroke makes a full disclosure of any disability when applying to renew or obtain a driving licence. If a medical report is required by the authority, the occupational therapist should discuss with the doctor any impairment in functional performance of tasks, which may not be obvious but which may affect safe driving.

If patients need practice to speed up driving reaction time, electronic driving games may be put to good use.

Negotiations with the employing body may need to be undertaken for the provision of a parking space close to the work situation.

(b) Being driven by a family member or work colleague may be a convenient and satisfactory solution to transport to and from work, especially if this is unlikely to become inconvenient or an unwanted chore for the driver.

(c) Public transport may be the only option. Patients should be given practice in managing the form of transport available to them. There are often problems with the depth of steps, absence of grab bars, and the fact that the vehicle may move before the patient is seated or standing braced against movement. For those with even slightly impaired balanced or less than perfect protective mechanisms there may be many problems, particularly in a crowded situation. Managing money to pay the fare may also be difficult, especially for the one handed who have to use a walking aid. A method of pre-organizing the fare which is acceptable to each patient, may be useful, as is exploring the possibility of season tickets. Some employers will allow flexible or reduced hours so that patients may travel at other than rush hours. The occupational therapist may help with such negotiations.

2. Architecture

Just as the architecture of the home may cause problems in independent functioning for patients, so may the design elements of work buildings. Steps, stairs, ramps, floor surfaces, doors, lights, ventilation andtoilet facilities may need consideration, and the occupational therapist may liaise early with employers to identify access problems and situations which will need practice and inclusion in retraining.

ATTITUDES

(a) Employers

Attitudes of employers to re-employing the patient should also be evaluated at an early date. If environmental changes are required, such as ramps or rails, or repositioning the actual job so that it is closer to necessary facilities, the employer must be sympathetic to and understanding of the problems, and willing to make the changes for the patient's benefit.

(b) Work colleagues

Employers and work colleagues may need assistance in understanding the nature of the patient's problems to prevent possible rejection or inappropriate responses, especially when there is impairment of language or facial musculature.

(c) The patient

The attitude of the patient towards work and disability should be considered (Ross, 1982), including whether his expectation of future potential and abilities is realistic, whether he is able to cope with other peoples' reaction to impairment, whether his ability to relate effectively with others has altered since stroke, and whether confidence, motivation and initiative are sufficient to overcome the problems to be faced.

WORK MODIFICATION AND SIMPLIFICATION

Careful job analysis is required, and information should be collected from the patient, work colleagues, employers, relatives, and from visits to the work situation, because even jobs with the same title may vary in working conditions and required skills (Rusk, 1964).

The job may be analysed using a similar method of work study to that described for homemaking, that is questioning why, what, and how are things done.

Working conditions should be analysed to determine special characteristics, such as the physical location, the temperature, atmosphere, lighting, presence of dangers, noise, smells, visual distractions, and whether the working arrangement demands close co-operation with others or independence and self-motivation.

When all the information regarding job procedures has been collected, alternatives may be considered, with only those which offer equal or more effective results being considered for a vocational situation. Modifications may lead to more effective procedures for the non-disabled (Rusk, 1964). The occupational therapist may be able to advise on simplifying techniques and procedures which may decrease stress or strain for workers and lead to increased productivity. Rationalizing job layout is preferable to the use of special devices which may make the patient feel different, slow down the job, or need carrying about. Changes may simply include altering work heights, seating, or the position of the telephone; or they may be more complex, for example, shifting a control or substituting leg for arm control, changing the telephone system so that holding the receiver is unnecessary, or building in special devices to stabilize materials.

ALTERNATIVES

For those who wish to return to some form of employment but do not appear to have the potential to return to a previous or new job, a sheltered workshop or voluntary occupation may be suitable. Alternatively, the occupational therapist may help the patient to explore the possibilities of self- or homebound employment, perhaps on the basis of previous skills or leisure interests which are still possible despite stroke, or using new skills learned during rehabilitation.

SUMMARY

For patients likely to return to employment, therapists working in acute rehabilitation should consider and bias retraining programs towards work and work-related skill development.

Accurate assessment of patient impairment and potential and job requirements is essential for realistic recommendations and relevant activity choices for programs.

Therapists need to develop skills to liaise with employers and work colleagues to discuss patient needs, access, attitudes, and possibilities for work modification.

REFERENCES

Alabama Rehabilitation Media Service 1971 Vocational evaluation and work adjustment: a book of readings. Materials and Information Centre, Alabama

Bottensbusch K F, Sax A B 1980 A comparison of commercial vocational evaluation systems. Menomonie, Wi

Hodges M, Schwartz A 1976 An office routine programme for use in treatment, assessment and work preparation in occupational therapy. Australian Occupational Therapy Journal 23.2: 51–57

Kester D 1983 Prevocational and vocational assessment. In: Hopkins and Smith (eds) Willard and Spackman's Occupational therapy, 6th edn. Lippincott, Philadephia, Ch 14

Robb J 1975 Returning the patient to work: an occupational therapy point of view. Australian Occupational therapy journal, 22.1: 37–40

Ross P J 1982 Basic work assessment and rehabilitation procedures. British Journal of Occupational Therapy, 45.8: 270–272

Rusk H A 1964 Principles of management of vocational problems. In: Rehabilitation medicine, a textbook on physical medicine and rehabilitation, 2nd edn. C V Mosby Co, St Louis

RECOMMENDED READING

Kester D 1983 Prevocational and vocational assessment. In: Hopkins and Smith (eds) Willard and Spackman's Occupational therapy, 6th edn. Lippincott, Philadelphia, Ch 14

Ross P J 1982 Basic work assessment and rehabilitation procedures. British Journal of Occupational Therapy 45.8: 270–272

Index